Radiology in Inflammatory Bowel Disease

Diagnostic Radiology Series

editors

Louis Kreel
Queen Mary's Hospital for the East End
and London Hospital Medical College
London, England

Morton A. Meyers
School of Medicine-Health Sciences Center
State University of New York at Stony Brook
Stony Brook, New York

Radiology in Inflammatory Bowel Disease

CLIVE I. BARTRAM, M.B.B.S., M.R.C.P., F.R.C.R.
Consultant Radiologist, St. Mark's Hospital for Diseases of the Rectum and Colon,
and St. Bartholomew's Hospital, London, England

with contributions by

James P. S. Thomson, M.S., F.R.C.S.
Consultant Surgeon and Dean of Postgraduate Studies, St. Mark's Hospital for Diseases of the
Rectum and Colon; Consultant Surgeon, Hackney Hospital; and Honorary Lecturer in Surgery,
St. Bartholomew's Hospital Medical College, London, England

and

Ashley B. Price, B.M., B.Ch., N.R.C.Path.
Consultant Histopathologist, Northwick Park Hospital, London, England

MARCEL DEKKER, INC.
BUTTERWORTHS

New York
London

Library of Congress Cataloging in Publication Data

Bartram, Clive I., [date]
  Radiology in inflammatory bowel disease.

  (Diagnostic radiology series; v. 2)
  Includes index.
    1. Colitis — Diagnosis — Addresses, essays, lectures.
2. Colon (Anatomy) — Radiography — Addresses, essays,
lectures.   3. Diagnosis, Radioscopic — Addresses,
essays, lectures.   4. Enteritis, Regional — Diagnosis —
Addresses, essays, lectures.   I. Thomson, James P. S.
II. Price, Ashley B.   III. Title.   IV. Series.   [DNLM:
1. Colitis, Ulcerative — Radiography.   2. Crohn disease —
Radiography.   W1 DI 258JR v. 2 / WI 522 B291r]
  ISBN 0-8247-1804-6

MARCEL DEKKER, INC.
270 Madison Avenue, New York, New York 10016

Current printing (last digit):
10 9 8 7 6 5 4 3 2 1

PRINTED IN THE UNITED STATES OF AMERICA

Series Introduction

The change in radiodiagnosis in the last ten years could not have been predicted even by a modern Nostradamus. Those who were conversant with computers saw the future in terms of the more rapid handling of data acquired from conventional radiography or to its use in administration in radiology departments. It took genius to use computers to invent totally new equipment, vastly more efficient in the utilization of x-rays, producing images of exquisite anatomical detail. Suddenly, computed tomography became the gold standard for contrast and spatial resolution.

Ultrasonography was not long in accepting the challenge. The lower cost, the possibility of real time images and the ease of manipulating the equipment were soon apparent but more importantly the modality uses a harmless form of non-ionizing energy.

Obstetrics soon yielded, followed shortly by the gallbladder and liver, and then, surprisingly, the neonatal brain. Ultrasonography produced a different kind of detail but with high accuracy and specificity. Even the diagnosis of thyroid and testicular disease became feasible.

The slow but inexorable march of nuclear medicine has been equally noteworthy if less dramatic. Diagnostic procedures in bone, lungs, kidneys, and the heart are providing invaluable information. New pharmaceuticals constantly expand the possible clinical uses of this discipline.

No sooner had these modalities reached maturity when radiology was faced with yet newer imaging methods, nuclear magnetic resonance and digital radiography. Shortly these techniques will also be added to our diagnostic armamentarium.

While imaging was thus progressing, remoreselessly and relentlessly from the administrative and financial viewpoint, angiography took on new dimensions, becoming therapeutic rather than diagnostic; angioplasty was born, balloon catheters became commonplace, bleeding was not only diagnosed but staunched, nor were radiologists slow to exploit the many other situations where needles, catheters, dilators and prostheses could be manipulated. Jaundice, gallstones, renal stones, abscesses, biopsies all became familiar as radiological problems for total patient management from diagnosis to treatment, from palliation to cure.

This may sound too dramatic a presentation of the last decade in radiology, but it is, if anything, an understatement when the individual patient is considered. How else is one to compare angioplasty with a bypass, percutaneous abscess drainage with laparotomy or needle biopsy with open operation?

Equally important is the totally new emphasis which has emerged, the problem-solving role of radiology as opposed to the mere demonstration of pathology. The diagnostic procedure is not merely a record of the previously known pathology, but must serve a definite role in patient management. Criteria for efficacy have been developed and applied to radiological procedures.

Hence, a new radiological series. The new diagnostic modalities will be assessed not only in their own right, but in relation to the newer techniques, not only as interesting physical signs, but as a contribution to patient management, not only as diagnostic procedures, but also in fulfilling a therapeutic role. In all, the patient must be paramount, rather than the technology.

Detection of tumors requires a special mention because of their common occurrence and unrelenting nature. The principle of using the least invasive and most accurate method is particularly important but diagnosis as such takes on a new meaning. In patients with tumor, the primary diagnosis is not the only important aspect, but staging the disease is crucial for management, as is the subsequent monitoring of treatment and planning radiotherapy when applicable. The detection of residual disease and any recurrence at the earliest possible time is equally important. Furthermore the diagnostic radiologist is now directly involved in the treatment of patients with malignant disease by undertaking tumor embolization, intra-arterial catheter localization for cytotoxic infusion, and even the introduction of radioactive material into tumors.

The modern radiologist is in the true sense a clinician, requiring technical expertise, diagnostic skills, a therapeutic and management commitment, and a thorough knowledge of anatomy and pathology. It is hoped that this series will fulfill the need of the modern radiologist.

Louis Kreel
Morton A. Meyers

Foreword

The needs of a patient with inflammatory bowel disease are best met when clinician and radiologist understand one another's problems. The questions posed by the clinician demand solution versatility and ingenuity on the part of the radiologist. Clive I. Bartram exemplifies these qualities to the full, as this book amply demonstrates. The interpretation of the radiographs requires a knowledge of pathological anatomy, and often of surgical technique. This volume draws on the experience of two busy gastroenterological units to present an unrivalled atlas of the variety of appearances seen in these disorders.

At times radiology reigns supreme, as in the examination of the small intestine, or in the demonstration of ramifying fistula tracks or abscesses. In certain situations, as in severe acute colitis, a simple abdominal radiograph, or an "air-enema," may answer all the questions a clinician needs to know about the extent and severity of the mucosal lesion. At other times, radiology and endoscopy are complementary. A diagnosis of colitis may be made by sigmoidoscopy and biopsy but an unprepared barium enema may be easier to perform, or more acceptable to the patient, than colonoscopy for demonstrating its extent or progress. Using a sophisticated air-contrast technique, the radiologist may be able to help the endoscopist by drawing attention to polypoid dysplastic lesions in colitis.

I have been privileged to work closely with my radiological colleagues and we have met weekly for many years to discuss the extraordinary variety of medical and surgical problems which develop in the course of ulcerative colitis and Crohn's disease. These meetings have been of inestimable value to me as a clinician. I am delighted that Dr. Bartram has brought together in this book the versatility of technique and almost uncanny skill in interpretation which characterize his work and I am confident that his unique experience will not only help all radiologists but also all clinicians concerned with the care of patients with inflammatory bowel disease.

J.E. Lennard-Jones
Professor of Medicine, St. Marks Hospital
and President of the British Society of Gastroenterology

Preface

Inflammatory bowel disease is now an important part of gastroenterology. The investigation and management of these patients can be extremely difficult, often requiring coordinated action from a number of disciplines. The radiologist has an important role to play, and to do this effectively it is not enough to have a basic knowledge of the radiological features of inflammatory bowel disease; the limitations and scope of various investigations and how these relate to the clinical problem must be appreciated.

This book provides a pragmatic approach to inflammatory bowel disease. The relevant radiological examinations are described, as the radiologist's ability to show the changes of inflammatory bowel disease depends on the techniques used. Also there are several examinations that are specific to patients with inflammatory bowel disease, and these are not widely known. The clinical detail given is minimal, as this is not intended to be a general medical study of inflammatory bowel disease. The pathology discussed is mainly macroscopic, as this relates directly to the radiological appearances. Emphasis is placed on areas where radiological interpretation is difficult and on the clinical relevance of the radiological findings.

Most of the principles of radiology in inflammatory bowel disease can be transferred from the adult to the pediatric age group, but the special problems that may be encountered in children are dealt with in a separate chapter. Chapters have also been allocated to the surgery of inflammatory bowel disease and rectal biopsy interpretation. These give an overview taken from the radiologist's standpoint, which is an emphasis lacking in most texts. Newer forms of imaging, such as ultrasonography, computerized axial tomography, and radioisotopes may be applied to inflammatory bowel disease, but their roles have not been fully evaluated and it is too early to judge their value. This book is intended for radiologists who wish to broaden their understanding and practical ability in dealing with these patients.

Clive I. Bartram

Acknowledgments

I am particularly grateful to Mr. James P. S. Thomson and Dr. Ashley B. Price for their contributions on subjects that were outside my sphere of competence, and for their efforts in relating their specialities to the needs of the radiologist.

I am fortunate to work in two specialized gastrointestinal units, in St. Mark's and St. Bartholomew's hospitals. This has provided me with wide experience of inflammatory bowel disease, which would, however, have been largely wasted without the support and interest of my clinical colleagues. I am indebted to many of the staff members of these hospitals, in particular to Prof. J. E. Lennard-Jones, Dr. C. B. Williams, Mr. J. P. S. Thomson, Mr. P. R. Hawley, and Dr. B. C. Morson at St. Mark's Hospital, and to Dr. A. M. Dawson and Dr. M. Clark at St. Bartholomew's Hospital, for their time and effort in participating in combined meetings. Over the years they have taught me a great deal, and their views have largely formulated my understanding of inflammatory bowel disease.

One of the easiest ways to improve one's understanding of colitis is to examine resected colons. Mr. N. Mackie of the photographic department at St. Mark's has taken outstanding photographs of these specimens, and I am grateful to Dr. B. C. Morson for giving me permission to reproduce a number of these.

I am particularly grateful to Carole Reeves of the Department of Medical Illustration at the Institute of Child Health, for her help with the photographic material, and all the contributors would like to thank the departments of medical illustration at St. Mark's, St. Bartholomew's, and Northwick Park hospitals (particularly Keith Bullock) for their excellent work in preparing the drawings and diagrams.

Finally, I would like to give public thanks, instead of many private ones, to my wife, Michele, for all her encouragement and for her help in typing the manuscript.

Contents

Radiology in Inflammatory Bowel Disease

Introduction

The term "inflammatory bowel disease" (IBD) is usually applied to two nonspecific forms of colitis: ulcerative colitis and Crohn's disease. Ulcerative colitis has been recognized for many years. The first description has been attributed to Wilks and Moxon in 1889 (1). In contrast, Crohn's disease is more recent, and although chronic transmural bowel disease was described by Dalziel in 1913 (2), the disease was not generally appreciated until its description in 1932 by Crohn et al. (3). They presented to the American Medical Association 14 cases of "terminal ileitis," in which granulomatous changes were present but no tuberculous bacillus was found. The term "regional ileitis" was suggested at the meeting, but has been superseded by a number of descriptions, such as granulomatous colitis or jejunitis. It is now known that this disease may affect any part of the gastrointestinal tract from mouth to anus, and as granulomas are found in only one-fourth of the cases, it would seem inappropriate to use either pathological or anatomical terms to describe the condition, and the eponym of "Crohn's disease" is preferred (4).

Epidemiological studies have failed to define an individual susceptibility to IBD, but have revealed groups more at risk. These include the following:

1. Western populations
2. Urban rather than rural populations
3. Whites more than blacks
4. Jews not living in Israel
5. Close relations of patients with IBD

The family history is a most significant factor, as about one-third of patients with IBD will have a positive family history and more than one member of a family will have IBD in approximately 8% of cases (5). The incidence of ulcerative colitis has remained relatively static over the years, but that of Crohn's disease has increased, to the point where the incidence of colonic involvement now equals that of ulcerative colitis (Table 1). Disease confined to the small intestine has become less common, and there is evidence that the overall incidence of Crohn's disease may be falling (6).

The radiology of IBD is difficult, as it embraces a number of examination techniques, which must be performed and interpreted with care if the radiologist is to make a worthwhile contribution to the patient's management. The clinical situations in which radiology may be helpful can be outlined as follows:

1. *Establishing the diagnosis.* A diagnosis of IBD is usually based on a combination of compatible clinical, endoscopic, radiological, and pathological findings. Of these the sigmoidoscopic appearances and rectal biopsy are the most important. These provide the basis for diagnosis in most patients with ulcerative colitis, but not in Crohn's disease, as rectal sparing is common. In these patients, if the disease is limited to the proximal colon or small intestine, the diagnosis may have to be made purely on the radiological findings without histological support unless endoscopic biopsies can be obtained from diseased areas.

2. *Classifying the type of colitis.* There is probably no specific pathognomonic sign of colitis which will enable the radiologist to state that the patient has a particular type of colitis, but there are a number of signs that in combination and distribution will indicate with a fair degree of certainty the type of colitis, or enable one form or another to be excluded.

3. *Assessing the extent and severity of the disease.* An instant enema will give the clinician an accurate guide, with a minimum of discomfort and risk to the patient, to the extent and severity of the mucosal lesions, which is helpful in planning the patient's management.

4. *In the acute attack.* Acute colitis is a life-threatening situation. Clinical assessment of the colonic state is difficult, and plain films provide an important means of demonstrating the extent and severity of the attack, as well as the possible development of acute complications such as toxic megacolon or perforation.

5. *Chronic complications.* IBD is a chronic condition, and particular complications may develop only after the disease has been present for many years. The most obvious is colonic cancer in ulcerative colitis. Endoscopy is now playing a major role in the investigation of risk, but radiology still has some value. In Crohn's disease strictures and fistulas are common problems in long-standing disease, and require radiological investigation.

The overall management of IBD requires a team approach, with the clinician, pathologist, and radiologist integrating their findings and investigations. Each patient requires individual assessment, so to fit into this scheme the radiologist must understand his or her role in the investigation of each patient.

Table 1 Incidence of IBD

Country	Crohn's disease (average incidence per 100,000 population)	Ulcerative colitis (average incidence per 100,000 population)	Reference
United Kingdom	0.8	6.5	Evans and Acheson, 1965 (7)
United States	1.8	4.6	Monk et al., 1967(8)
Denmark	1.29	7.3	Bonnevie et al., 1968 (9)
United States	3.7	4.7	Garagliano et al., 1973 (11)

Source: Modified from Ref. 10.

REFERENCES

1. Wilks, S., Moxon, W. (1889). *Lectures on Pathological Anatomy*. Longmans, Green, London, 3rd ed., p. 434.
2. Dalziel, T.K. (1913). Chronic intestinal enteritis. Br. Med. J. 2; 1068.
3. Crohn, B.B., Ginzberg, L., Oppenheimer, G.D. (1932). Regional ileitis. A pathologic and clinical entity. JAMA 19; 1328.
4. Morson, B.C. (1972). Pathology of Crohn's disease. Clin. Gastroenterol. 1 (2); 265.
5. Framer, R.G., Michiner, W.M., Mortimer, E.A. (1980). Studies of family history among patients with inflammatory bowel disease. Clin Gastroenterol. 9 (2); 271.
6. Kyle, J., Stark, G. (1980). Fall in the incidence of Crohn's disease. Gut 21; 340.
7. Evans, J.G., Acheson, E.D. (1965). An epidemiological study of ulcerative colitis and regional enteritis in the Oxford area. Gut 6; 311.
8. Monk, M., Mendeloff, A.I., Siegel, C.I., et al. (1967). An epidemiological study of ulcerative colitis and regional enteritis among adults in Baltimore. 1. Hospital incidence and prevalence 1960–1963. Gastroenterology 53; 198.
9. Bonnevie, O., Riis, P., Anthonisen, P. (1968). An epidemiologic study of ulcerative colitis in Copenhagen County. Scand. J. Gastroenterol. 3; 432.
10. Mendeloff, A.I. (1980). The epidemiology of inflammatory bowel disease. Clin. Gastroenterol. 9 (2), 259.
11. Garagliano, C.F., Mendeloff, A.I., Lilienfeld, A.M. (1980). First hospitalization rates for ulcerative colitis and Crohn's disease in Baltimore 1963–73, and for 16 other areas in 1973. In preparation.

1
Radiological Techniques

Patients with inflammatory bowel disease (IBD) require careful examination to show early changes of disease, and their general condition may necessitate modification of standard radiological investigations to provide diagnostic information with minimal disturbance to the patient. This chapter does not contain a complete description of all the possible investigations, but highlights the technical and interpretive considerations of the most relevant ones.

PLAIN FILMS   The basic supine abdominal view gives a lot of information about the colon, and is particularly important in the assessment of an acute attack. It might almost be considered part of the clinical examination, in the same way that the chest x-ray is part of the examination of the chest. The distribution of the fecal residue gives some indication as to the extent of disease, and the gas within the bowel will outline the mucosa revealing the severity of the colitis (Fig. 1).

In an acute attack the supine view should be supplemented by an erect or decubitus film with a horizontal tube to exclude free air and show air-fluid levels. In the noncolitic bowel the residue is subject to wide variations of distribution (1,2). However, it is rare for some residue not to be visible in the cecum. In colitis the inflamed mucosa prevents a buildup of formed residue, so that where this can be seen it may be assumed that the mucosa is not actively inflamed. There is therefore a loose relationship between the distal extent of the residue and the proximal extent of the colitis. If a colitic shows no residue, the colitis is most likely to be total (Fig. 2), whereas if the residue extends to the splenic flexure, the colitis will be distal to this.

Gas in the bowel is derived partly from swallowed air, but mainly from bacterial fermentation in the small bowel. Small pockets of gas may collect in the colon, and in about one-third of noncolitics (1) this is sufficient to outline the following (3) (Fig. 3):

1. *The mucosal edge.* Should be smooth.

2. *The haustral pattern.* The clefts should be sharp with narrow walls.

3. *The width of the colon.* The upper limit of normal for the transverse colon is 5.5 cm (4). On a supine view, this part of the colon is highest, so that gas rises up into it. In colitics gas in the colon tends to be present more frequently and is more extensive, although it may still be absent even with an extensive active colitis (Fig. 2).

It may be possible to outline the bowel wall thickness, where the mucosa is shown by gas and the serosa by properitoneal fat (Fig 4). Normally, the wall is 2 mm or less in thickness. An apparent increase in thickness is common due to incomplete distension of the bowel. This is shown by lack of parallelism between the mucosa and serosa (Fig. 5) (5).

Plain films provide only a general appraisal of the state of the colon. This may be adequate in certain clinical circumstances, such as a severe attack, but a contrast examination is required to obtain a detailed and reliable picture of the mucosa.

INSTANT ENEMA

This is a modification of the double-contrast enema, devised by Young (6) for use in patients known to have ulcerative colitis. Its objectives are to provide a double-contrast examination of the abnormal colon without submitting the patient to bowel preparation. The actual risk of bowel preparation in patients with ulcerative colitis is difficult to assess. The barium enema has been implicated in the development of toxic megacolon (7), but whether the risk relates to bowel preparation or the barium enema itself is not established. Most authors advise a less stringent bowel preparation for colitics. Some have suggested the use of two water washouts without colonic activator (8), whereas others advocate supplementing this with just a mild laxative the day before (9). Whatever the danger, bowel preparation is certain to cause discomfort and some aggravation of symptoms. If sufficient diagnostic information can be obtained without the use of bowel preparation, this is obviously a considerable advantage.

The instant enema has now been in use at St. Mark's Hospital for 17 years and at least 8000 examinations have been performed. The examination causes minimal disturbance to the patient, and rarely has there been any suggestion that it has caused any deterioration in a patient's condition. The information it provides is perfectly adequate for the clinician as long as the examination is used within its designated limits (10).

There is no preparation for an instant enema. The patient remains on his or her normal diet and therapeutic regime. A preliminary plain abdominal film is taken to exclude toxic megacolon or perforation, and should be checked before proceeding with the barium enema. The barium suspension used is similar to that for any double-contrast examination. It is run in with the patient prone and the colon filled to the splenic flexure or until residue is reached. The rectum is then drained and air gently insufflated with the patient prone and then on the right side. Enough air should be given to obtain an adequate double-contrast view of the affected colon. It is unnecessary to attempt a complete double-contrast demonstration of the entire colon. Only the colon free of residue needs delineating. Once residue is encountered the mucosa should be inactive and technically becomes difficult to visualize. The success of the instant enema depends on ulcerative colitis being a disease that remains in continuity with its distal extent (Fig. 6).

The following overcouch films are taken (Fig. 7): prone, left lateral pelvis, and erect. These are sufficient to obtain the maximum information from the instant enema. The lateral view is useful to show the configuration of the rectum and the postrectal space (Fig. 8). The erect view gives the optimum double-contrast views of the flexures and transverse colon

(Fig. 7d). A complete film series is recommended for the patient's initial investigation. However, if the patient is young, or for follow-up, the instant enema should be limited to a single prone view with barium and air, which provides practically all the necessary information for the minimum of radiation. The preliminary film is vital only if the patient is in an acute attack.

The indications for an instant enema are as follows:

1. To show the extent and severity of mucosal disease in a patient found to have proctitis on sigmoidoscopy.

2. To provide a reliable assessment of the severity and extent of disease in a patient in an acute attack, when the plain films are inconclusive but exclude perforation or toxic megacolon.

3. To document the patient's progress in follow-up.

The contraindications are as follows:

1. Toxic megacolon or perforation.

2. In patients with long-standing relatively quiescent disease where there is a risk of cancer. The presence of residue could hide a small tumor, so patients in a high-risk group should have a full double-contrast barium enema.

3. There is some danger in performing an instant enema immediately after a rectal biopsy. The risk is small and in some centers a barium enema is often performed after a biopsy. The site and depth of the biopsy affect the risk. Suction biopsies from the anterior wall could lead to an intraperitoneal perforation, whereas from the posterior wall the perforation would be extraperitoneal (Fig. 9). Our policy is to wait 10 days after a rectal biopsy, although this is not regarded as an absolute rule. If the information is required sooner, it is obviously worth the small risk and better to go ahead with the instant enema.

4. In other forms of colitis the examination may not work as well. For an example, with a patchy disease such as Crohn's colitis, residue may accumulate adjacent to small areas of mucosal disease, which will then be obscured. However, if the disease is active and extensive, the examination will work well and save the patient having bowel preparation (Fig. 10).

Therefore, where the type of colitis is unknown or uncertain and the patient has only minimal symptoms, a full double-contrast examination is warranted to obtain the optimum information. However, if the patient has an acute attack, the instant enema will usually give sufficient information whatever the type of colitis and should be attempted first.

AIR ENEMA The main problem with assessing the mucosal state from plain films is that there is often insufficient gas in the colon to outline the bowel. Rather than bringing the patient to the x-ray department for an instant enema, a simpler expedient is to supplement the colonic gas if the plain film shows this to be inadequate (11).

About 10 contractions of the bulb of a Higginson's syringe will introduce about 600–800 ml of air. The nozzle of the syringe is inserted per rectum, with the patient in the left lateral position, and the air then pumped in gently with the patient supine. Colitics often find rectal distension painful. The supine position helps reduce this as the air rises rapidly into the sigmoid and descending colon. The amount of air needed to fill the right colon depends on the size of the colon. The passage of air can be monitored by placing the palm of the hand over the right side of the abdomen. Air can be felt gurgling through the bowel, and insufflation should be stopped when air is felt in the proximal colon. A supine abdominal film is then taken. Unless the patient expels the air, reabsorption is slow, so there is no undue haste to take this film.

The air enema can show the general contour of the bowel: the state of the mucosa in general terms as to whether it is normal, granular, or ulcerated (Figs. 11–14). It is obviously not as precise as an instant enema. Its use is to provide a rough guide regarding the state of the mucosa during an acute attack. The technique is so simple that it can be performed by anyone. No special equipment is needed, so it could be performed on the ward.

D-C BARIUM ENEMA   The double-contrast barium enema has been the routine method of colonic examination in some centers for many years, but its general acceptance has been slow. There are a number of studies confirming its value in the detection of the early changes of colitis (3,8,9,12), and personal experience leaves no doubt that colitis in its early stages is more reliably shown on the double-contrast enema.

A successful examination requires proper bowel preparation, the correct barium suspension, adequate filling of the bowel, sufficient air distension, and good radiography. Many different regimes for bowel preparation have been suggested (13,14). The following has been in use for many years at St. Mark's Hospital:

1. The patient is placed on a low-residue diet 48 hr before the examination.
2. The low-residue diet is replaced by clear fluids only 24 hr before the barium enema. Once a purgative has been given, the patient should be encouraged to drink copiously.
3. The afternoon before the examination, 30 ml of castor oil or sennosides A and B (X prep*) should be given.
4. On arrival at the department on the day of the examination, the patient is given 0.1 mg of atropine orally unless there is a contraindication such as glaucoma. This reduces spasm and is claimed to reduce mucus in the colon (15). Just how successfully it does this is a matter of debate, but it certainly makes the whole procedure easier for the patient to tolerate.
5. At least one cleansing enema of 2 liters of tap water should be given 1 hr before the barium enema. Agents such as Clysodrast or oxyphenisatin may be added to aid complete evacuation. Not everyone recommends the use of these agents (13). They may cause spasm and prevent complete filling of the colon. At St. Mark's Hospital, 3 g of oxyphenisatin is used in a second cleansing enema.

The volume of enema required to fill the colon varies. Ideally, the abdomen should be palpated and water run in until the cecum is felt to be distended. Two liters represents an average volume and has been found satisfactory provided that the entire enema is always administered (13).

This represents a meticulous approach to bowel preparation which will guarantee a clean colon. Other regimes may be employed (16). Those that do not use a cleansing enema will always have a certain failure rate, although in some countries these are very successful. If the patient does not receive dietary restriction and purgation, the cleansing enema becomes more difficult to perform and has to be repeated several times before a clear return is obtained. The minimal acceptable bowel preparation would therefore include clear fluids on the day before with a purgative such as castor oil, and one 2-liter cleansing water enema before the barium enema.

Technique   The barium is run in with the patient prone until the splenic flexure is reached. This usually requires 400–600 ml. The rectum is then drained and air insufflated. The actual method depends on the equipment being used. With the E-Z-M bags,† the bag itself may

*Napp Laboratories Ltd., Hill Farm Ave., Watford WD2 7RA, U.K.

be blown up with air prior to use, or air pumped in via a Miller air tip.† The way the patient is moved during air insufflation is most important. If the patient has a redundant sigmoid it may be helpful to start this with the patient on the left side, but usually air insufflation can be started with the patient prone. This has the effect of driving the barium column from the descending colon into the transverse. If more air is pumped in with the patient prone, it will bubble through the barium and distend the cecum. This could lead to an air-block situation (17), but is easily overcome by turning the patient onto the right side so that the barium falls into the proximal colon.

The following overcouch films are taken:

Prone

Left lateral pelvis

Right and left supine 35-degree obliques (Fig. 15)

Anterioposterior and posterioanterior decubitus films with horizontal tube

Erect (to include the flexures)

Spot films should be taken of any area not clearly shown on the foregoing series or when there is any doubt as to the presence of an abnormality.

The contraindications for a full double-contrast barium enema in inflammatory bowel disease are the following:

Severe active disease (use the instant enema)

Toxic megacolon

Perforation

Colonic obstruction

The type of barium suspension used and method of bowel preparation affects the nature of the mucosal layer. Using cleansing enemas necessitates a thick suspension to obtain a layer of sufficient radiographic density. This is probably because fluid is retained in the colon, which dilutes the barium and impairs coating. In such circumstances the innominate grooves are rarely seen. Williams showed these in about 25% of barium enemas (18). Japanese studies show that they are not seen at all in over half the examinations where a cleansing enema or castor oil is given (19). The optimum bowel preparation was found to be a combination of dietary restriction, magnesium citrate, and a contact laxative such as bisacodyl. Using a barium suspension of 60–70% wt/vol with films taken at 100 kV, the innominate grooves were shown throughout the colon in 33%, partially in 54%, and not at all in only 11%.

The innominate grooves are thin transverse lines that may branch, forming a network pattern (Fig. 16). At the mucosal line the grooves are seen on edge as a short peglike projection (Fig. 17) which is sometimes referred to as spiculation. The grooves have been related to thinning of the mucosa over lymphoid follicles which are arrayed transversely (20). The significance of the innominate grooves in inflammatory bowel disease is that they may be confused with ulceration, or that their loss could represent the earliest change of colitis, or alternatively, that their accentuation due to edema is the earliest manifestation of Crohn's disease (12). The significance of the innominate grooves in the diagnosis of colitis has yet to be determined.

Spiculation is usually distinguished from superficial erosions by the sharpness and symmetry of the peglike projections (Fig. 19). Irregular spikes 1–3 mm deep have been noted in ulcerative colitis when the bowel is contracted, and to disappear on distention (21). Changes in profile may be confusing, and more reliance should be placed on the en face view, where the thin interbranching lines of the grooves can be seen clearly.

†E-Z-EM, 7 Portland Ave., Westbury, N.Y. 11590.

SMALL
BOWEL

Endoscopists are now able to examine the duodenal loop and distal part of the terminal ileum, but the overall examination of the small bowel remains the perogative of the radiologist. Comparisons in the colon with endoscopy have shown the importance of high-quality examinations in the diagnosis of inflammatory bowel disease, and similarly in the small bowel the diagnosis of IBD may depend to a large extent on the standard of examination. It is unfortunate that small bowel examinations are frequently poorly performed. This may result in failure to diagnose Crohn's disease, which in the pediatric age group can have serious consequences in growth retardation; or the converse may occur and a fallacious diagnosis is made and the patient placed on steroids. Radiologists should remember that unless a laparectomy is performed it may be impossible to obtain histological confirmation of the diagnosis of IBD, which may depend largely on the radiologist's opinion.

Small Bowel Meal The small bowel meal is a standard method of examination in which the patient drinks the barium suspension and films are taken at intervals as the barium passes through the small bowel. A major drawback of this method has been the time that the barium takes to reach the cecum. With less stable suspensions slow transit can result in flocculation and loss of mucosal definition. Many factors can affect the rate of gastric emptying and transit through the small bowel; the volume of contrast given and the use of accelerating agents are two that the radiologist can control. Golden recommended giving 250 ml of contrast, but Marshak (22) increased this to 480 ml which reduced the transit time and improved mucosal defintion. Metoclopramide is now widely used and is of proven value in speeding up gastric emptying (23). Film timing is important to avoid missing areas of the small bowel. To begin with, films should be taken at short intervals, and then longer when the rate of transit can be assessed.

About 10 minutes before the examination, 20 mg of metoclopramide is administered orally. A typical examination would include the following:

1. 300 ml of barium suspension is administered and the esophagus, stomach, and duodenal loop quickly screened.
2. Prone overcouch films are taken after 10 and 30 min.
3. Further films are taken at 30- to 45-min intervals depending on the rate of transit.
4. The terminal ileum is screened and spot films taken routinely.

Compression views are particularly important to show small ulcers (Fig. 18). Careful compression studies can show aphthoid ulcers in the small bowel in up to 52% of patients with Crohn's disease (24) (Fig. 20). Such ulcers are usually not seen unless compression views are taken.

Per oral pneumocolon is a useful method of obtaining double-contrast views of the distal small bowel. The terminal ileum is often deep in the pelvis and cannot be compressed (Fig. 21), or where there is doubt as to abnormality (Fig. 22), this method offers an alternative approach with the advantages of distension to show strictures, and double contrast to show the mucosal surface in detail. The technique is very simple (25). Air is insufflated into the colon and refluxed into the small bowel. Incompetence of the ileocecal valve may be aided by intravenous relaxants (Fig. 22b).

Small Bowel Enema A number of methods exist for giving a small bowel enema, but the common aim is to introduce a large volume of low-density contrast agent into the small bowel. The following advantages are claimed:

Flocculation is avoided, so there is optimum visualization of the mucosa.
The bowel is distended, so strictures are readily apparent.

The valvulae conniventes are clearly shown, so small mucosal lesions can be identified. Using a low-density suspension with high-kilovolt films allows superimposed loops to be "seen through." A double-contrast effect can be achieved by the infusion of water or air.

Sellink advocates the enteroclysis technique (26). The duodenum is intubated with a Bilbao-Dotter tube, and 600 ml of barium suspension of specific gravity 1.25 is infused at a rate of 80–100 ml/min. If the distal small bowel has not filled, an additional 600 ml can be given. This can be followed by 600 ml of water to achieve a double-contrast effect. Herlinger's modification (27) of this involves an initial infusion of about 200 ml of 85% wt/vol barium suspension, followed by a large volume of an aqueous suspension of methyl cellulose. This is prepared by dissolving 10 g of methyl cellulose powder in 2 liters of water. This is infused at a rate of 100 ml/min until the distal ileum is filled. The methyl cellulose prevents the mixing of barium with water. An excellent double-contrast image is created which, unlike the water infusion in enteroclysis, last for a considerable time (Fig. 23).

Miller's technique of the complete reflux small bowel examination does not involve duodenal intubation (28). The colon is filled with 2 liters of a 20% wt/vol suspension, followed by 2–2.5 liters of near-normal saline (1 teaspoonful of salt to 1 liter of tap water). Reflux into the small bowel is aided by intravenous relaxants. The colon is drained once sufficient barium has refluxed into the small bowel.

Overcouch high-kilovolt films with spot views under compression are taken whatever the method of examination. The reflux method avoids intubation, but the colonic distension can cause considerable discomfort and has not found widespread acceptance.

Superimposition of ileal loops in the pelvis is a common problem. Sigmoid distension tends to push these loops out of the pelvis, so the distal ileum is visualized better by the reflux method, as colonic distension is an integral part of the examination. However, a similar effect can be achieved during intubation studies by air insufflation per rectum.

The dilution of the barium suspension by the small bowel intestinal contents can degrade visualization of the distal small bowel. This is largely overcome by using relatively large volumes of suspension, but better-quality views of the ileum may be obtained by the reflux technique. A loaded cecum will slow transit in the ileum (29) and cause difficulties demonstrating the terminal ileum on intubation studies, so a laxative should be given the day before.

Proponents of the small bowel enema claim a higher diagnostic yield in IBD (30–34). Certainly, strictures are more clearly defined, and the higher pressures involved may reveal fistulas that would not fill on a small bowel meal, but the highest reported incidence of aphthoid ulceration in Crohn's disease has been achieved by careful compression studies during a standard small bowel meal (24). Preoperative assessment of Crohn's involvement of the small bowel is probably best performed by small bowel enema to show strictures.

ILEOSTOMY ENEMA

Patients with an ileostomy may be examined by a small bowel meal or enema, but the distal small bowel immediately under the site of the ileostomy is often not well shown. Palpation is impossible and this segment is obscured by barium filling the ileostomy bag. A different approach is therefore required to show this segment of the bowel.

A medium-sized Foley catheter is inserted into the ileostomy. The balloon is inflated with 10 ml of air and the catheter withdrawn so that the balloon rests gently against the abdominal wall. This forms a seal, which is useful to prevent spillage of barium but not sufficient to allow undue pressure to build up or to cause enough expansion of the balloon to endanger the bowel at any narrowing. It is helpful if the patient uses a disposable bag for the examination. A hole can be made in this and the catheter introduced through it. Some spillage is inevitable, and this will then collect in the bag and not spread all over the skin to obscure the small bowel.

The patient is then given an intravenous relaxant, usually 20–40 mg of Buscopan.* This is an essential part of the examination. Any attempt to fill the small bowel retrogradely causes intense peristalsis and rapid emptying. Peristalsis must be inhibited if a reasonable segment of bowel is to be visualized and a persistent narrowing (i.e., a stricture) demonstrated. Barium suspension of 100% wt/vol is injected with a syringe. It is often only possible to use about 50–150 ml. Air is then insufflated with a Higginson's syringe and several spot films taken to show double-contrast views of the distal small bowel and area immediately under the ileostomy (Fig. 24).

SINOGRAPHY

Sinography is probably the most neglected radiological investigation in gastroenterology and is usually regarded as an unpleasant chore. Unfortunately, a number of patients with Crohn's disease develop numerous abscesses, tracks, sinuses, and fistulas such that the anterior abdominal wall is a battleground of openings. The management of these patients is obviously extremely difficult and surgeons require detailed sinography to decide what should be done. On many occasions sinography is an extremely important investigation and deserves greater consideration than it usually receives.

Sinography should be performed before any barium study, as residual barium may obscure a small track. The sinus opening should be inspected, then gently probed, to determine the direction of the track. A soft rubber catheter is then introduced with forceps along the path of the sinus and directed as far in as possible without using force. The contrast agent is injected under screening control using moderate pressure. Spot films are taken. If any track is shown, the direction of the track has to be determined by taking a film at right angles to the original one, which is usually supine. This means turning the patient onto his or her side, but if it would be difficult to move the patient, a supine decubitus film with a horizontal tube could be used instead. A water-soluble contrast medium is recommended, as oily contrast can persist for a long time and interfere with subsequent investigations. The density of the agent should not be too low; otherwise, a thin track could be missed. Some of the tracks are very narrow. It may not be possible to introduce a probe into these. If there is evidence of recent discharge, an attempt should be made to enter the track with a fine polyethylene catheter.

RETENTION ENEMA

Topical corticosteroids are a successful method of treating colitis. The patient self-administers the steroid enema using a disposable plastic bladder syringe and rubber catheter. The volume of the enema can be varied from 50 to 200 ml and is altered to suit the extent of the colitis. To check that sufficient volume is being given, a "retention enema" may be performed.

Five percent by volume of barium suspension is added to the enema, which the patient administers in the usual fashion. The patient then lies prone on the x-ray table for 5 min, after which a plain film is taken (Fig. 25a). This will show how far the enema has filled the colon, and the efficacy of the enema can be judged by comparing this to the extent of the colitis on the instant enema (Fig. 25b). For a given volume of enema, there is considerable variation between individuals as to how far the enema extends, but little variation for any given individual on repeat studies (35). For most distal colitis, 100 ml is adequate, but larger volumes are needed for more extensive disease, and it is mainly in these patients that a retention enema is advised to ensure that an adequate volume is being given.

*Hyoscine butylbromide, 20 mg/ml, Boehringer Ingelheim Ltd., Southern Industrial Estate, Bracknell, Berks, U.K.

REFERENCES

1. Bartram, C.I.(1976). The plain abdominal X-ray in acute colitis. Proc. R Soc. Med. 69; 617.
2. Connell, A.M., Lennard-Jones, J.E., Madanagopalan, N. (1964). The distribution of faecal X-ray shadows in subjects without gastrointestinal disease. Proc. R. Soc. Med. 57; 894.
3. Bartram, C.I. (1977). Radiology in the current assessment of ulcerative colitis. Gastrointest. Radiol. 1; 383.
4. Hywel-Jones, J., Chapman, M. (1969). Definition of megacolon in colitis. Gut 10; 562.
5. Bartram, C.I., Herlinger, H. (1979). Bowel wall thickness as a differentiating feature between ulcerative colitis and Crohn's disease of the colon. Clin. Radiol. 30; 5.
6. Young, A.C. (1963). The instant enema in proctocolitis. Proc. R. Soc. Med. 56; 491.
7. Roth, J.L.A., Valdes-Dapena, A., Skin, G.A., Bockus, H.L. (1959). Toxic megacolon in ulcerative colitis. Gastroenterology 37; 239.
8. Simpkins, K.C., Stevenson, G.W. (1972). The modified Malmo double contrast barium enema in colitis: an assessment of its accuracy in reflecting sigmoidoscopic findings. Br. J. Radiol. 45; 486.
9. Welin, S., Brahme, F. (1961). The double contrast method in ulcerative colitis. Acta Radiol. 55; 257.
10. Thomas, B.M. (1979). The instant enema in inflammatory disease of the colon. Clin. Radiol. 30; 165.
11. Preston D., Bartram, C.I., Thomas, B.M., Lennard-Jones, J.E. (1980). Air introduced per rectum can be used to give radiological contrast in severe acute colitis: the "air enema." Gut 21; 1914.
12. Hildell, J., Lindstrom, C., Wenckert, A. (1979). Radiographic appearances in Crohn's disease. 1. Accuracy of radiographic methods. Acta Radiol. Diagn. 20; 609.
13. Miller, R.E. (1975). The cleansing enema. Radiology 117; 483.
14. Dodds, W.J., Scanlon, G.T., Shaw, D.K., et al. (1977). An evaluation of colon cleansing regimes. Am. J. Roentgenol. 128; 57.
15. Welin, S. (1958). Modern trends in diagnostic roentgenology of the colon. Br. J. Radiol. 31; 453.
16. De Lacey, G., Benson, M., Wilkins, R., et al. (1982). Routine colonic lavage is unnecessary for double-contrast barium enema in outpatients. Br. Med. J. 284; 1021.
17. Miller, R.E. (1979). Solution for the "air block" problem during fluoroscopy. Am. J. Roentgenol. 132; 1020.
18. Williams, I. (1965). Innominate grooves in the surface of mucosa. Radiology 84; 877.
19. Matsura, K., Nakata, H., Takeda, N., et al. (1977). Innominate lines of the colon. Radiology 123; 581.
20. Cole, F.M. (1978). Innominate grooves of the colon: morphological characteristics and etiologic mechanisms. Radiology 128; 41.
21. Paterson, D. (1979). Ulcerative colitis, innominate pits and faecal retention. Aust. Radiol. 22; 242.
22. Marshak, R.M., Lindner, A.E. (1970). *Radiology of the Small Intestine*. Saunders, Philadelphia, p. 2.
23. Howarth, F.H., Cockel, R., Roper, B.W., Hawkins, C.F. (1969). The effect of metoclopramide upon gastric motility and its value in barium progress meals. Clin. Radiol. 20; 294.
24. Engelholm, L., Haingnet, P., Potulige, P. (1976). Radiology in early Crohn's disease of the small intestine. In *Proceedings of the Workshop on Crohn's Disease*. Leiden, p. 73.

25. Kellet, M.J., Zboralske, F.F., Margulis, A.R. (1977). Per oral pneumocolon examination of the ileocaecal region. Gastrointest. Radiol. 1; 361.

26. Sellink, J.L. (1976). *Radiological Atlas of Common Diseases of the Small Bowel.* Stenfert Kroese, Leiden.

27. Herlinger, H. (1978). A modified technique for double contrast small bowel enema. Gastrointest. Radiol. 3; 201.

28. Miller, R.E. (1969). Reflux examination of the small bowel. Radiol. Clin. N. Am. 7; 175.

29. Nolan, D.J. (1979). Rapid duodenal and jejunal intubation. Clin. Radiol. 30; 183.

30. Nolan, D.J., Piris, J. (1980). Crohn's disease of the small intestine: a comparative study of the radiological and pathological appearances. Clin. Radiol. 31; 591.

31. Vallance, R. (1980). An evaluation of the small bowel enema based on an analysis of 350 consecutive examinations. Clin. Radiol. 31; 227.

32. Skjennald, A., Smaset, J.H., (1980). Duodeno-jejunal intubation in examination of the small intestine. Clin. Radiol. 31; 221.

33. Ekberg, O. (1977). Crohn's disease of the small bowel examined by double contrast technique: a comparison with the oral technique. Gastrointest. Radiol. 1; 355.

34. Saunders, D.E., Ho, C.S. (1976). The small bowel enema: experience with 150 examinations. Am. J. Radiol. 127; 743.

35. Swarbrick, E.T., Loose, H., Lennard-Jones, J.E. (1974). Enema volume as an important factor in successful topical corticosteroid treatment of colitis. Proc. R. Soc. Med. 67; 753.

FIGURES 1 THROUGH 25

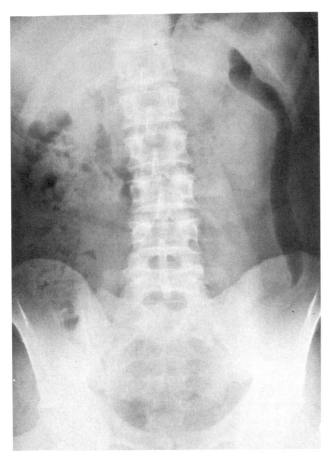

Figure 1 Ulcerative colitis with a granular mucosa as judged from the extent of the formed fecal residue and abnormal gas shadow.

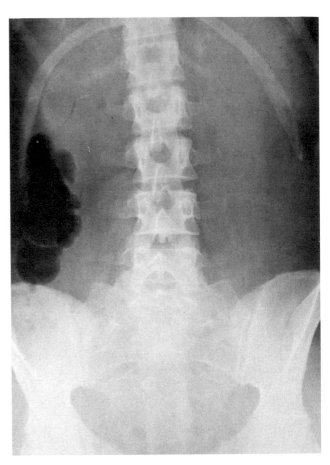

Figure 2a No formed residue, suggesting a total active colitis. The bowel contains very little gas.

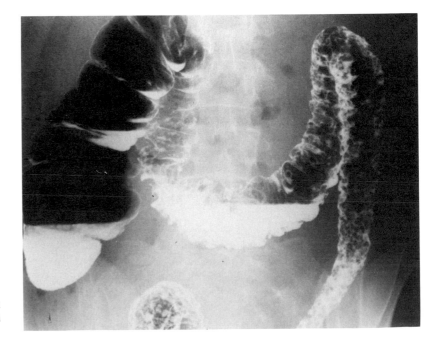

Figure 2b Severe colitis with ulceration extending to the hepatic flexure confirmed on an instant cnema.

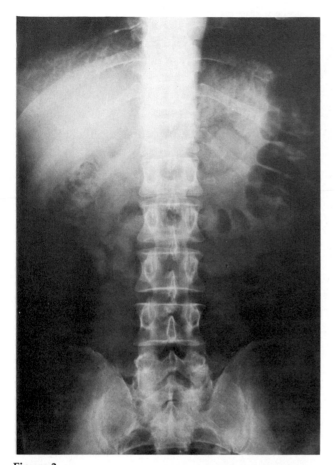

Figure 3

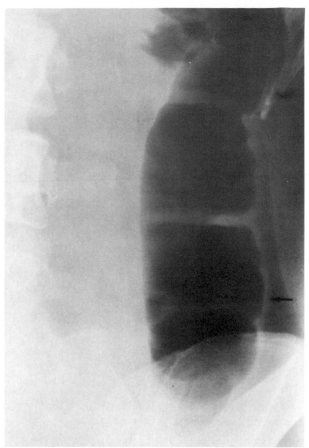

Figure 4

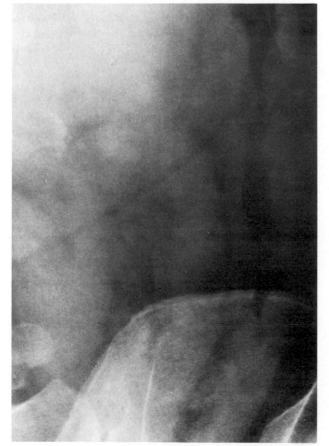

Figure 3 Noncolitic patient, showing a normal distribution of residue and bowel gas, with well-defined sharp haustral clefts and a smooth mucosal edge in the distal transverse colon. (From Ref. 36.)

Figure 4 Normal bowel wall thickness of 2 mm. The serosa is outlined by properitoneal fat (arrow) and the mucosa by intracolonic gas.

Figure 5 The bowel is poorly distended and the wall appears grossly thickened. Gas in the lumen shows a wavy outline that does not follow the serosal edge. On barium enema the bowel wall thickness was seen to be normal.

Figure 5

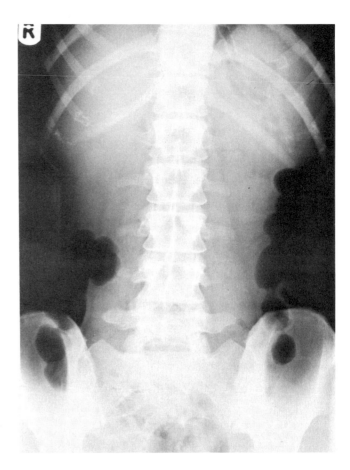

Figure 6a Instant enema—preliminary film. No residue. The gas that is present shows a rather tubular bowel but no mucosal irregularity.

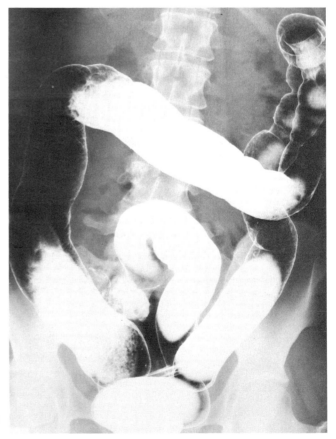

Figure 6b Prone view after barium and air confirms total colitis with a granular mucosa.

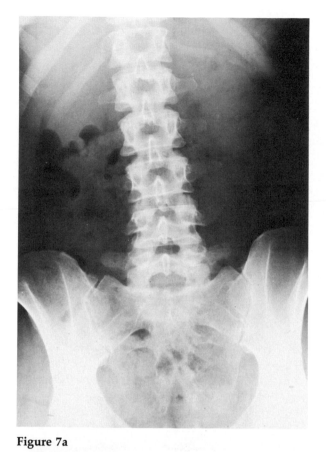

Figure 7a

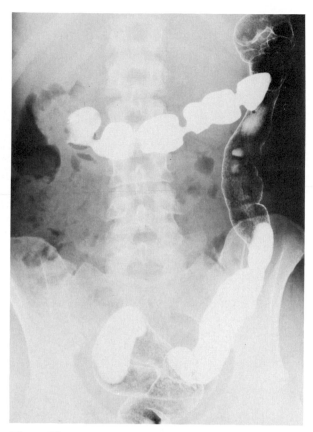

Figure 7b

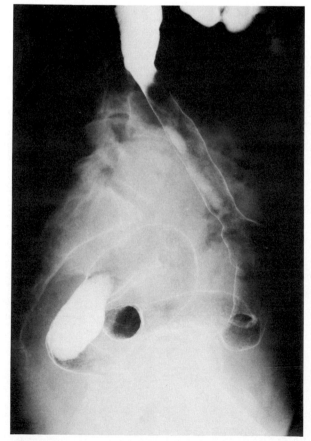

Figure 7c

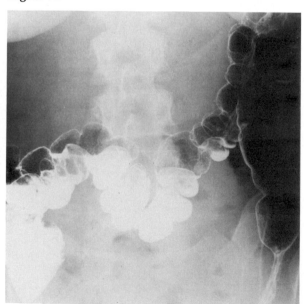

Figure 7d

Figure 7 Instant enema—complete series. (a) Preliminary film. (b) Prone. (c) Left lateral pelvis. (d) Erect.

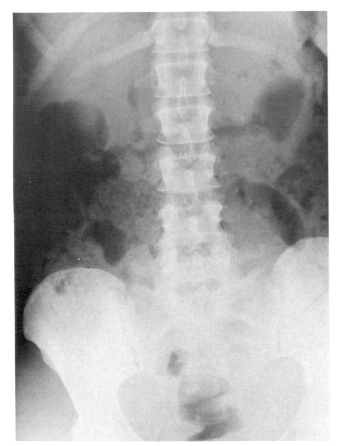

Figure 8a

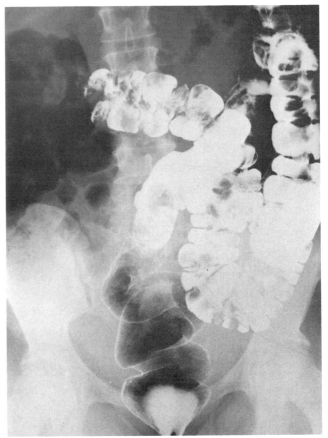

Figure 8b

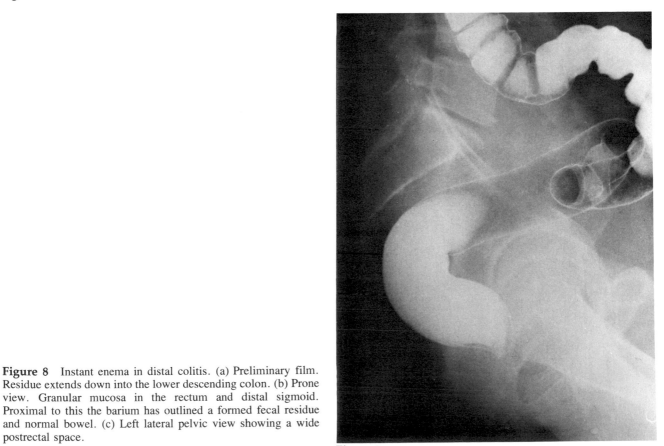

Figure 8c

Figure 8 Instant enema in distal colitis. (a) Preliminary film. Residue extends down into the lower descending colon. (b) Prone view. Granular mucosa in the rectum and distal sigmoid. Proximal to this the barium has outlined a formed fecal residue and normal bowel. (c) Left lateral pelvic view showing a wide postrectal space.

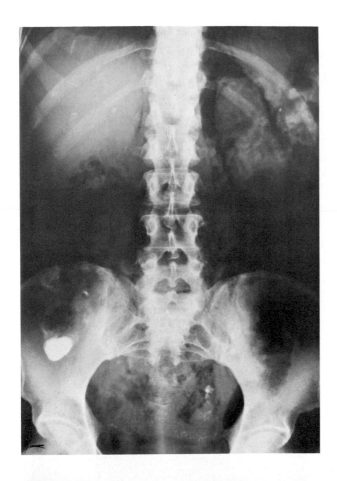

Figure 9 Retroperitoneal air following perforation of the rectum due to rectal biopsy at sigmoidoscopy.

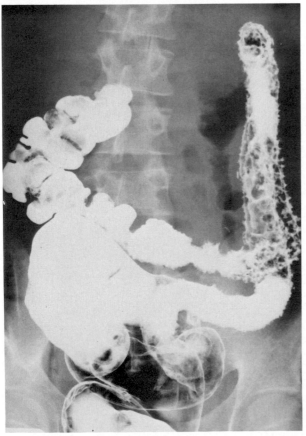

Figure 10 Instant enema in Crohn's disease. Rectal sparing with extensive ulceration in the transverse and descending colons. Residue has prevented demonstration of the proximal colon, but the extent of gross disease has been shown.

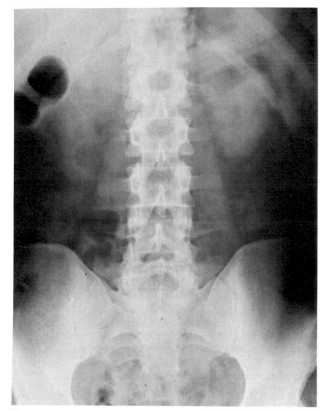

Figure 11a

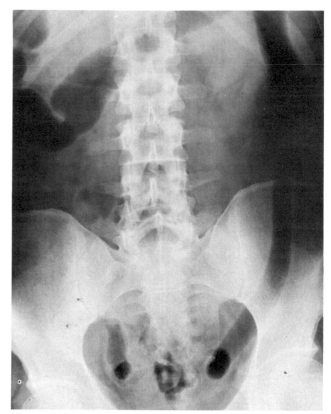

Figure 11b

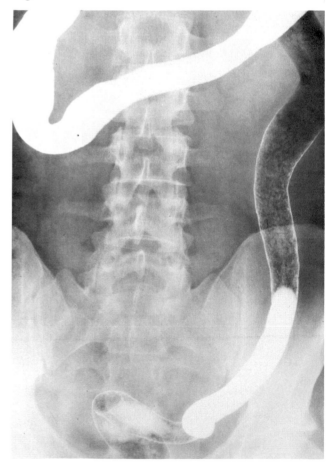

Figure 11c

Figure 11 Air enema. (a) The plain films show no gas or residue in the colon. (b) After air insufflation a tubular smooth-edged bowel is outlined, suggesting total colitis with a granular mucosa. (c) This is confirmed on an instant enema performed within 24 hr of (b).

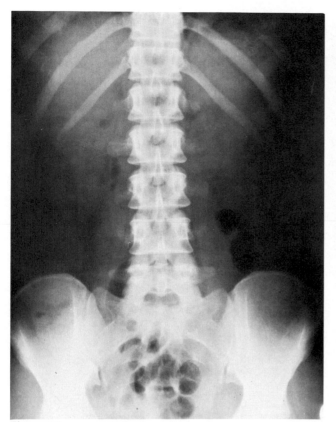

Figure 12a

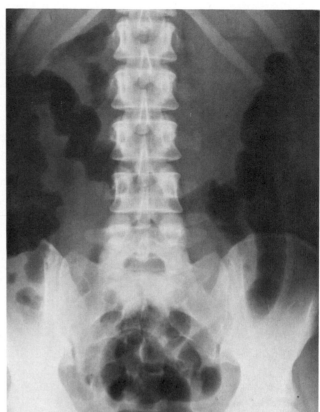

Figure 12b

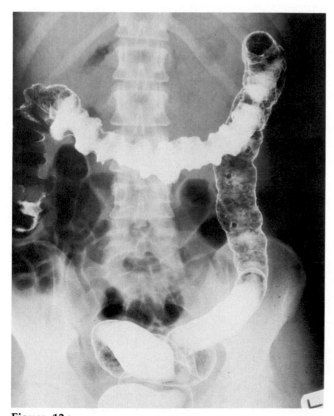

Figure 12c

Figure 12 Air enema. (a) The plain film shows no gas or residue in the colon. (b) After air insufflation the entire colon is outlined. There is no mucosal irregularity. Some blunted haustration is present. The appearances again suggest a total colitis with a granular mucosa. (c) This is confirmed by an instant enema. Some superficial ulceration is noted in the descending colon. This degree of detail is not visible on the air enema.

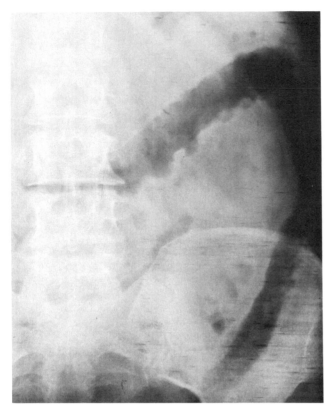

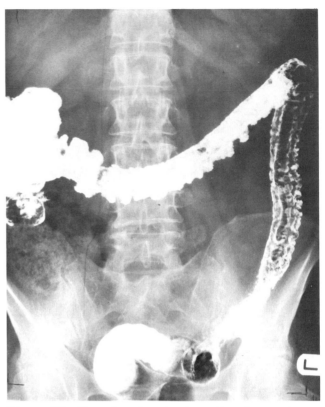

Figure 13 Air enema. (a) Film after air insufflation. The preliminary view did not show any gas in the colon, so the mucosal state could not be assessed. Coarse irregularity of the mucosal edge indicates ulceration.

Figure 13b Extensive ulceration is confirmed on an instant enema performed within 24 hr of (a).

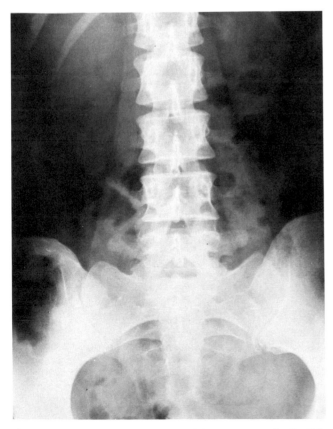

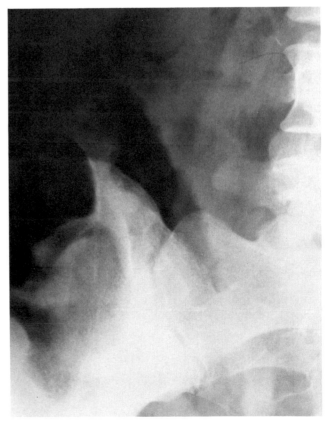

Figure 14a Plain film in a patient with an acute attack of colitis. The volume of gas in the bowel is inadequate to assess detail.

Figure 14b A close-up view of the air enema showing ulceration in the transverse colon.

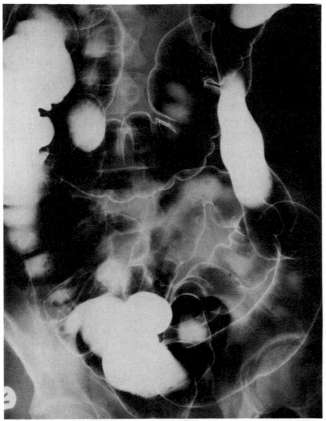

Figure 15 Double-contrast barium enema, supine oblique view (LPO). Note the smooth coating of barium en face and the thin even mucosal line.

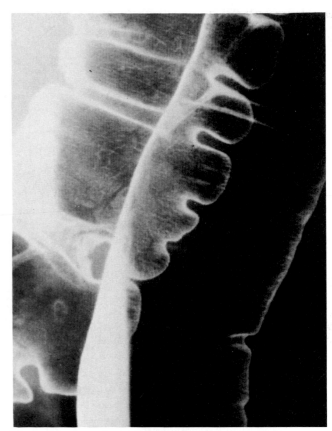

Figure 16 Innominate groove pattern.

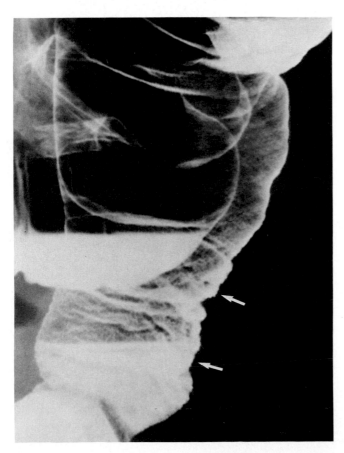

Figure 17 The innominate grooves in profile present as small peglike projections (arrows).

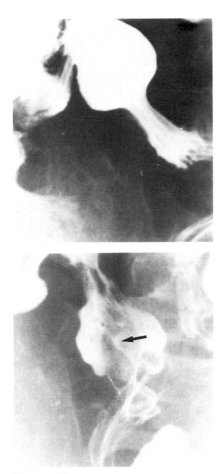

Figure 18

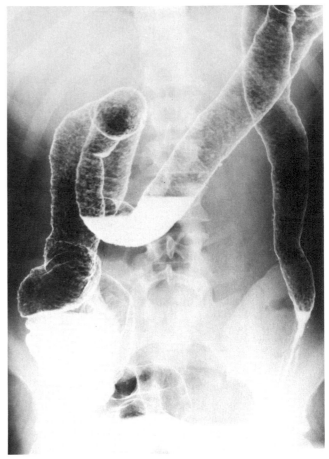

Figure 19

Figure 18 Compression showing a small linear ulcer in the terminal ileum in Crohn's disease (arrow).

Figure 19 Total colitis with a granular mucosa and some superficial ulceration causing small irregular projections from the mucosal line, which do not follow a linear pattern like the innominate grooves. (From Ref. 36.)

Figure 20 Aphthoid ulcers seen in the jejunum with compression (arrows).

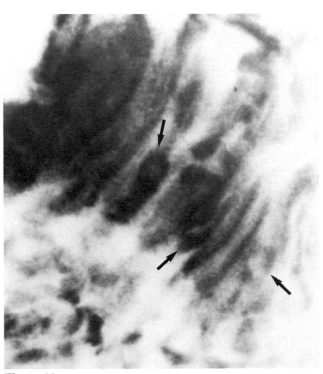

Figure 20

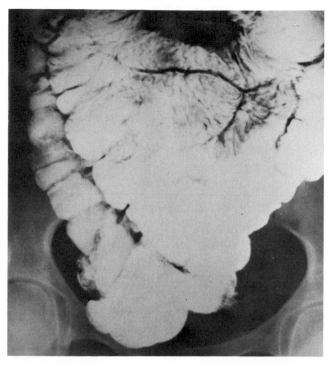

Figure 21a The terminal ileum lies deep in the pelvis and was impossible to compress.

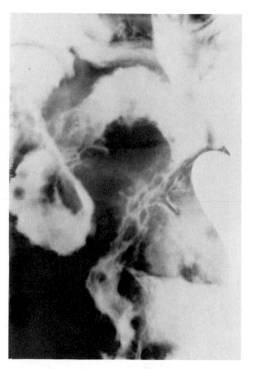

Figure 21b Following rectal air insufflation the distended sigmoid has pushed the cecum up into the right iliac dossa and the terminal ileum was clearly visible.

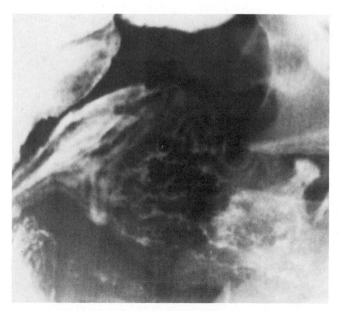

Figure 22a Compression views of the terminal ileum in a patient suspected of having Crohn's disease. The fold pattern is irregular.

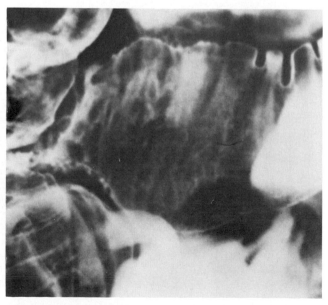

Figure 22b Air insufflation and reflux into the terminal ileum (after intravenous relaxant) showed a normal mucosal surface. This was confirmed endoscopically.

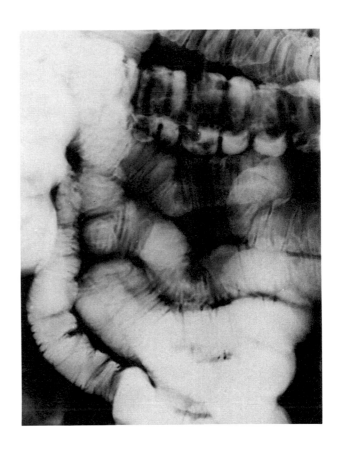

Figure 23 Small bowel infusion using the Herlinger technique.

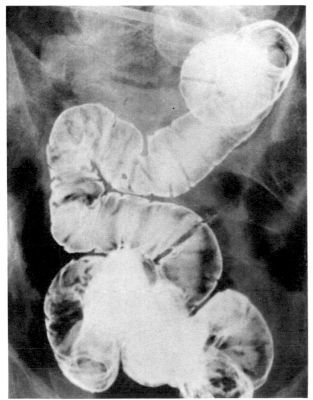

Figure 24a Ileostomy enema with Foley catheter in situ showing normal distal small bowel.

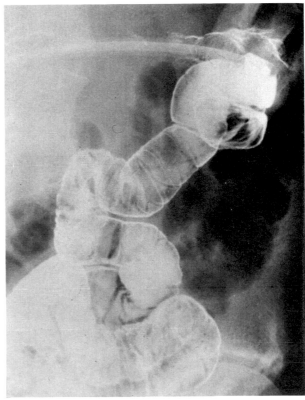

Figure 24b Ileostomy enema. Oblique view of normal distal small bowel.

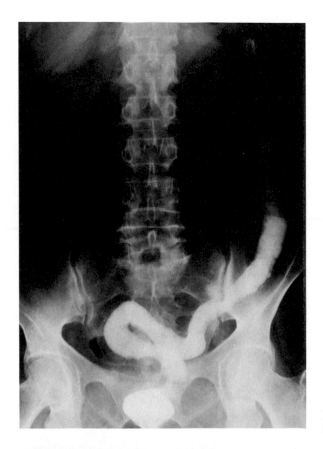

Figure 25a Contrast mixed with the retention enema to show how far proximally the enema reaches.

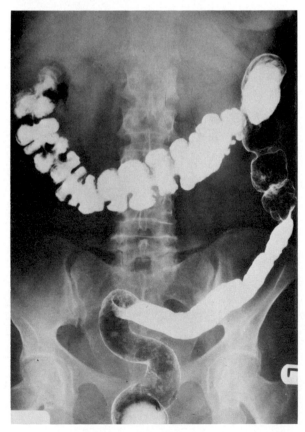

Figure 25b Comparison with the instant enema indicates that the extent of active colitis is being adequately covered by the retention enema.

2

Ulcerative Colitis

This nonspecific form of colitis is characterized by involvement of the rectum, spreading in continuity to its proximal extent. A diffuse granular mucosa is typical. The nomenclature regarding ulceration is misleading, as this is seen only in acute attacks.

The symptoms of ulcerative colitis are diarrhea, rectal bleeding, and constitutional disturbance. These may be gradual or sudden in onset. The disease is often severe in its first year, with acute episodes in which hemorrhage is profuse. Compared to Crohn's disease there is increased mortality and need for surgery in the first year (1). A few patients will have a single attack and then go into either complete or partial remission, with low-grade continuous disease. The majority suffer a chronic course with intermittent flare-ups. Four out of five have a second attack within 1 year of the first, and after 15 years only 4% escape a second attack (2).

The diagnosis is suggested from the history and findings at sigmoidoscopy. There are a number of other causes of proctitis, for example:

Idiopathic   Salmonella
Ulcerative colitis   Amebiasis
Crohn's disease   Mucosal prolapse
Ischemia   Antibiotic therapy
Radiation   Chronic diarrhea
Gonorrhea

Thus the demonstration of proctitis at sigmoidoscopy does not imply a diagnosis of ulcerative colitis unless supported by rectal biopsy (Chap. 8). About 10% of patients with idiopathic proctitis develop ulcerative colitis (3), and it is now accepted that this should be regarded as ulcerative colitis limited to the rectum.

Various other terms have been used to describe ulcerative colitis, such as idiopathic proctocolitis, mucosal colitis, or rectocolite hemorrhagique. Although these may be more correct descriptively than "ulcerative colitis" (4), they have not found routine usage.

RADIO-LOGICAL PATHOLOGY

The appearance of the mucosa reflects the duration and severity of the colitis. The changes can be divided roughly into "active disease" or "disease in remission" (4). In active disease the mucosa is granular and hemorrhagic (Fig. 1). The capillaries in the mucosa and submucosa are congested and dilated. There is edema and an inflammatory cell infiltrate, which may extend into the submucosa. Inflammatory changes in ulcerative colitis are limited to the mucous membrane, and involve only the muscularis propria and serosa in fulminating states. This is a fundamental difference from Crohn's disease, where the inflammation is always transmural.

Cellular debris tends to block the crypts of Lieberkühn, leading to the formation of microabscesses in the mucous membrane. These are usually called "crypt abscesses" and are a frequent finding in ulcerative colitis but not specific to this condition, as they may be seen in Crohn's disease and the dysenteries. Crypt abscesses may discharge into the lumen, giving pus in the feces, or rupture. The contents then tend to track longitudinally in the loose submucosal tissues, thus separating the mucosa from its supporting submucosa. Part of the mucosa sloughs, leaving an undermined ulcer. The ulcers often have a linear configuration, related to the attachment of the taeniae (Fig. 2). Ulceration may be very extensive and involve all the affected colon and rectum, or localized, when the sigmoid and descending colon are involved most commonly.

When the colitis goes into remission, the mucosa loses its hemorrhagic component. The mucous membrane becomes atrophic, and the surface may be quite smooth (Fig. 3). Histologically, it is still abnormal. Inflammatory polyps are a common residue from a previous acute attack with ulceration (Fig. 4). A consistent feature of ulcerative colitis is the shortening and narrowing of the bowel, with loss of haustration. This is not due to fibrosis, which is almost entirely absent in ulcerative colitis, but to hypertrophy of the muscle. Thickening of the muscularis propria is said to be responsible for the generalized changes in contour of the large bowel, with thickening of the muscularis mucosae, causing localized strictures (5). As there is no fibrosis, these changes are reversible and the bowel can revert to its normal shape and size in remission (6).

The rectum is always involved in ulcerative colitis. The disease spreads into the colon in continuity. The intensity may vary, which can rarely give the appearance of a skip lesion (4,7) (Figs. 5 and 6), but there is no histological discontinuity. In a similar fashion the rectum can heal and seem normal radiologically (Fig. 7) or sigmoidoscopically, but a biopsy will still be abnormal. "Rectal sparing" and "right-sided colitis" are macroscopic descriptions only and do not imply a different histological distribution of the colitis. To assess this requires biopsy, as it is possible for a microscopic abnormality to be present when the mucosa appears normal macroscopically.

Visual comparisons between the surface appearance of the resected colon and that on barium enema, demonstrates the detailed view of the mucosa that is possible using double contrast (8) (Figs. 8 and 10).

PLAIN FILM CHANGES

There is much information to be gained from plain abdominal x-rays in assessment of ulcerative colitis, particularly in an acute attack. While concentrating on the colon it is important not to forget other abnormalities, such as renal calculi or sacroiliitis, or that many of the changes are relatively nonspecific (Fig. 9).

The following features are used to assess the extent and severity of the colitis (7,9):

1. The extent of formed fecal residue
2. The appearance of the mucosal edge
3. Any alteration of haustration
4. The width of the colon

Features 2 to 4 require the presence of intracolonic gas. The colon may be quite devoid of gas, even during an acute attack, so that the plain film will show only the extent of the residue. If none is present, the abdomen will appear completely "empty" (Fig. 11). This situation can be rectified by use of the air enema (Chap. 1), (Fig. 12).

Colonic Residue There is no absolute relationship between the distal extent of the formed fecal residue and the proximal extent of the colitis. However, provided that some limitations are accepted, it will provide a good guide to the extent of the colitis.

In patients with proctitis there is considerable variation in the extent of the residue (Fig. 13), which is indistinguishable from that in noncolitics (10). However, where a substantial part of the colon is involved, the distal extent of the residue gives a good indication of the proximal extent of the colitis. It is possible that the extent of the colitis may be overestimated, but not underestimated, as comparisons with instant enemas indicate that active mucosal disease does not extend past formed residue. The following conclusions may be drawn from the extent of the residue:

1. If there no residue is visible, the patient probably has a total active colitis (Fig. 11).
2. If the residue extends down into the sigmoid colon, the colitis is distal to this (i.e., only a proctitis is present). Where there is doubt as to the upper limit of the disease on sigmoidoscopy but residue is present in the sigmoid, a proctitis is confirmed and there is no need to perform an instant enema.
3. If residue is visible only in the proximal colon, the colitis is most likely to extend to this level, but could be more distal.
4. If the upper limit of disease is seen on sigmoidoscopy but only a little formed residue is present in the colon, this is still in keeping with a proctitis.

Mucosa The normal mucosal edge is smooth (Fig. 14). An active granular mucosa causes the mucosal line to become indistinct and somewhat fuzzy (7) (Fig. 15), although it remains an intact line. This is difficult to judge, and changes in haustration are more reliable to show early involvement. Ulceration disrupts the mucosal line and causes a coarse irregular edge (8) (Fig. 16). Where there is extensive ulceration, only edematous mucosal "islands" (11) are left, which are visible in profile and en face (Fig. 17). Speckled gas shadows in the bowel wall may present in fulminating colitis with necrosis of the bowel wall (Fig. 18). Linear streaks of gas in the wall suggest either very deep ulceration or extraperitoneal perforation with gas trapped alongside the bowel wall (Fig. 19).

Haustration The haustral cleft is clearly identified on barium enemas as two lines that turn in from the edges of the saccules to run in parallel, about 2–4 mm apart across one-third of the bowel (Fig. 21). The haustral cleft can also be seen when the colon is distended by gas (Fig. 14). Widening of the cleft with loss of the parallel lines is the earliest alteration (Figs. 15 and 20). It accompanies a granular mucosa and is more obvious than the mucosal abnormality on plain films.

Unfortunately, it is easy to confuse blunting with underdistension. This will also cause a rounding of the bowel edge at the site of the cleft, but there is no evidence of lines into the cleft (Fig. 22). Blunting should not be diagnosed when there is only a little gas in the bowel.

In most patients with a granular mucosa on instant enema, the haustra are absent, but the progression to ulceration always causes complete loss of the haustral clefts (Fig. 16). Changes in the haustra reflect alteration in the tone of the smooth muscle in the bowel wall, and appear, pari passu with narrowing and shortening of the colon.

Colonic Width The colon becomes narrowed and tubular with active colitis, so that it is usually considerably less than 5.5 cm wide, which is the upper limit of normal for the transverse colon in the noncolitic bowel (12). Dilatation of more than 5 cm implies deep ulceration down to the muscle layer. In ulcerative colitis this means that the inflammation has become transmural and that the patient has a fulminating colitis and is at risk from perforation or toxic megacolon (Chap. 3) (Fig. 23).

Haustral and mucosal changes should really be viewed in conjunction, as this will improve diagnostic accuracy. It is unwise to place too much reliance on some of the early changes, but a possibly abnormal mucosa becomes a definite abnormality if there is blunting of the haustral clefts as well (Fig. 15). On the other hand, if the haustral clefts are absolutely normal, the mucosa is almost certainly normal and there may be some other explanation, such as adherent liquid residue, to account for the mucosal change. Ulceration with loss of haustration is the most definite change (Fig. 23). It should be noted that none of these features is specific for ulcerative colitis and may be found in any form of diffuse colitis.

BARIUM ENEMA CHANGES There should be no difference in the radiographic features between an instant and a formal barium enema with full bowel preparation, as in both the mucosa is visualized in double contrast. Artifacts are more common in an instant enema. A liquid residue may smear the mucosa with debris, creating the impression of inflammatory polyps or ulceration (Figs. 24 and 25). This can usually be distinguished from true ulceration, as the mucosal line remains intact. With a little experience artifacts may be excluded with confidence.

The interpretation of barium enema changes should be based on two factors: analysis of the mucosal lesions, which show the primary mucosal disease, and alteration in the configuration of the bowel, which reflects changes in the smooth muscle tone associated with the mucosal inflammation (13).

Mucosal Abnormalities Mucosal abnormalities include granularity, ulceration, and inflammatory polyps.

Granularity This is the earliest abnormality that can be recognized on double-contrast studies (14). The normal smooth coating of barium is replaced by an amorphous texture. This varies considerably; it may be fine or coarse, or contain a stippled component (Fig. 26). Fine granularity has been associated with mucosal edema and hyperemia and stippling with small pools of barium in superficial erosions (15). There is usually a gradual transition between normal and abnormal mucosa, extending over several centimeters. Granularity is best appreciated by its en face appearance. The mucosal line remains intact, although becoming slightly thickened with ill-defined edges (Fig. 26). A chronic atrophic mucosa may cause a fine granular change, but can be smooth and appear normal radiologically (Fig. 27).

Ulceration In contrast to granularity, ulceration is recognized most easily by looking at the mucosal line where the barium-filled ulcers project out from and disrupt the line (Fig. 28). En face the difference between coarse granularity and superficial ulceration may not be so readily apparent, and where there is doubt the problem is easily resolved by inspecting the mucosal line.

Ulceration in ulcerative colitis is typically shallow (i.e., less than 3 mm deep) and confluent. The ulcers are said to have a linear configuration, frequently related to the taeniae, but with undercutting of the mucosal edges the result is more pleomorphic (Fig. 29). The undercutting is seen in profile as small T-shaped projections from the mucosal line (Fig. 30).

Ulceration is a sign of severe disease in ulcerative colitis and is found only in an acute attack. It is always symmetrical across the bowel and in continuity longitudinally. It may be localized to a segment of the involved colon. This is often the sigmoid and descending colon. The rectum may be ulcerated (Fig. 9a), but is more often spared (Fig. 31).

The "double-tracking" sign (16) may be seen in severe states where there is extensive ulceration. It has been suggested that this is due to submucosal tracking, but it is more likely to be related to linear ulceration with undermining of the mucosal edges trapping a thin line of barium (Fig. 32).

A discrete ulcer surrounded by normal mucosa is never seen in ulcerative colitis. Occasionally, discrete ulcers are present, but these are always in an area of abnormal mucosa (Figs. 33–35).

Alteration in Colonic Configuration   Changes in the configuration of the colon include (a) widening of the postrectal space, (b) narrowing and shortening of the colon, (c) blunting or loss of the haustral clefts, and (d) loss of the rectal valves. These are due to alteration in tone of the smooth muscle in the bowel wall (Fig. 36), and provide useful supportive evidence of active disease. This is particularly so where the mucosa is atrophic and not obviously abnormal (Figs. 37 and 38a). If the colitis goes into complete remission, the colonic configuration may revert to normal.

The normal postrectal space is ≤ 1 cm at the 4th sacral segment. In ulcerative colitis there is an inverse relationship between the size of the rectum and the postrectal space (17). This helps distinguish widening of the postrectal space due to ulcerative colitis from other causes (18), where the rectum would be of normal size. In colitis no correlation has been found with the duration of symptoms or extent of disease, except that the earlier the onset of colitis, the smaller the rectum and so the wider the postrectal space (17) (Fig. 38b).

The haustra are created by the action of the taeniae coli shortening the colon. Proximally the circular muscle is fused to the taeniae, so the haustra are fixed anatomical landmarks. This is not so in the distal colon, where the haustra are formed by active contraction of the taeniae. Distension of the bowel during double-contrast barium enema can obliterate the haustra in the distal colon, so it is quite normal for the colon up to the midtransverse part to be devoid of haustration (Figs. 39 and 40). Haustral abnormalities in the proximal colon are always abnormal. Early changes are widening or blunting of the clefts. Complete loss of haustration is typical of chronic ulcerative colitis, but may be found in a variety of lesions:

Inflammatory: ulcerative colitis, ischemia, Crohn's disease, and specific forms of colitis
Cathartic colon
Scleroderma
Amyloid
Dermatomyositis
Myotonic dystrophy
Fabry's disease

Any condition that alters the smooth muscle tone or diffusely infiltrates the bowel wall will affect its normal contours.

In acute colitis a corrugated outline to the colon has been noted (19) on single-contrast barium enema and termed the "indenture sign" (20) (Fig. 41). The suggestion that this is due to swollen mucosal folds is probably inaccurate, as such a change causes "thumbprinting," as in ischemic colitis. It is more likely to be due to a mixture of ulceration and deformed haustration. It is not a common finding on double-contrast examinations, although there should not be any difference in the outline of the bowel between single- or double-contrast studies. A more likely explanation is that contrast examinations are now seldom performed on patients with very active colitis.

The rectal valves can cause confusion, as these are subject to some normal variation. At least one fold should be visible, usually in the lateral view at about the 3rd–4th sacral segment level. This corresponds to the plica transversalis of Kohlrausch (21). The fold should be less than 5 mm thick. In active proctitis narrowing of the rectum, widening of the postrectal space, and thickening or loss of the rectal folds tend to be interrelated changes (22). It is therefore helpful to interpret the rectal folds in conjunction with the presacral space. If the postrectal space is widened to more than 1.5 cm, and the folds are thickened or absent, proctitis is almost certainly present. However, if the folds are absent but the presacral space is normal, this may be a normal variant. Proctitis should not be diagnosed on such a change alone. If the folds are more than 6.5 mm thick and the postrectal space is normal, this is suggestive of proctitis (21).

The rectal ampulla is frequently narrowed in proctitis. The diameter of the normal ampulla should be more than half that of the pelvic cavity. If it is less than a third, proctitis is the most likely cause (22), and other signs sought to support the diagnosis.

The columns of Morgagni are folds in the anorectal junction, usually three to four in number, that taper into the anal canal. The folds are appreciated best on after-evacuation films, but may be seen in double-contrast examinations (Fig. 42). The folds become irregular, thickened (Fig. 43), ulcerated, or obliterated in proctitis (22). Internal hemorrhoids can cause polypoid expansion of the columns. Irregular thickening may be seen in some patients with chronic diarrhea, whatever the cause (Fig. 44).

REFLUX ILEITIS The terminal ileum is abnormal in about 10% of colons removed for chronic ulcerative colitis (23). The distal 5–25 cm of ileum is inflamed with a granular surface. Small superficial ulcers may be present. The ileocecal valve is patulous and rigid (24) (Figs. 45 and 46). The pathogenesis of the ileitis is uncertain. It has been suggested that it is due to the reflux of colonic contents. Certainly, once the colon has been removed the ileal changes disappear. This is not a primary inflammation of the ileum, and it is quite safe to use affected ileum in the formation of an ileostomy, as the mucosa reverts to normal within 1–2 weeks (25).

Reflux ileitis develops only when a total colitis is present. Radiologically, the colon usually shows typical changes of chronic total disease, with a narrowed tubular bowel and granular mucosa. The ileocecal valve is widened and fixed so that reflux occurs readily. The terminal ileum is dilated for 10–20 cm and does not contract. Probably for this reason there is no fold pattern. The mucosa may appear granular (Fig. 47).

It is easy to overdiagnose reflux ileitis. The terminal ileum can appear dilated and featureless during a double-contrast barium enema and yet be normal endoscopically (Fig. 48). Alternatively, the mucosa may seem granular due to the reflux of colonic contents (Fig. 49). This is demonstrated during small bowel enema, when flushing a large volume of fluid through the small bowel will clear out the terminal ileum and confirm it to be normal (26).

The diagnosis of reflux ileitis may be made when total colitis is present, the ileocecal valve is patulous, and the terminal ileum dilated. Clinically, the diagnosis is not important. It is a stigma of total colitis, and its presence may be helpful to confirm total involvement, but it should not be used as a primary feature by which to diagnose colitis.

ASSOCIATED DIVER-TICULAR DISEASE Ulcerative colitis will modify the radiological presentation of diverticular disease by altering the smooth muscle tone in the bowel wall. The increased tone has two effects: the necks of the diverticula are closed off, and as the bowel becomes narrowed the typical interdigitating fold pattern of diverticular disease is obliterated (Fig. 50). The overall effect is to suggest that the diverticular disease has disappeared. This is not so, as the examination of surgically resected specimens shows that the diverticula are still present, and in some cases when the colitis goes into remission the diverticular disease reappears. This sequence may occur in any diffuse form of colitis and has been reported in Crohn's disease (27). Although the diverticula may not fill, the mouths of the diverticula may remain patent (Fig. 51), creating odd, conical-shaped projections (Fig. 52) (28).

REFERENCES

1. Lennard-Jones, J.E., Ritchie, J.K. (1976). Proctocolitis and Crohn's disease of the colon: a comparison of the clinical course. Gut 17; 477.
2. Edwards, F.C., Truelove, S.C. (1963). The course and prognosis of ulcerative colitis. Gut 4; 299.
3. Newell, A.C., Avery-Jones, F. (1958). Observations on the management of idiopathic proctitis. Pro. R. Soc. Med. 51; 431.
4. Morson, B.C. (1980). Pathology of ulcerative colitis. In *Inflammatory Bowel Disease*, Kirsner, J.B., Shorter, R.G. (Eds.). Lea & Febiger, Philadelphia, 2nd ed., p. 281.
5. Goulston, S.J.M., McGovern, V.J. (1969). The nature of benign strictures in ulcerative colitis. N. Engl. J. Med. 281; 290.
6. Kirsner, J.B., Palmer, W.L., Klotz, V. (1951). Reversibility in ulcerative colitis, clinical and roentgenological observations. Radiology 57; 1.
7. Bartram, C.I. (1977). Radiology in the current assessment of ulcerative colitis. Gastrointest. Radiol. 1; 383.
8. Bartram, C.I., Walmsley, K. (1978). A radiological and pathological correlation of the mucosal changes in ulcerative colitis. Clin. Radiol. 29; 323.
9. Halls, J., Young, A.C. (1964). Plain abdominal films in colonic disease. Proc. R. Soc. Med. 58; 859.
10. McMann, M., Bartram, C.I. (1980). The extent of ulcerative colitis as judged from the faecal residue. Submitted for publication.
11. Brooke, B.N., Sampson, P.A. (1964). An indication for surgery in acute ulcerative colitis. Lancet 11; 1272.
12. Hywel-Jones, J., Chapman, M. (1969). Definition of megacolon in colitis. Gut 10; 562.
13. Morson, B.C. (1980). Pathology of ulcerative colitis. In *Inflammatory Bowel Disease*, Kirsner, J.B., Shorter, R.G. (Eds.). Lea & Febiger, Philadelphia, p. 284.
14. Welin, S., Brahme, F. (1961). The double contrast method in ulcerative colitis. Acta Radiol. 55; 257.
15. Laufer, I., Mullens, J.E., Hamilton, J. (1976). Correlation of endoscopy and double contrast radiography in the early stages of ulcerative and granulomatous colitis. Radiology 118; 1.
16. Dick, A.P., Berridge, F.R., Greyson, M.J. (1959). The pathological basis of the radiological changes in ulcerative colitis. Br. J. Radiol. 32; 432.
17. Farthing, M.J., Lennard-Jones, J.E. (1978). Sensibility of the rectum to distension and the anorectal distension reflex in ulcerative colitis. Gut 19; 64.
18. Kattan, K.R., King, A.Y. (1979). Presacral space revisited. Am. J. RAdiol. 132; 437.
19. Anton, H.C., Palmer, J.H. (1962). Corrugation of the colon: its significance in ulcerative colitis. Br. J. Radiol. 35; 762.

20. Poppel, M.H., Beranbaum, S.L. (1957). The identure sign in acute exudative colitis. Am. J. Dig. Dis. 2; 382.

21. Cohen, W.N. (1968). Roentgenographic evaluation of the rectal valves of Houston in the normal and in ulcerative colitis. Am. J. Roentgenol. 104; 580.

22. Fennessy, J.J., Sparberg, M., Kirsner, J.B., (1966). Early roentgen manifestations of mild ulcerative colitis and proctitis. Radiology 87; 848.

23. Golligher, J.C. (1954). Primary excisional surgery in the treatment of ulcerative colitis. Ann. R. Coll. Surg. Engl. 15; 316.

24. Counsell, B. (1956). Lesions of the ileum associated with ulcerative colitis. Br. J. Surg. 44; 276.

25. Hawley, P.R., Ritchie, J.K. (1979). Complications of ileostomy and colostomy following excisional surgery. Clin. Gastroenterol. 8(2); 406.

26. Sellink, J.L. (1976). *Radiological Atlas of Common Diseases of the Small Bowel*. Stenfert Kroese, Leiden, pp. 94 and 202.

27. Berridge, F.R. (1976). Effect of Crohn's disease on colonic diverticula. Br. J. Radiol. 49; 926.

28. Beranbaum, S.L., Yaghmai, M., Beranbaum, E.R. (1965). Ulcerative colitis in association with diverticular disease of the colon. Radiology 85; 880.

FIGURES 1 THROUGH 52

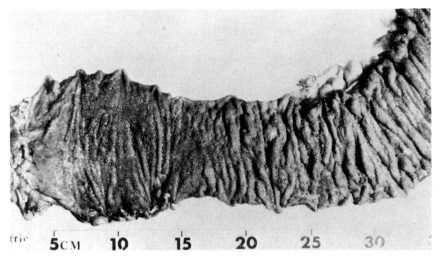

Figure 1 Active colitis with a granular mucosa. (From Ref. 8.)

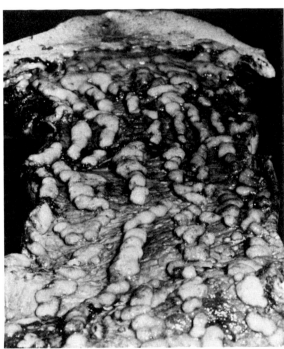

Figure 2 Extensive ulceration, mainly linear in configuration, with undermining of the residual mucosa creating a pseudopolypoid surface.

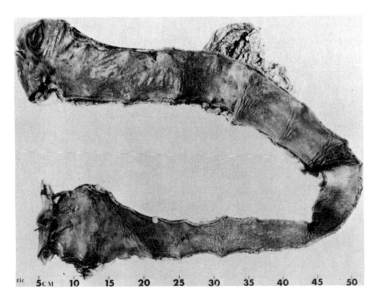

Figure 3 Smooth atrophic mucosa in chronic colitis.

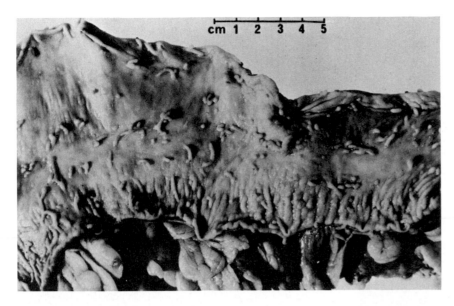

Figure 4 Following an acute attack, the colitis went into remission, leaving a normal background mucosa but a number of inflammatory polyps. (From Ref. 29.)

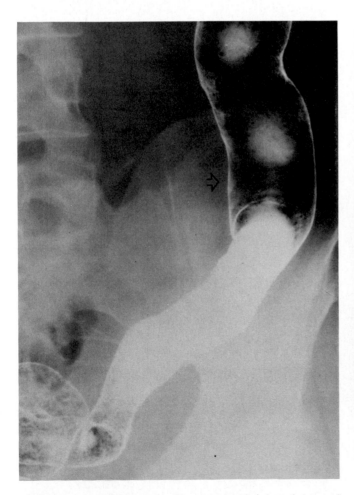

Figure 5 A short segment of normal-looking bowel (arrows) suggests discontinuity. Histologically, the colitis was in continuity, so that this represents an unusual variation in the activity of ulcerative colitis. (From Ref. 7.)

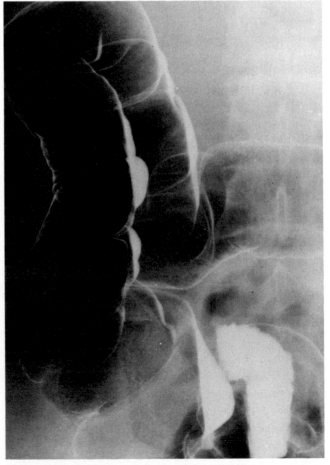

Figure 6 Ulcerative colitis with minimal radiological changes. A segment of the ascending colon appears normal, but as in Figure 5 this represents only macroscopic variation in the activity of the colitis.

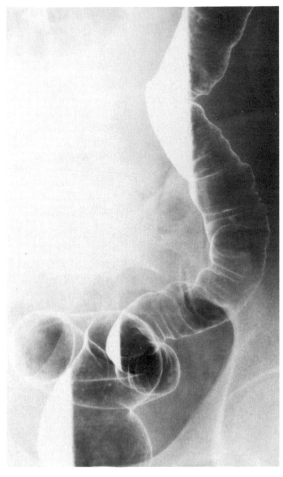

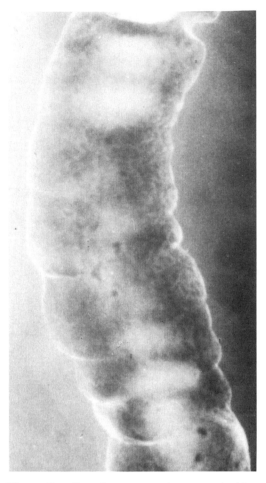

Figure 7 Treatment with predsol enemas has healed the mucosa in the rectosigmoid, creating a colitis with "rectal sparing." This is only true macroscopically; histologically, the rectum remained abnormal.

Figure 8a Granular mucosa shown on double-contrast barium enema in a patient with ulcerative colitis.

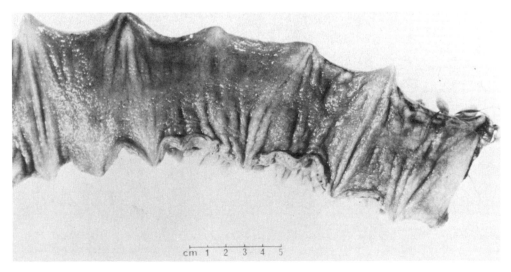

Figure 8b The colon was resected and this segment corresponds to that seen in Fig. 8a. Note the coarse velvety surface texture of the mucosa that creates the "granular" appearance radiologically.

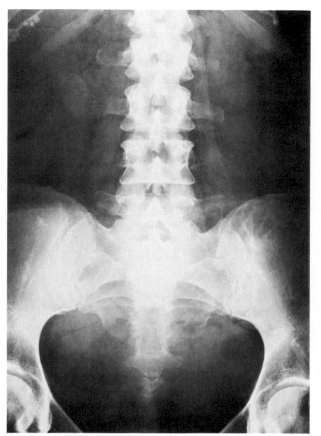

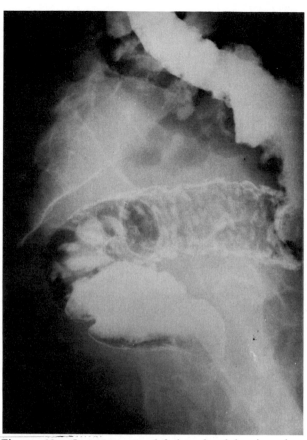

Figure 9 Bilateral sacroiliitis in a patient with colitis.

Figure 10a Instant enema, left lateral pelvic view, in a patient with an acute attack of ulcerative colitis. Extensive ulceration is seen in the rectum.

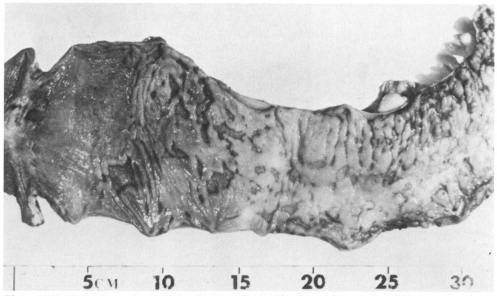

Figure 10 b Ulceration—comparisons between the double-contrast image (a) and the macroscopic appearance of the resected specimen (b) (From Ref. 8.)

43

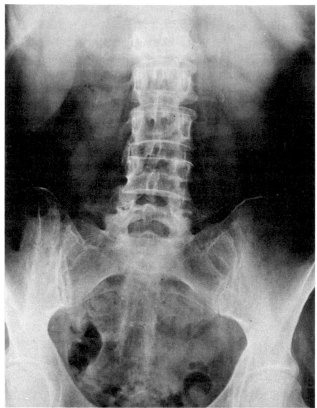

Figure 11a "Empty abdomen" with no residue or gas in the colon.

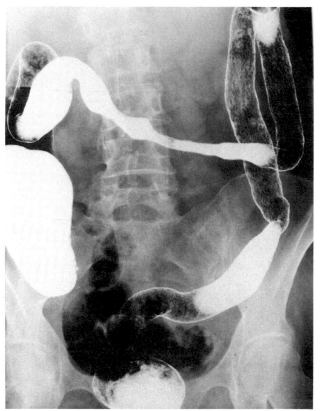

Figure 11b An instant enema confirms the presence of a total active colitis.

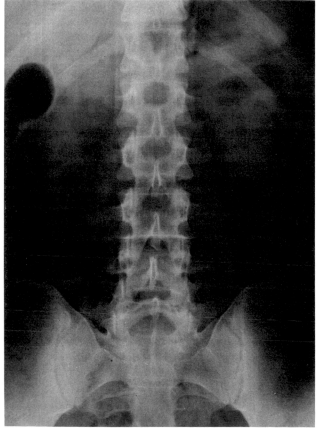

Figure 12a "Empty abdomen" in a patient presenting with acute colitis.

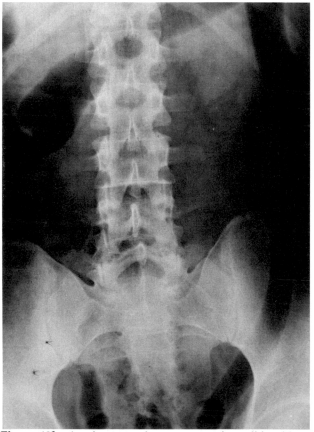

Figure 12b An air enema shows an extensive colitis without significant ulceration.

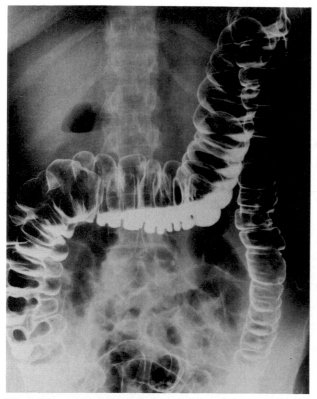

Figure 13 Erect view from an instant enema in a patient with proctitis. Note that the colonic mucosa is normal, but there is no residue.

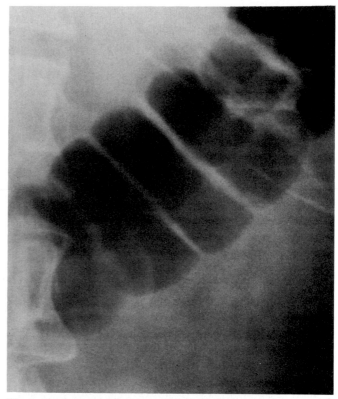

Figure 14 Normal colon — sharply defined mucosal edge and haustral clefts.

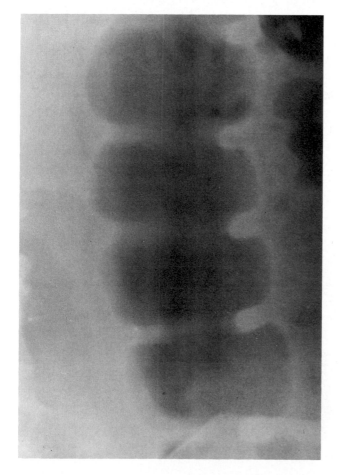

Figure 15 Granular mucosa—blunting of the haustral clefts. The mucosal edge may appear fuzzy, but this is difficult to judge.

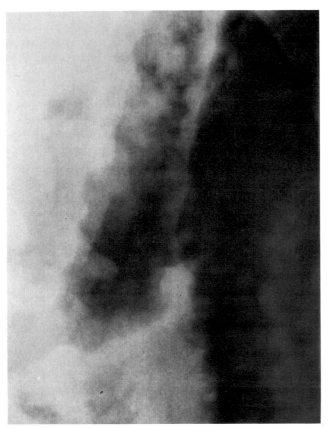

Figure 16 Ulceration—coarse irregularity of the mucosal edge.

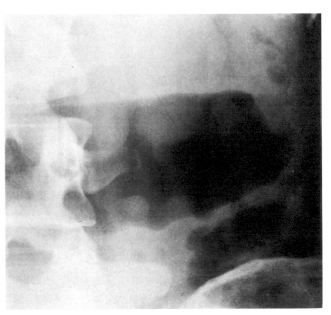

Figure 17 Mucosal islands—large polypoid lesions clearly defined and separated from each other.

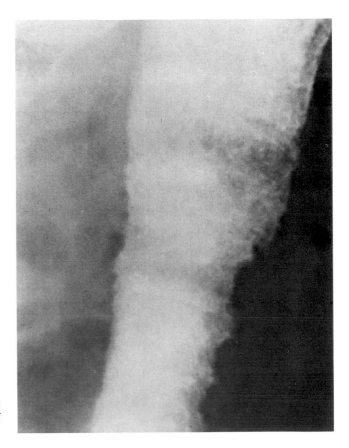

Figure 18 Necrotizing enterocolitis—residual barium outlines the lumen. Numerous small gas bubbles are present in the wall of the bowel.

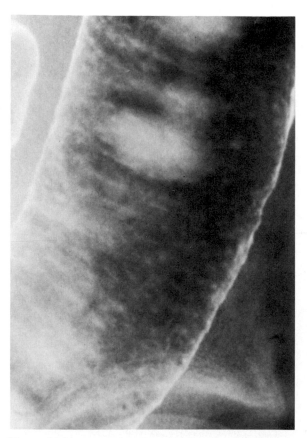

Figure 26d

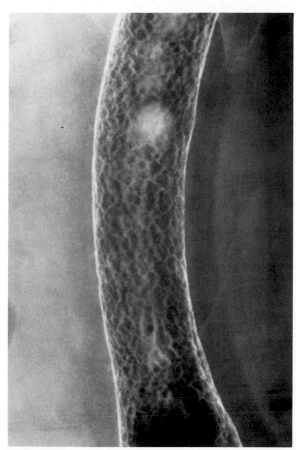

Figure 26e

Figure 26 (continued)

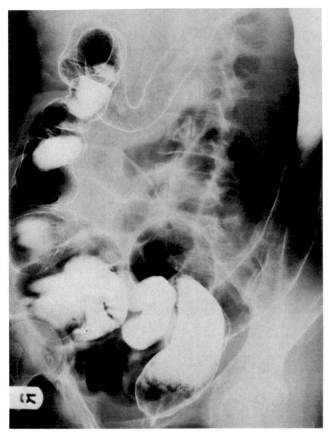

Figure 27 Chronic ulcerative colitis with an atrophic mucosa. The surface texture is within the technical limits of normality.

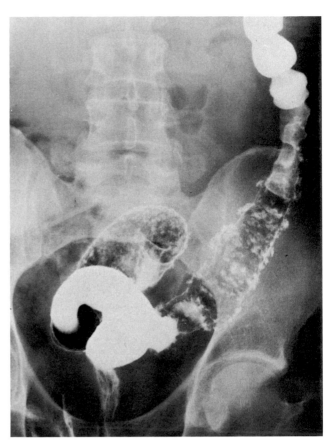

Figure 28 Ulceration in an acute attack. The ulcers are seen projecting outward from the mucosal line.

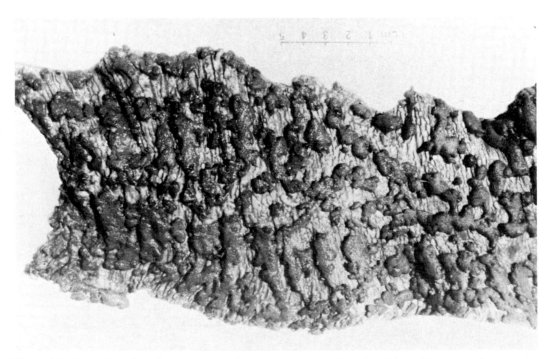

Figure 29 Extensive ulceration not conforming to any pattern with undermining of the mucosal remnants.

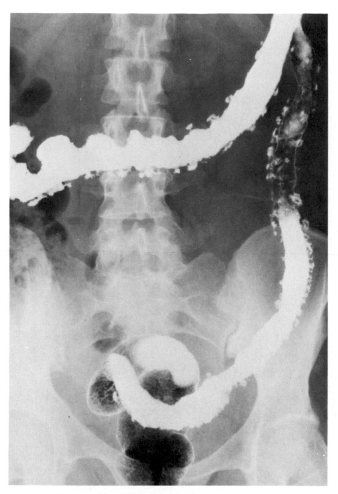

Figure 30 Undercutting T-shaped ulceration.

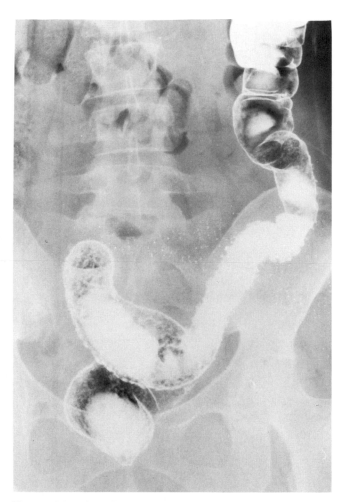

Figure 31 Ulceration in the sigmoid and lower descending colon, with rectal sparing.

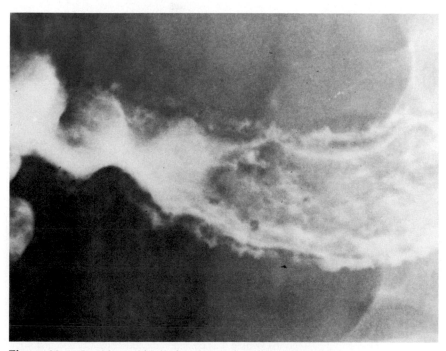

Figure 32 ''Double-tracking'' sign due to deep linear ulceration.

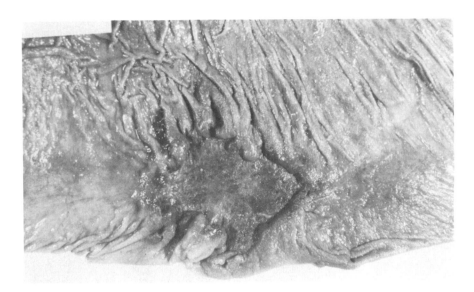

Figure 33 Large solitary ulcer within an area of granular mucosa in ulcerative colitis.

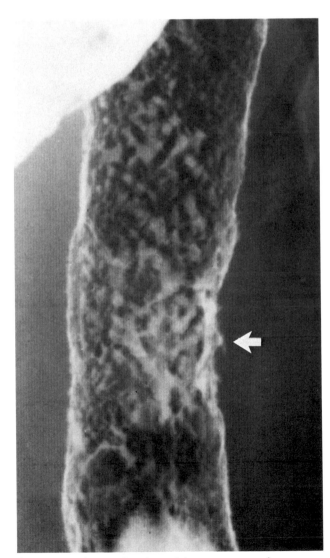

Figure 34 Discrete ulcer (arrow) in a coarse granular mucosa.

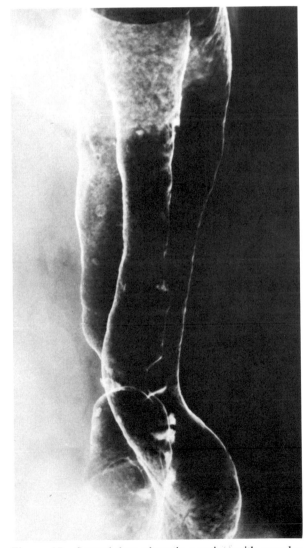

Figure 35 Several deep ulcers in a patient with granular colitis, which was considered endoscopically and histologically to be ulcerative colitis.

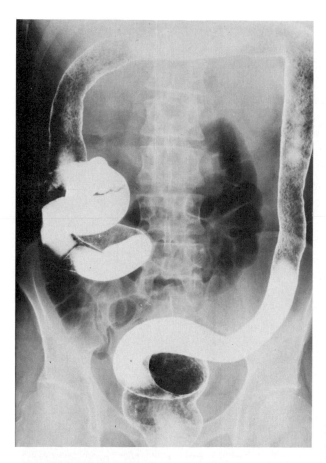

Figure 36 Total colitis on instant enema, showing a typically narrow tubular colon.

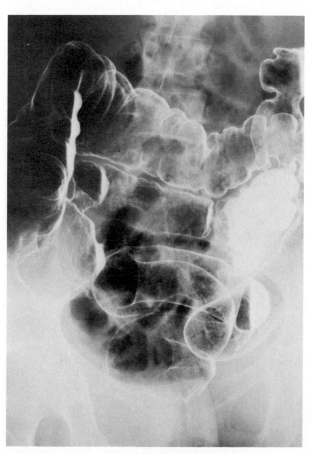

Figure 37 Chronic total colitis. The mucosa is atrophic and the presence of a total colitis is suggested from loss of normal haustration in the proximal colon and a dilated patulous ileocecal valve.

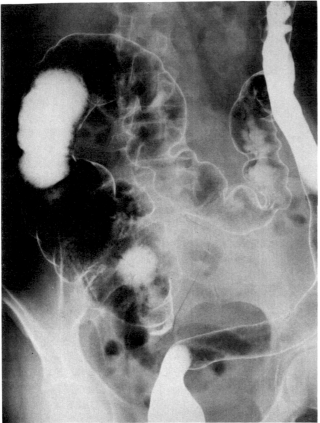

Figure 38a Chronic colitis with an atrophic mucosa. Note the absence of normal haustration in the proximal colon.

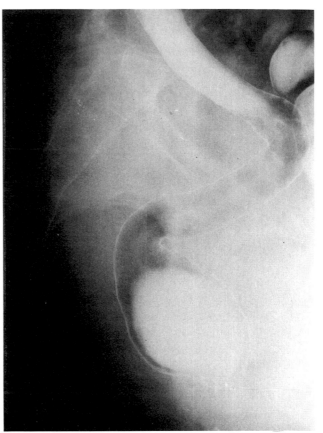

Figure 38b Wide postrectal space. The rectal mucosa appears radiologically normal.

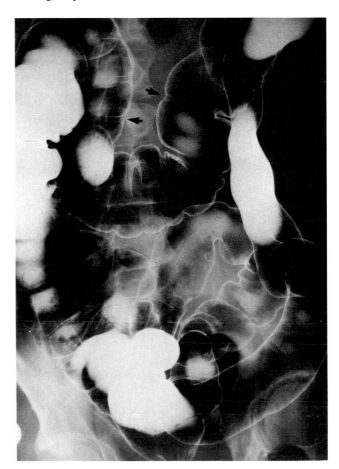

Figure 39 Double-contrast barium enema. No haustration in the descending colon, but normal clefts are seen in the transverse colon (arrows), a common normal variant.

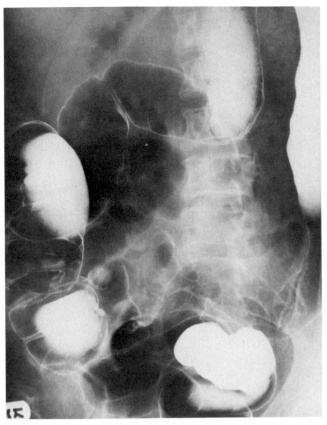

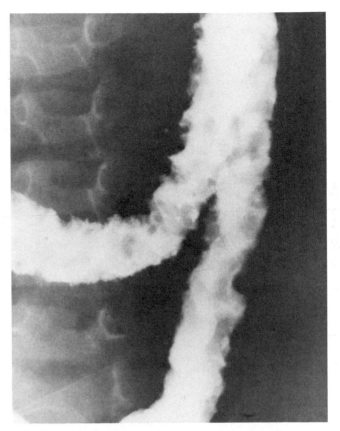

Figure 40 No haustration in the transverse colon and only a few clefts were seen in the ascending colon. Colitis was excluded on colonoscopy.

Figure 41 "Indenture sign" on a single-contrast barium enema.

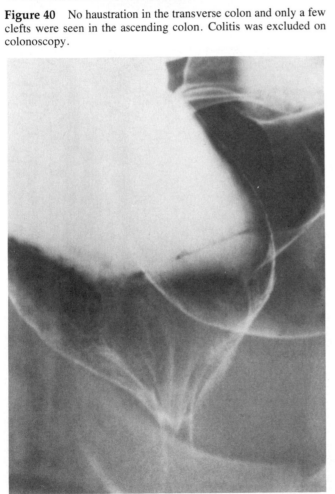

Figure 42 Columns of Morgagni—normal appearances.

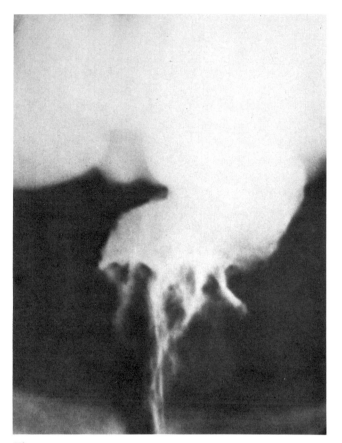

Figure 43

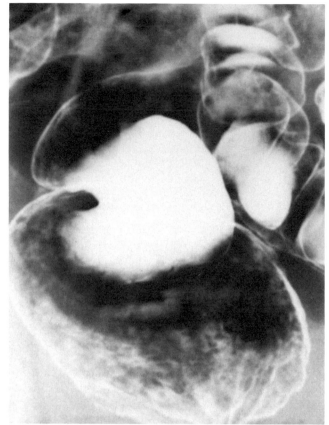

Figure 44

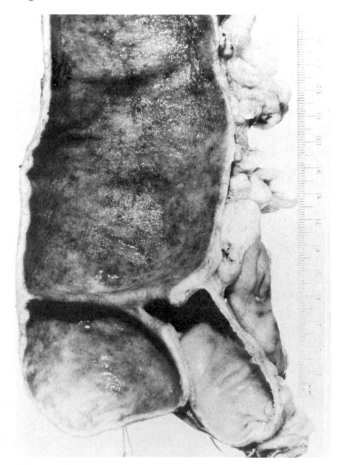

Figure 45

Figure 43 Irregular thickening of the columns of Morgagni in proctitis.

Figure 44 Slightly thickened columns in a patient with the irritable bowel syndrome and diarrhea.

Figure 45 Reflux ileitis; the ileocecal valve is rigid and patulous.

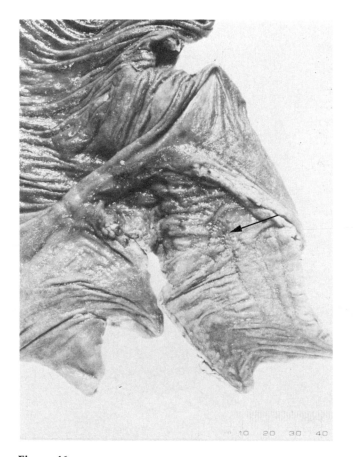

Figure 46

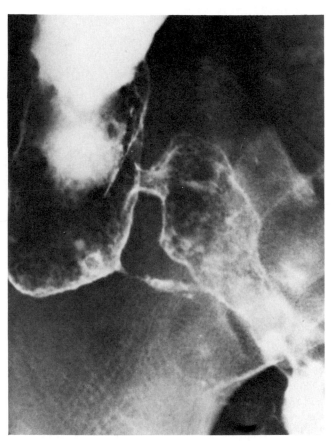

Figure 47

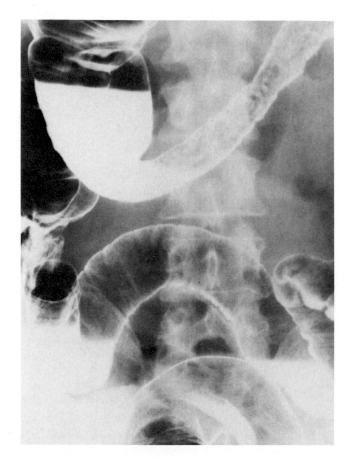

Figure 46 Reflux ileitis with patchy superficial ulceration in the terminal ileum (arrow) and a granular mucosa.

Figure 47 Reflux ileitis on double-contrast barium enema. The ileocecal valve is thickened and patulous. The terminal ileum is dilated with a granular mucosa similar to that in the cecum.

Figure 48 Dilated featureless terminal ileum on double-contrast barium enema. No evidence of colitis.

Figure 48

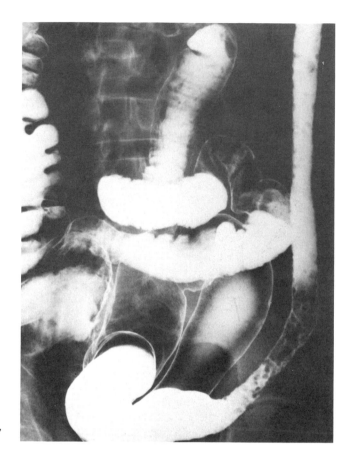

Figure 49 Reflux of colonic residue into the terminal ileum, giving a granular effect.

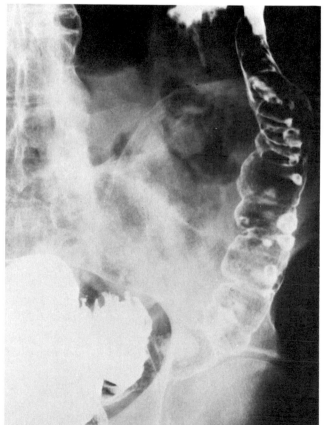

Figure 50a Ankylosing spondylitis with ulcerative colitis and diverticular disease. Note the muscle thickening in the sigmoid and diverticula in the descending colon.

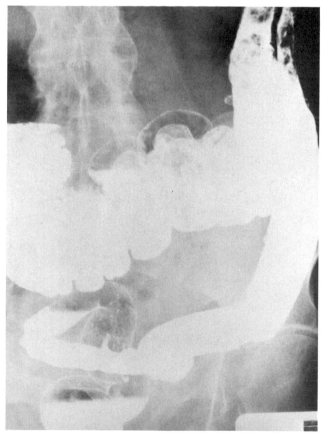

Figure 50b Two years later the colitis is more pronounced. The colon has narrowed and most of the diverticular changes are not apparent.

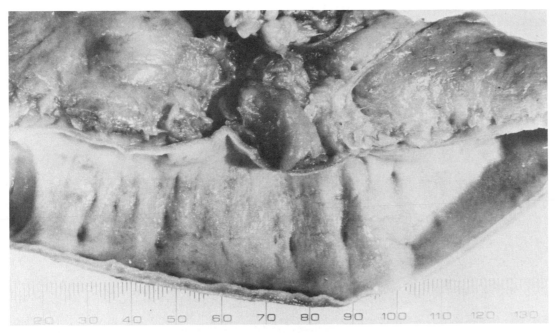

Figure 51 Macroscopic view of the lumen showing a granular mucosa with the mouths of the diverticula still visible.

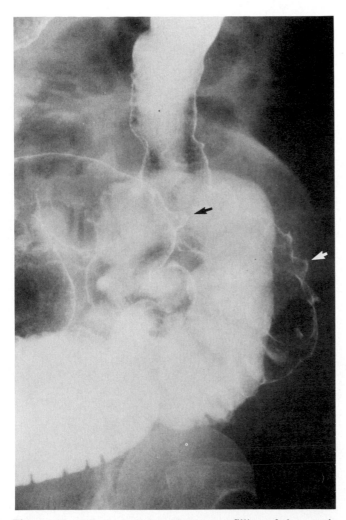

Figure 52 ''Conical'' deformities due to filling of the mouths of the diverticula (arrows). (From Ref. 29.)

3

Complications of Ulcerative Colitis

The complications of ulcerative colitis create difficult management problems and are a most important facet of radiological investigation in inflammatory bowel disease (IBD). In acute complications the emphasis is on plain film interpretation. The complications, loosely classified as "chronic," have a more insidious presentation, usually in well-established disease, and require investigation by double-contrast barium enema. The role of the double-contrast barium enema in the problem of large bowel cancer has yet to be fully determined. This subject remains controversial, and the opinions expressed portray the current views at St. Mark's Hospital. To avoid repetition Crohn's disease has been included in the sections on arthritis, liver, and biliary tract abnormalities.

TOXIC MEGACOLON

Toxic megacolon is a fulminating form of colitis, which may develop either during the first attack or in an acute relapse. It is the commonest cause of death related to ulcerative colitis (1), and is an indication for emergency surgery. Toxic megacolon may complicate other forms of colitis, such as Crohn's disease (2,3) (Fig. 1) ischemia (4), amebiasis (5), or pseudomembranous colitis (6).

Although the pathogenesis of toxic megacolon is not understood, the appearances are distinctive. The entire colon may be involved (Fig. 2), but the rectum, cecum, and ascending colon are often spared (7). The involved colon, which usually includes the transverse part, is dilated and thinned. There is extensive sloughing of the mucosa, leaving only isolated remnants—the mucosal islands (Fig. 3). The external surface shows an intense serositis and the omentum is edematous and inflamed. Small sealed perforations are common, and fibropurulent exudate is present on the peritoneal surface (8). The bowel is extremely easy to perforate during manipulation, having the consistency of wet blotting paper. Histologically, there is transmural inflammation, fissuring ulceration deep into the muscle layer with degeneration of the ganglion cells in the myenteric plexus, and myocytolysis of the muscularis propria, with an intense vascular dilatation (9). Once developed it may be very difficult to establish the nature of the underlying colitis, as in fulminating colitis the accepted criteria for Crohn's disease and ulcerative colitis overlap (10).

The incidence of toxic megacolon is about 1.6–13% in ulcerative colitis (11–14). It may develop over a period of several hours (Fig. 4). The patient becomes toxic and is prostrate with abdominal distension and reduced bowel sounds. The presence of abdominal tenderness with guarding suggests peritonitis, but a precise clinical definition of toxic megacolon is difficult. A number of parameters, such as pyrexia, tachycardia, increased bowel frequency, anemia, raised erythrocyte sedimentation rate (ESR), leucocytosis, and low albumin have been compared to the severity of the colitis (14). The temperature, pulse rate, bowel frequency, presence of blood in the stools, hemaglobin, and ESR may be used to grade the severity of the attack and predict the outcome regarding the response to medical treatment (11). A simpler method of prediction is possible using the maximum body temperature and stool frequency after 24 hr in the hospital (15).

Such parameters reflect different systemic effects of the disease. For example, the ESR indicates the inflammatory response; the albumin, the protein loss. Clinical parameters are important factors in assessing an acute attack, but the critical factor is the depth of the ulceration. Ulceration in an acute attack becomes dangerous once it penetrates the muscle layer. Dilatation of the colon is related to this and perforation with full-thickness ulceration (16). Correlation between clinical and laboratory features, and the width of the colon shown on plain abdominal x-ray, have shown that radiology provides the most accurate indication of the depth of ulceration (16).

The interpretation of the plain film in fulminating colitis is difficult but probably represents the most important role that the radiologist has in the overall management of IBD. Failing to take plain films, or ignoring the findings on them, is the commonest cause of death related to colitis (1).

A number of features should be noted:

1. *Dilatation.* Where the colon contains gas, its width can be measured. In toxic megacolon mean diameters for the segment of colon maximally dilated, of between 8.2 and 9.2 cm (17,18), have been reported (Figs. 5 and 6). Dilatation in excess of 5 cm correlates with ulceration penetrating the muscle layer (16) and should be considered as the threshold for dilatation in fulminating colitis (Fig. 7). Plain films usually show gas in the transverse colon. This is partly because this is a common site for toxic megacolon, but also that this is the highest point of the colon when the patient is supine, so that gas tends to collect in this segment. Radiologically, this may overemphasize its frequency of involvement. The descending colon and sigmoid are the next most common segments to be affected. Dilatation of the rectum is unusual. In advanced cases the entire colon is involved, but earlier in the process the dilatation may be quite localized, so that only a short segment of the colon is dilated.

2. *The mucosa.* Mucosal islands (19) (Figs. 8 and 9) indicate extreme disruption of the mucosa and are a common finding in toxic megacolon. Compared to the resected specimen their presence and extent may be underestimated radiologically (20). This can be due to the large volume of gas in the dilated colon, blackening out the bowel so that there is insufficient contrast to show the islands (Fig. 10). Also, the mucosal damage may be so extensive that there is no mucosa left and therefore no mucosal island (Fig. 11). A nodular or cobblestoned edge has been reported, but is probably best termed "coarse irregularity" (20) and represents severe ulceration (Fig. 7). The distinction between severe ulceration and mucosal islands can be arbitrary and the terms should not be applied too rigidly. In coarse irregularity there is no flat area around the elevated mucosal remnant as there is with a mucosal island. Confusion

can arise when a patient with inflammatory polyps develops an acute attack. Sessile polyps can look like mucosal islands (Fig. 12), and the distinction is impossible unless the presence of the polyps is known beforehand.

3. *Haustration.* The presence of normal haustra excludes toxic megacolon (Fig. 13). The extensive ulceration and inflammation of toxic megacolon always causes the loss of haustration.

4. *Bowel wall.* Although this is thinned pathologically, radiologically it appears thickened (12, 21). This is due to subserosal or omental edema (Fig. 14). A radiolucent stripe has been noted running parallel to the wall. This has been ascribed to gas tracking in the wall, but probably represents the pericolic fat line (21).

5. *Small bowel changes.* Gaseous distension of the small bowel, possibly with some free fluid (causing increased separation of bowel loops), is a feature of severe colitis (12, 22). Gastric atony has been reported (12).

6. *Decubitus or erect view.* Long fluid levels may be seen in the colon which are in keeping with an ileus. Free air indicates a perforation. Excess intestinal gas is an interesting feature of severe colitis and has been studied by Vernia et al. (22), who showed that the volume of small bowel gas did not vary between controls and those with mild or moderate ulcerative colitis, but was significantly increased in severe colitis or toxic megacolon. Colonic gas showed a definite increase in toxic megacolon. The total volume of intestinal gas correlated with the arterial pH and less well with the ESR and body temperature. It was concluded that small bowel distension and a metabolic alkalosis may be a sign of impending toxic megacolon.

Plain films should form an integral part of the examination of a patient with an acute attack of colitis. Radiologically patients tend to fall into three broad categories:

1. There is no dilatation. The mucosa may be granular or ulcerated. If the mucosa is granular, this patient is not at risk from perforation. The presence of ulceration means that the patient will require more careful observation; if the ulceration starts to penetrate the muscle layer, dilatation or perforation may result.

2. Part of the colon is dilated to about 5 cm. Irrespective of the appearance of the mucosa, this is a worrying feature. In addition, severe ulceration and small bowel distension place the patient in a high-risk group, and urgent surgery must be considered.

3. Mucosal islands, or more than 5 cm dilatation, indicates that toxic megacolon is established.

During the critical phase, a supine abdominal x-ray should be taken daily, and may be needed even more frequently. Recovery is indicated by a reduction in the diameter of the colon, the presence of gas in the rectum, and a return of haustration (23).

Occasionally, cases of toxic megacolon are seen that have been managed medically. Extensive adhesions may form, as small sealed perforations and a fibropurulent exudate are common in toxic megacolon. Although the patient may get over the fulminating state, continued ill health often necessitates surgery, which is then complicated by numerous adhesions. Rarely, the bowel may remain dilated following neuronal damage (24). The development of post inflammatory polyps is common (25) (Fig. 15).

The barium enema has often been incriminated as a precipitating factor in toxic megacolon (13). In a critical review of the literature, Goldberg (26) did not find that any causal relationship had been proved. There is only one case reported where a patient with minimally active disease developed toxic megacolon, and that was 11 days after the barium enema (27). In most cases the barium enema had been performed during an acute attack of colitis, but some time before the onset of toxic megacolon. The experience at St. Mark's does not suggest that there is significant danger in active colitis to deter a clinician from requesting an instant enema. The air enema is a useful alternative. Toxic megacolon is a plain film diagnosis, and once developed a barium enema is unnecessary to clarify the diagnosis, and dangerous owing to the risk of perforation. It is therefore an absolute contraindication to an instant enema.

Toxic megacolon is really a condition in its own right. When fully developed it has a high mortality. The plain film is extremely valuable in demonstrating those patients most at risk and in revealing the early stages of this condition.

Dilatation of the colon may occur in conditions other than fulminating colitis, and it is important that these are considered in the differential diagnosis of toxic megacolon. The more important causes are the following:

Generalized peritonitis

Acute cholecystitis, pancreatitis, appendicitis

Idiopathic megacolon, intestinal pseudo-obstruction

Hirschsprung's disease

Amyloid

Drug-induced: atropine, propantheline, morphine, ganglion blocking agents

Endocrine: myxedema, Addison's disease, diabetic coma

Congestive cardiac failure

Electrolyte imbalance

Trauma

Reflex: urinary calculous, myocardial infarction, retroperitoneal hematoma, spinal cord lesion, pneumonia

Vascular

Porphyria

Celiac disease

Scleroderma

The distinction between ileus and chronic obstruction is not always easy (27a). In an ileus there is usually continuous gaseous distension of the colon, minimal fluid with preservation of the haustra, and a smooth mucosal outline. In obstruction the findings may be more variable. Gaseous distension in the colon proximal to the obstruction is not always continuous, the right colon may be filled with fluid, the haustra closely packed, and retained fecal residue may cause some irregularity of the mucosal edge. If the colon is dilated but the mucosal edge smooth and the haustration normal, there is no problem in excluding toxic megacolon as in Figure 13. Dilatation with retained residue may simulate toxic megacolon (Fig. 16), and in such cases the clinical picture must be taken into consideration when making the diagnosis.

PERFORATION Perforation is the result of full-thickness ulceration. In ulcerative colitis this implies a fulminating colitis. When this is extensive, as in toxic megacolon, multiple perforations are indeed common. However, perforation can occur in localized severe disease without dilatation. An incidence of 3.2% has been reported (11), where perforation was associated with dilatation in only 1 in 20. The sigmoid colon is the commonest site of perforation, which is most likely to happen during the first attack of colitis (Fig. 17).

Perforation may be free, when air is present intraperitoneally (Fig. 18), or sealed, when there will not be any free air to show that the perforation has occurred. The exact diagnosis of a sealed perforation from plain films is really impossible (20). The presence of a coarse mucosal edge indicates ulceration. Dilatation to 5 cm is a further warning of deep ulceration (16). If the mucosal surface appears flat, ulceration cannot be completely excluded, as it may have been so widespread that the entire surface has sloughed off. In these circumstances the colon would be dilated and toxic megacolon present. If the sigmoid colon is of normal diameter and the edge smooth, ulceration—and perforation—can be excluded. There is often not enough gas in the involved colon to show the mucosal edge. If the patient is very ill, an air enema may be preferred to an instant enema (Chap. 1). The presence of dilated small bowel loops cannot be taken to indicate an abscess, as this change is seen in severe colitis without perforation (20, 22). Dilatation of an apparently normal looking proximal colon may be associated with very severe distal disease, and as perforation is common in this state, the presence of a dilated right colon is a worrying feature (Fig. 19).

When interpreting the plain film, the following statements can be made with regards to perforation:

1. Free air obviously indicates perforation.

2. Air tracking along the edge of the bowel wall may mean very deep ulceration or a localized extraperitoneal collection of air (Figs. 18b and 20) and should be taken to indicate that free perforation is imminent (28).

3. Proximal colonic dilatation, with no gas to show the distal colon and distended small bowel loops on the left side of the abdomen, is highly suspicious of a sealed perforation.

4. Coarse irregularity of the mucosal edge means ulceration, and this places the patient at risk from perforation. Conversely, a smooth edge excludes ulceration, so ulceration is not a risk in that segment of bowel.

Perforation is an indication for emergency surgery, and was present in 15 of 43 such operations in one series (1), with the perforation being free in 10 and sealed in 5 cases. Perforation leads to sepsis (Figs. 21,22) and adhesions, which are major factors in the operative mortality for ulcerative colitis (19). Clinicians are therefore very concerned to exclude perforation in a patient with a severe attack of colitis. Careful analysis of the plain films, possibly supplemented by an instant (Figs. 21–23) or air enema, and monitoring the changes with repeat plain films can provide very helpful information as to the risk of perforation.

INFLAMMATORY POLYPS

The term "polyp" may be used to desribe any lesion that is raised above the flat mucous membrane. It does not imply any histological diagnosis (29).

In colitis there are a number of situations where the mucosal surface may become grossly uneven or mamillated (30). In acute colitis ulceration causes loss of mucosa. What remains may appear "polypoid," although this is not an accurate use of the term, as the lesions are not raised up above the mucosal surface; instead, parts of the surface are depressed from ulceration (Fig. 24). "Pseudopolyposis" has been used to describe these residual areas of mucosa in ulceration (31) (Fig. 25). The most extreme form of pseudopolyps are the mucosal islands in toxic megacolon (19).

Exuberant masses of granulation tissue may develop in the ulcerated areas to form true polyps (Fig. 26) (32). During the healing phase granulation tissue covering ulcers may prevent smooth reepithelization of the mucosa. Ulceration is typically undermining, and this lifts up tags of mucosa. The presence of granulation tissue is thought to prevent these tags reforming with the mucosa. Although the mucosa may heal completely, its architecture remains distorted by these tags, which are true polyps because they are elevated above the normal surface. Histologically, they are cylinders of muscularis and submucosa with a variable inflammatory infiltrate that reflects the general state of the colitis (33). Their origin from acute colitis makes the term "postinflammatory polyps" appropriate (34) (Fig. 27).

Being elevated lesions, polyps should cause filling defects in the barium layer, as opposed to ulceration, where the barium pools in the ulcers. This distinction can be difficult from the en face view with extensive pseudopolyps, and it is usually easiest to refer to the mucosal line. With acute ulceration small undermining T-shaped ulcers project out from the mucosal line (Fig. 28), leaving no doubt as to the nature of the mucosal irregularity. Inflammatory polyps are seen often when the colitis is inactive, so that the mucosal line is normal (Fig. 29).

As the ulceration heals there may be an intermediate stage of nodular regeneration in the mucosa (Fig. 30). En face the mucosa shows a confluent polypoid appearance which the mucosal line reflects in a wavy outline, possibly with some slight irregularity from residual ulceration, but not the T-shaped undermining ulcers of acute colitis. Further healing may result in a mass of small sessile polyps. The background mucosa will then be intact, so that the mucosal line is normal (Fig. 31).

Inflammatory polyps composed of granulation tissue may be single or multiple and are usually sessile. They tend to be found with active disease and have an irregular surface, in keeping with the granular background mucosa (Fig. 32). Radiologically, there is no certain way of distinguishing them from adenomas (Fig. 33) or cancers, and in the case of a solitary lesion the latter will be of particular concern. Fortunately, their composition of granulation tissue is readily apparent on direct vision during endoscopy. If there is any doubt as to the nature of the polyp, it can be biopsied rather than excised, as the presence histologically of granulation tissue is diagnostic. These types of polyps are a marked feature of colitis due to schistosomiasis.

Postinflammatory polyps are found in 10–20% of patients with ulcerative colitis (11, 33–37) (Fig. 29) but are less common in Crohn's disease (33) (Figs. 34 and 35). They are usually situated in the left hemicolon and are uncommon in the rectum. Their distribution merely reflects that of the ulceration. Total involvement is rare, probably because most of these patients required surgery during the acute stage. The polyps may be seen soon after an acute attack, and once formed tend to remain unchanged for many years, even though the colitis becomes inactive (Fig. 26b,c). The polyps may be sessile or filiform, single or multiple (Figs. 36 and 37). Filiform polyps are common (38). These are long fronds and not truly pedunculated, as there is no distinction between the head and stalk (Fig. 38). They may be mobile, like a mass of seaweed (Fig. 39), form bridges across the bowel lumen (Figs. 40 and 41) (39), or run along the surface of the mucosa. A pathognomonic feature is adherence, where some part of the polyp is fused to another polyp (Fig. 42). Radiologically, this provides conclusive evidence that the polyps are inflammatory in nature. The background mucosa is often normal radiologically and haustration may be present (Fig. 39). Postinflammatory polyps can be diagnosed with confidence radiologically, so endoscopy is not required.

The superimposition of active disease on postinflammatory polyps may cause problems. One patient developed severe protein-losing enteropathy due to exudation from the inflamed mucosa, which was greatly increased in surface area by the massive filiform polyposis (Fig. 43). Sessile polyps may be confused with mucosal islands on plain films. Toxic megacolon is excluded by the absence of ulceration and colonic dilatation.

Inflammatory polyps have been reported in the small bowel (Fig. 44) (38,40) and stomach (38) in patients with Crohn's disease. They are probably more common in the small bowel than is generally realized, as their demonstration requires a small bowel enema.

Complications due to the polyps themselves are uncommon. Localized dense masses of filiform polyps have been reported as causing obstruction (41) or preventing filling during barium enema (41,42) (Figs. 45 and 46). Inflammatory polyps are not premalignant and there is a low incidence of dysplasia in patients with these polyps (43). However, in certain circumstances diagnostic problems may arise. A solitary sessile inflammatory polyp cannot be distinguished radiologically from an adenoma, and if large might be thought malignant (37). A localized segment of sessile or frondlike inflammatory polyps may simulate a villous adenoma or annular mass (44,45). Air distension in a double-contrast examination will usually show normal mucosa in between the polyps. Any problem may be easily resolved by endoscopy.

Inflammatory and adenomatous polyposis have been considered radiologically similar (45). In typical cases there is a clear distinction on double-contrast barium enema between these two conditions. In familial adenomatous polyposis coli, the polyps are sessile and present throughout the colon and rectum (Fig. 47). The polyps are never frondlike, adherent, or localized to part of the colon, as in inflammatory polyposis. However, the development of the adenomas in familial polyposis is not uniform, so that in the early stages it is possible that only a few polyps are present which might simulate inflammatory polyposis. As in every patient with familial polyposis the diagnosis depends on the histological demonstration of adenoma.

In most colitics inflammatory polyps do not cause any problem in diagnosis or management. Their presence is really only a reminder of a previous severe episode, from which they have made a good recovery. It is rare for inflammatory polyps to be pedunculated (Figs. 48 and 49), so that apart from the fear of neoplasia in a solitary lesion, this is the only direct indication for endoscopy.

The nature of polypoid mucosal changes in ulcerative colitis and the appearance of the mucosal line are summarized in Fig. 50. Radiologically, three main categories of polypoid mucosa should be considered:

1. *Pseudopolyposis:* undermining ulceration in acute colitis.

2. *Inflammatory polyps composed of granulation tissue:* sessile lesions with a granular mucosa.

3. *Postinflammatory polyps:* small mucosal tags often filiform and adherent in quiescent colitis.

STRICTURES Strictures have been considered uncommon in ulcerative colitis (47) and more likely to be malignant than benign (48). Neither is true; strictures are common in ulcerative colitis and most are benign.

About a third may be apparent within 5 years of the onset of the colitis (11), but most are seen after the colitis has been established for many years. Incidences between 6.3 and 11.2% are quoted (11,35). Seventeen percent of patients with total colitis (35) have strictures, so that this complication appears to be commoner with extensive disease. Most strictures have been diagnosed from barium enema by the presence of a constant narrowing. Narrowing from spasm can be abolished with intravenous relaxants (49), but in practice this is seldom a problem in colitis. Strictures on resected colons have been defined as a reduction in the caliber of the lumen by two-thirds or more. Using this definition strictures have been reported in 12% of resected specimens (50). Endoscopists tend to underdiagnose strictures compared to radiologists, as minor changes in the caliber of the bowel are difficult to appreciate at colonscopy and there is no rigidity of the bowel wall to help confirm deformity (51).

A typical stricture involves the rectosigmoid, is only a few centimeters long, and is symmetrical with a fusiform configuration (50). About 10% of them are multiple (Fig. 51), and occasionally long strictures up to 30 cm in length may be seen (Fig. 52) (35). The strictures in ulcerative colitis are not fibrotic in origin. Fibrosis is minimal and the narrowing is the result of localized thickening of the muscularis mucosae (50). The absence of fibrosis means that theoretically the stricture is reversible. The long-term follow-up of patients suggests that this may occur, although only one case has been reported (52). Changes in strictures may be underestimated, as patients tend to be investigated radiologically only during the acute phase and are unlikely in the early years of the colitis to be followed up when quiescent.

Strictures are often an incidental finding. The risk of malignancy in a typical stricture is very low, but the possibility must be considered. Features that suggest malignancy and would indicate colonoscopy are as follows:

1. Shouldering at the ends of the stricture.
2. Irregularity of the mucosa within the stricture that differs from that either side of the stricture (Fig. 53).
3. A stricture in the proximal colon, even if it appears benign, should be viewed with considerable suspicion, as benign strictures are rare in this location (Fig. 54).

Strictures may be difficult to assess. Benign strictures can look malignant (Figs.55 and 56), and vice versa. Endoscopy easily resolves any problem. Many patients with strictures will have had extensive disease for more than 10 years, and so require endoscopy to search for dysplasia. This is often convenient for the radiologist, as endoscopy will be performed irrespective of the possible nature of the stricture.

FECAL STASIS   The patient with a distal colitis who is passing liquid stools may have some fecal residue in the proximal colon if this is not inflamed, but the amount of residue is not excessive and comparable to that seen in normals. A paradoxical situation can develop, where there is a marked buildup of residue as though the patient was constipated, although liquid stools are still passed. This has been termed fecal stasis (53). For it to occur, there has to be active distal disease but with the proximal colon relatively normal. The active disease causes a degreee of functional holdup. The proximal colon, being relatively normal, continues to reabsorb water, thereby impacting the retained residue.

Fecal stasis may produce a sense of constipation with the passage of hard masses in the liquid stool. Subacute obstruction is a rare complication. Excess buildup of residue should be noted (Fig. 57), as fecal stasis can be treated by a reduction of opiates and judicious use of laxatives.

CANCER   The incidence of large bowel cancer in ulcerative colitis is about 3–5% (54), which causes a significant problem in the long-term management of the disease (see Table 1). Compared to large bowel cancers in noncolitics, the cancers in colitis tend to be infiltrative plaques rather than annular lesions, are more often multiple, and are histologically of a higher grade (Fig. 58). The cancers still predominate in the left side of the colon and rectum (55). Proctocolectomy may abolish the risk of cancer, but may not be warranted in all patients, as not every patient has the same risk of developing cancer (43). The following are important factors in determining the risk of cancer:

1. *The duration of the disease*. If this is taken from the onset of the patient's symptoms, there is no excess risk of colorectal cancer, compared to the general population, within the first 10 years. After 10–20 years there is a 23-fold excess risk, which rises to a 32-fold risk after 20 years. The patient would then have a 1 in 60 chance of developing cancer during the subsequent year (Fig. 59).

2. *The presence of extensive colitis*. This is a radiological description. It is applied to a colitis that extends proximally, at least to the hepatic flexure, on instant enema (Fig. 60). Radiologically, extensive colitis implies total histological colitis (56). Total colitis is an important factor in the development of cancer (35,54,57,58), but whether the colitis has to be total for the entire course of the disease or only of the duration is not clear.

Table 1   Flow Chart for the Investigation of Cancer in Ulcerative Colitis

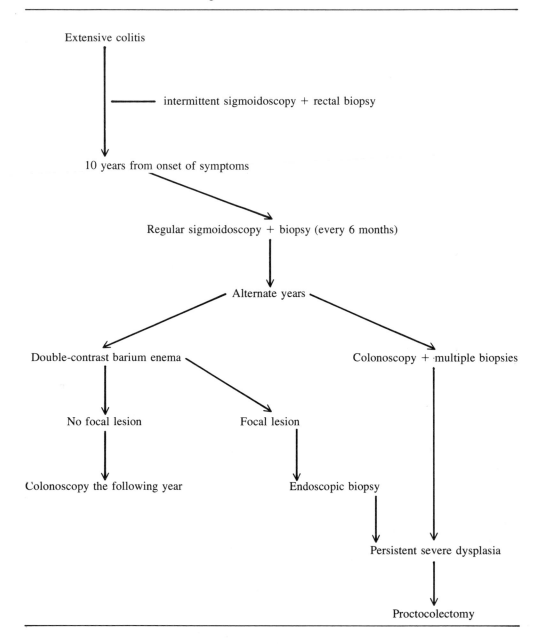

3.   *The presence of dysplasia.* Dysplasia may be defined as disordered cell growth, indicative of neoplastic transformation. It is a morphologically identifiable precursor of cancer. In the noncolitic bowel dysplasia is associated with adenomatous polyps (59), but in colitis the dysplasia develops within the abnormal mucosa. Dysplasia may be graded histologically as mild, moderate, or severe. Morphologically, it may occur in a flat mucosa, but with the adenomatous type the surface is velvety or nodular, due to a villous or tubular

pattern of dysplasia (55) (Fig. 61). When severe, slightly elevated, poorly circumscribed lesions may be seen which resemble small villous adenomas (Figs. 62–64). Reactive hyperplasia in the recovery stage following active inflammation simulates dysplasia. To avoid confusion, dysplasia should be considered significant only if it is persistent (60). Dysplasia is patchy in distribution. Sigmoidoscopy and rectal biopsy will detect only about 60–80% of dysplasia (43), so that the entire colon must be examined with multiple endoscopic biopsies. Not all of these will show dysplasia, even in the presence of a cancer (60).

4. *A macroscopic mucosal abnormality.* In a review of all the cancers associated with ulcerative colitis seen at St. Mark's Hospital, a macroscopic mucosal abnormality was always visible in the resected specimen (61). An area of slightly elevated nodularity or infiltrative plaque were the commonest lesions (Figs. 65 and 66). Endoscopic biopsy of such lesions may show only dysplastic changes (60), and the presence of invasive cancer is most easily appreciated on palpation of the resected colon. Infiltration causes thickening and rigidity of the wall, which are easier to feel than to see (Fig. 67).

There is no excess risk of cancer within the first 10 years of the disease. After that, and if the colitis is extensive, the risk of cancer starts to become significant. It is obviously undesirable to wait until an overt tumor presents, but it is also undesirable to perform a procto-colectomy on a patient who may be relatively well and with no evidence of cancer just because the disease has been present for a certain time. The present policy at St. Mark's Hospital relies on a search for dysplasia to monitor this high-risk type of patient (43). Rectal and endoscopic biopsies are performed at regular intervals. If severe dysplasia persists for several months, consideration is then given to procto-colectomy.

Until recently, radiology has had no role in this program other than to demonstrate the extent of the colitis, or an overt tumor mass. However, it has been shown that severe adenomatous dysplasia can be recognized on double-contrast barium enema (62). The dysplastic lesions are slightly elevated with rather polygonal edges (Figs. 68 and 69). The distinction from inflammatory polyps can be difficult (Fig. 70), as these may be localized and of pleomorphic shape. Filiform shapes or branching are confirmatory signs of an inflammatory nature.

Radiology remains unable to detect dysplasia in a flat mucosa, but in these circumstances the dysplasia is likely to be only mild or moderate, and the absence of any macroscopic abnormality makes the presence of carcinoma most unlikely. The double-contrast barium enema can therefore can therefore be used to separate patients with long-standing extensive colitis into two groups.

A. Where the colitis shows typical radiological changes but there is no localized lesion.

B. Where a localized abnormality is present. This could be a polyp, an area of nodularity, a plaque, or a focal deformity (i.e., not a symmetrical stricture, but indrawing of part of the bowel wall, which may be associated with one of the above (Fig. 71).

A polyp could be a solitary inflammatory lesion or an adenoma. Adenomas are uncommon in ulcerative colitis (Fig. 72) and their presence may increase the risk of cancer (61). To some extent this will depend on the patient's age. In an elderly patient with a short history of colitis, an adenoma would be an incidental finding, whereas in a young patient with a long history of colitis it would represent a significant risk factor (60). An elevated lesion with an indrawn base is probably the most definite sign of early invasive cancer (Fig. 73). All lesions in this group require endoscopic examination and biopsy for histological clarification. Colectomy must never be contemplated from the radiological appearances alone.

In the follow-up of high-risk patients, a double-contrast barium enema can be used as a screening technique, perhaps alternating each year with colonoscopy (Table 1). Patients in group A would not need further investigation, but those with a focal lesion in group B would require endoscopy. The value of this is yet to be established, but endoscopy must not be considered the final arbiter, as overt cancer can be missed (61), and the ability of the radiologist to highlight an area for scrutiny may prove valuable.

Carcinoma in the Rectal Stump in Patients with an Ileorectal Anastomosis The rectal stump can be examined at sigmoidoscopy, and as the ileum does not seem to be at risk from cancer, radiology is not required for the particular problem. In a large series of patients with ileorectal anastomosis for ulcerative colitis, cancer developed in the rectal stump in 6% (63). This did not occur in less than 10 years from the onset of symptoms, and almost all the patients who develop rectal cancer had a total colitis at the time of colectomy, so that the pattern of cancer in the rectal stump follows that for the colon. The majority of tumors are poorly differentiated and survival is poor.

Malignant Lymphoma in Ulcerative Colitis Primary malignant lymphoma of the large bowel is a rare complication in ulcerative colitis, and only about 20 cases have been reported (63). Although the bowel contains a considerable volume of lymphoid tissue in chronic ulcerative colitis, no association or increased risk of lymphoma has been established. Any irregular mass is more likely to be a carcinoma, but the possibility of a lymphoma must be borne in mind (Fig. 74).

ARTHRITIS Arthritis is the commonest extracolonic complication of IBD. There are three types of arthropathy:

1. *Peripheral arthropathy.* A mild migratory synovitis affecting mainly large joints, usually the knees or ankles and sometimes the hands or feet, is found in 6.6–22% of cases (64,65). It is seronegative to rheumatoid factor. Radiologically, the involved joint appears normal, without erosion or joint space narrowing. Soft tissue swelling may be noted (66). The arthropathy may fluctuate with the activity of the colitis and will be cured by colectomy (67). Rarely, the arthritis may precede the colitis (68).

2. *Sacroiliitis.* Early changes affect the iliac bone more and may be unilateral. There is patchy osteoporosis and loss of definition at the joint margins, with some erosions and areas of subchondral bone sclerosis (Fig. 75). Progression of the sacroiliitis with further erosion leads to widening of the joint space. Eventually, ossification within the joint may lead to bony trabeulae transversing the joint space (69). In the elderly inflammatory changes in the sacroiliac joints must be distinguished from degenerative disease (69). Sacroiliitis may be seen in 10.1–15.8% of cases and is often asymptomatic (64,70).

3. *Ankylosing spondylitis.* This may be diagnosed radiologically when syndesmophyte changes are seen in the spine in association with sacroiliitis (Fig. 76). The incidence of ankylosing spondylitis is between 3 and 17% (70–72). Unlike peripheral arthropathy, it is not affected by the state of the colitis and may manifest before the colitis. The association between the antigenic phenotype HLA-B27 and ankylosing spondylitis is well known (70) and has been investigated in IBD. There is no significant difference in the incidence of this phenotype in IBD, but patients who do have IBD and the B27 phenotype seem to have a higher chance of developing ankylosing spondylitis. Patients with a peripheral arthropathy may be B27 negative, but those with ankylosing spondylitis are usually positive (73).

Avascular Necrosis of the Femoral Head This is known to be a complication of steroid therapy, but in practice it is a rare problem. Only the occasional patient presents with an abnormal hip joint, but when this happens the changes tend to be severe (Figs. 77 and 78).

LIVER AND BILIARY TRACT

Abnormal liver function tests are found in 15% of ulcerative colitis patients (74), and there is one report of 30% in Crohn's disease (75). Liver biopsies are frequently abnormal. Seventy-seven percent of wedge biopsies taken at the time of colectomy showed significant histological changes (76), with pericholangitis (the presence of portal zone inflammation on liver biopsy) in 50%, fatty change in 35%, cirrhosis in 4%, and granulomas in 7%.

Fatty change in the liver is very common and is related to the malnutrition of severe colitis. Cirrhosis is found in 5% (77). Chronic active hepatitis tends to present with or precede the colitis (77), whereas cirrhosis may predominate only after many years of colitis. The end stage of pericholangitis may be macronodular cirrhosis (78). Colectomy has no effect on the course of cirrhosis.

Pericholangitis has been reported in up to 50% (76) of biopsies from patients with ulcerative colitis, and in 78% of patients with Crohn's disease (75). The relationship between pericholangitis and sclerosing cholangitis is not clear (79), as in most of these reports cholangiography was not performed. Ulcerative colitis is an important cause of sclerosing cholangitis, and in one series accounted for 72% of the cases (79). It appears to be rare in Crohn's disease (80). The colitis is likely to be total, but was only distal in 10%. Colectomy does not appear to influence sclerosing cholangitis.

Colitics who have persistent abnormal liver function tests may have sclerosing cholangitis. To confirm this would require cholangiography. This may be performed endoscopically or percutaneously (79), but is probably not justified unless the patient is jaundiced. This will show the extent of the duct involvement (Figs. 79 and 80) and whether surgical bypass is feasible. Interventional studies, with the insertion of splints to drain strictured ducts, is a possible method for treatment. Sclerosing cholangitis is not rapidly progressive, and the patient may survive for several years after the onset of jaundice.

Another indication for cholangiography in jaundiced colitic patients is the exclusion of bile duct carcinoma. The cholangiographic changes may simulate sclerosing cholangitis, but typically a centrally placed tumor will cause sudden stenosis of the dilated ducts, producing the "carrot sign" (Fig. 81). Tumors in the extrahepatic bile ducts produce an irregular stricture or occlusion (Fig. 82). Laparotomy and biopsy is often the only certain method for diagnosing bile duct cancers, which colitics have an eightfold increased risk of developing (81).

Most studies indicate that hepatobiliary abnormalities are common in ulcerative colitis, although these do not frequently cause clinical problems. There are reports that the problem is similar in Crohn's disease, although most indicated that it is rare. In the National Cooperative Crohn's Disease Study (82), only 1% of patients were excluded for known liver disease. Of those in the study, only 3.9% showed abnormal liver function tests. However, until there is a large series with liver biopsies in ulcerative colitis and Crohn's disease, the relative frequency of liver disease remains unproven.

REFERENCES

1. Ritchie, J.K. (1974). Results of surgery for inflammatory bowel disease: a further survey of one hospital region. Br. Med. J. 1; 264.
2. Javett, S.L., Brooke, B.N. (1970). Acute dilatation of the colon in Crohn's disease Lancet 2; 126.
3. Schacter, H., Goldstein, M.J., Kirsner, J.B. (1967). Toxic dilation complicating Crohn's disease of the colon. Gastroenterology. 53; 136.
4. Marston, A., Pheils, M.Y., Lea Thomas, M., Morson, B.C. (1966). Ischaemic colitis. Gut 7; 1.
5. Cardoso, J.M., Kimura, K., Stoopen, M. et al. (1977). Radiology of invasive amebiasis of the colon. Am. J. Roentgenol. 128; 935.

6. Rosen, I.B., Cooter, N.B., Ruderman, R.L. (1973). Necrotizing colitis. Surg. Gynecol. Obstet. 137; 645.

7. Lennard-Jones, J.E., Vivian, A.B. (1960). Fulminating ulcerative colitis. Recent experience in management. Br. Med. J. 11; 96.

8. Klein, S.H., Edelman, S., Krischner, P.A., et al. (1960). Emergency cecostomy in ulcerative colitis with acute toxic dilatation. Surgery 47; 399.

9. Ripstein, C.B., Weiner, E.A. (1973). Toxic megacolon. Dis. Colon Rectum, 16; 402.

10. Price, A.B. (1978). Overlap in the spectrum of non-specific inflammatory bowel disease — ''colitis indeterminate.'' J. Clin. Pathol. 31; 567.

11. Edwards, F.C., Truelove, S.C. (1964). The course and prognosis of ulcerative colitis. Part III. Complications. Gut 5; 1.

12. McInery, G.T., Sauer, W.G., Baggenstos, A.H., Hodgson, J.R. (1962). Fulminating ulcerative colitis with marked colonic dilatation. A clinico-pathologic study. Gastroenterology. 42; 244.

13. Roth, J.L.A., Valdes-Dapena, A., Stein, G.N., et al. (1959). Toxic megacolon in ulcerative colitis. Gastroenterology. 37; 239.

14. Jalan, K.N., Sircus, W., Card, W.I., et al. (1969). An experience of ulcerative colitis:1. Toxic dilation in 55 cases. Gastroenterology 57; 68.

15. Lennard-Jones, J.E., Ritchie, J.K., Hilder, W., Spicer, C.C. (1975). Assessment of severity in colitis: a preliminary study. Gut 16; 579.

16. Buckell, N.A., Williams, G.T., Bartram, C.I., et al. (1980). Depth of ulceration in acute colitis. Gastroenterology 79; 19.

17. Jones, H.J., Chapman, M. (1969). Definition of megacolon in colitis. Gut 10; 562.

18. Neschis, M., Siegelman, S.S., Parker, J.G. (1968). Diagnosis and management of the megacolon of ulcerative colitis. Gastroenterology 55; 251.

19. Brooke, B.N., Sampson, P.A. (1964). An indication for surgery in acute ulcerative colitis. Lancet 2; 1272.

20. Bartram, C.I. (1976). The plain abdominal X-ray in acute colitis. Proc. R. Soc Med. 69; 617.

21. McConnel, F., Hanelin, J., Robbins, L.L. (1958). Plain film diagnosis of fulminating ulcerative colitis. Radiology 71; 674.

22. Vernia, P., Colaneri, O., Tomei, E., Caprilli, R. (1979). Intestinal gas in ulcerative colitis. Dis. Colon Rectum 22; 346.

23. Fazio, V.W. (1980). Toxic megacolon in ulcerative colitis and Crohn's colitis. Clin. Gastroenterol. 9, 2; 389.

24. Marshak, R.H., Lester, L.J., Friedman, A.I. (1950). Case reports: megacolon, a complication of ulcerative colitis. Gastroenterology 16; 768.

25. Jalan, K.N., Walker, R.J., Sircus, W., McManus, J.P.A. (1969). Pseudopolyposis in ulcerative colitis. Lancet 2; 555.

26. Goldberg, H.I. (1975). The barium enema and toxic megacolon: cause-effect relationship. Gastroenterology 68; 617.

27. Wrable, L.D., Bronstein, M.W. (1968). Toxic dilatation of the colon following barium enema examination during the quiescent stage of ulcerative colitis. Am. J. Dig. Dis. 13; 918.

27a. Bryk, D., Soong, K.Y. (1967). Colonic ileus and its differential roentgen diagnosis. Am. J. Roentgenol. 101; 329.

28. Bartram, C.I. (1977). Radiology in the assessment of ulcerative colitis. Gastrointest. Radiol. 1; 383.

29. Morson, B.C., Dawson, I.M.P. (1979). *Gastrointestinal Pathology*. Blackwell Scientific Publications, Oxford, p. 607.

30. Young, A.C. (1969). *Inflammatory Disease of the Colon — A Textbook of X-ray Diagnosis,* Vol. IV, Shanks, S.C., Kerley, P. (Eds.). H.K. Lewis, London, 6th ed., p. 459.
31. Schacter, W. (1975). Definitions of inflammatory bowel disease of unknown etiology. Gastroenterology 68; 591.
32. Dukes, C.E. (1954). The surgical pathology of ulcerative colitis. Ann. R. Coll. Surg. Engl. 14; 389.
33. Price, A.B. (1978). Benign lymphoid and inflammatory polyps. In *Pathogenesis of Colorectal Cancer,* Morson, B.C. (Ed.). Saunders, Philadelphia, p. 33.
34. Bartram, C.I. (1979). Inflammatory bowel disease. In *Double Contrast Gastroentestinal Radiology,* I. Laufer, Saunders, Philadelphia, p. 620.
35. DeDombal, F.T., Watts, J., Watkinson, G., Goligher, J.C. (1966). Local complications of ulcerative colitis, stricture, pseudopolyposis and carcinoma of the colon and rectum. Br. Med. J. 1; 1442.
36. Jaln, K.N., Walker, R.J., Sircus, W., et al. (1969). Pseudopolyposis in ulcerative colitis. Lancet 2; 555.
37. Teague, R.H., Read, A.E. (1975). Polyposis in ulcerative colitis. Gut 16; 792.
38. Zegel, H.G., Laufer, I. (1978). Filiform polyposis. Radiology 127; 615.
39. Hammerman, A.M., Sahtz, B.A., Susman, N. (1978). Radiographic characteristics of colonic "mucosal bridges": sequelae of inflammatory bowel disease. Radiology 127; 611.
40. Nolan, D.J., Gourtsoyiannis, N.C. (1980). Crohn's disease of the small intestine: a review of the radiological appearances of 100 consecutive patients examined by a barium infusion technique. Clin. Radiol. 31; 597.
41. Jones, B., Abbruzzese, A.A. (1978). Obstructing giant pseudopolyps in granulomatous colitis. Gastrointest. Radiol. 3; 437.
42. Keating, J.W., Mindell, H.J. (1976). Localized giant pseudopolyposis in ulcerative colitis. Am. J. Roentgenol. 126; 1178.
43. Lennard-Jones, J.E., Morson, B.C., Ritchie, J.K., et al. (1977). Cancer in colitis: assessment of the individual risk by clinical and histological criteria. Gastroenterology 73; 1280.
44. Joffe, N. (1977). Localised giant pseudopolyposis secondary to ulcerative or granulomatous colitis. Clin. Radiol. 28; 609.
45. Martinez, C.R., Siegelman, S.S., Saba, G.P., et al. (1977). Localized tumor-like lesions in ulcerative colitis and Crohn's disease of the colon. J. Hopkins Med. J. 140; 249.
46. Marshak, R.H., Lindner, A.E., Maklansky, D. (1977). Familial polyposis. Am. J. Gastroenterol. 67; 177.
47. Marshak, R.H., Lindner, A.E. (1980). Radiologic diagnosis of chronic ulcerative colitis and Crohn's disease. In *Inflammatory Bowel Disease,* Kirsner, J.B., Shorter, R.G. (Eds.). Lea & Febiger, Philadelphia, 2nd ed., p. 351.
48. Fenessy, J.J., Sparsberg, M.B., Kirsner, J.B. (1968). Radiological findings in carcinoma of the colon: complications of chronic ulcerative colitis. Gut 9; 388.
49. Ferruci, J.T., Benedict, K.T. (1971). Anticholinergic aided study of the gastrointestinal tract. Radiol. Clin. N. Am. 9; 23.
50. Goulston, S.J.M., McGovern, V.J. (1969). The nature of benign strictures in ulcerative colitis. N. Engl. J. Med. 281; 290.
51. Deliwari, J.B., Parkinson, C., Ridell, R.H., et al. (1973). Colonoscopy in the investigation of ulcerative colitis. Gut 14; 426.
52. Koloday, M. (1970). Reversible right colonic strictures in chronic ulcerative colitis. Radiology 97; 83.
53. Lennard-Jones, J.E., Langman, M.J.S., Avery-Jones, F. (1962). Faecal stasis in proctocolitis. Gut 3; 301.

54. Edwards, F.C., Truelove, S.C. (1964). The course and prognosis of ulcerative colitis. Part IV. Carcinoma of the colon. Gut 5; 15.

55. Morson, B.C., Dawson, I.M.P. (1979). *Gastrointestinal Pathology*. Blackwell, Scientific Publications, Oxford, p. 536.

56. Lennard-Jones, J.E., Misiweicz, J.J., Parrish, J.A., et al. (1974). Prospective study of outpatients with extensive colitis. Lancet 1; 1065.

57. MacDougall, I.P.M. (1964). The cancer risk in ulcerative colitis. Lancet 2; 655.

58. Hinton, J.M. (1966). Risk of malignant change in ulcerative colitis. Gut 7; 427.

59. Muto, T., Bussey, II.J.R., Morson, B.C. (1975). The evolution of cancer of the colon and rectum. Cancer 36; 2251.

60. Riddell, R.H. (1980). Dysplasia in inflammatory bowel disease. Clin. Gastroenterol. 9, (2); 439.

61. Butt, J., Konishi, F., Morson, B.C., et al. (1981). Macroscopic features of cancer and dysplasia in chronic ulcerative colitis. In preparation.

62. Frank, P.H., Ridell, R.H., Feczko, P.J., Levin, B. (1978). Radiological detection of colonic dysplasia (precancer) in chronic ulcerative colitis. Gastrointest. Radiol. 3; 209.

63. Baker, W.N.W., Glass, R.E., Ritchie, J.K., Aylett, S.O. (1978). Cancer of the rectum following colectomy and ileo-rectal anastomosis for ulcerative colitis. Br. J. Surg. 65; 862.

64. Ansell, B.M., Wigley, R.A.D. (1964). Arthritic manifestation in regional enteritis. Ann. Rheum. Dis. 23; 64.

65. Greenstein, A.J., Janowitz, H.D., Saclar, D.B. (1976). The extra-intestinal complications of Crohn's disease and ulcerative colitis. Medicine 55; 401.

66. Clark, R.G., Muhletaler, C.A., Margulies, S.I. (1971). Colitic arthritis. Radiology 101; 585.

67. Brooke, B.N. (1956). Outcome of surgery for ulcerative colitis. Lancet 2; 532.

68. McCullock, D.K., Fraser, D.M., Turner, A.L. (1980). Arthritis preceding fulminant ulcerative colitis and responding to colectomy. Br. Med. J. 281; 839.

69. Resnik, D., Niwayama, G., Gocrgen, T.,G. (1977). Comparison of radiographic abnormalities of the sacroiliac joint in degenerative disease and ankylosing spondylitis. Am. J. Roentgenol. 128; 189.

70. Dekker, S., Agenant, B.J., et al. (1978). Ankylosing spondylitis and inflammatory bowel disease. Ann. Rheum. Dis. 37; 30.

71. Wright, V., Watkinson, G., (1965). Sacro-iliitis and ulcerative colitis. Br. Med. J. 2; 675.

72. Jayson, M.I.V., Salmon, P.R., Harrison, W.J. (1970). Inflammatory bowel disease in ankylosing spondylitis. Gut 11; 506.

73. Mallen, E.G., Mackintosh, P., Asquith, P., et al. (1976). Histocompatible antigens in inflammatory bowel disease. Gut 17; 906.

74. Perrett, A.D., Higgins, G., Johnston, H.H., et al. (1971). The liver in ulcerative colitis. Q. J. Med. 158; 211.

75. Cohen, S., Kaplan, M., Gottlich, L. (1971). Liver disease and gallstones in regional enteritis. Gastroenterology 60; 237.

76. Eade, M.N. (1970). Liver disease in ulcerative colitis. 1. Analysis of operative liver biopsy in 138 consecutive patients having colectomy. Ann. Intern. Med. 74; 518.

77. Holdsworth, C.D., Hall, E.W., Dawson, A.M., Sherlock, S. (1965). Ulcerative colitis in chronic liver disease. Q. J. Med. 34; 211.

78. Sherlock, S. (1975). *Disease of the Liver and Biliary System*. Blackwell Scientific Publications, Oxford, 5th ed., p. 656.

79. Chapman, R.W.G., Marborgh, B.A., Rhodes, J.M., et al. (1980). Primary sclerosing cholangitis: a review of its clinical features, cholangiography, and hepatic histology. Gut 21; 870.

80. Atkinson, A.J., Carroll, W.W. (1964). Sclerosing cholangitis — association with regional enteritis. JAMA 188; 183.

81. Ritchie, J.K., Allan, R.N., Macartney, J., et al. (1974). Biliary tract carcinoma associated with ulcerative colitis. Q. J. Med. 43; 263.

82. Rankin, G.B., Watts, D., Clifford, S., et al. (1979). National Cooperative Crohn's Disease Study: extraintestinal manifestations and perianal complications. Gastroenterology 77; 914.

FIGURES 1 THROUGH 82

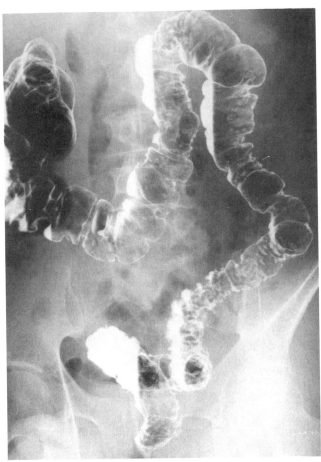

Figure 1a Typical changes of Crohn's colitis with patchy ulceration.

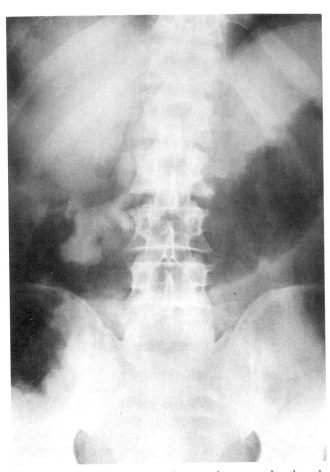

Figure 1b Twenty-five days later toxic megacolon has developed with perforation; note the free air under the liver.

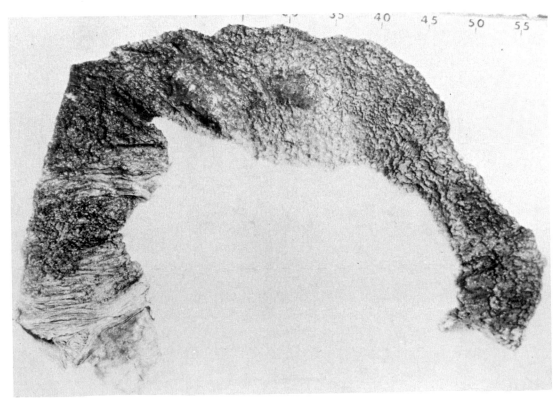

Figure 2 Total colitis with extensive ulceration and dilatation in the transverse colon.

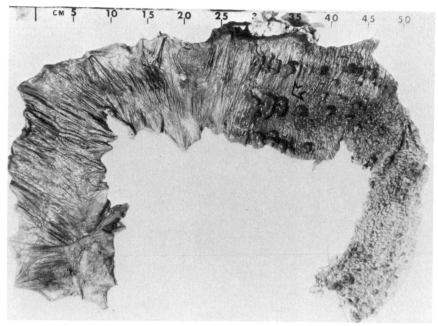

Figure 3 Toxic megacolon limited to the splenic flexure. Note the presence of mucosal islands (arrow). (From Ref. 83.)

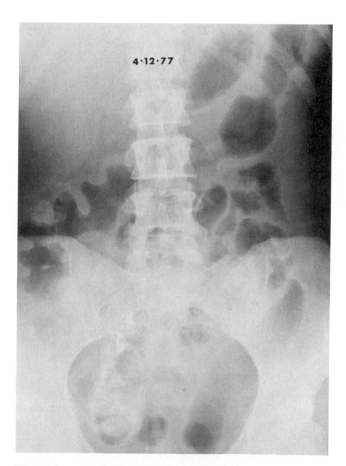

Figure 4a Total colitis but no evidence of dilatation.

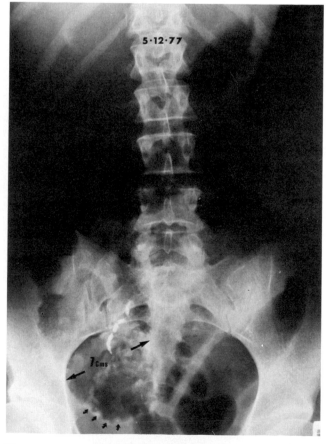

Figure 4b One day later toxic megacolon has developed in the cecum and ascending colon (arrow).

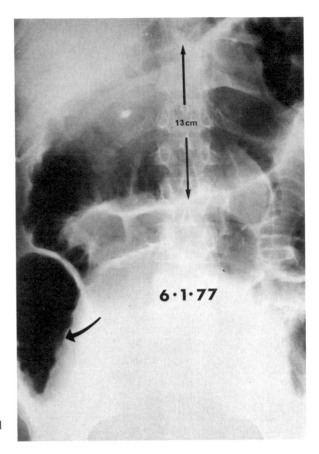

Figure 5a Gross dilatation of the transverse colon. Mucosal islands visible in the ascending colon.

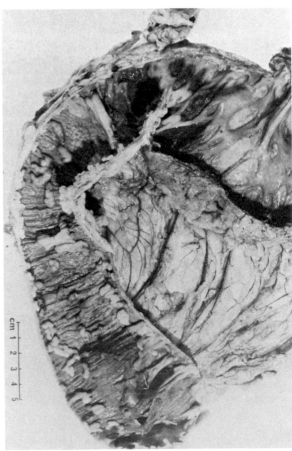

Figure 5b Mucosal islands clearly demonstrated on the resected specimen.

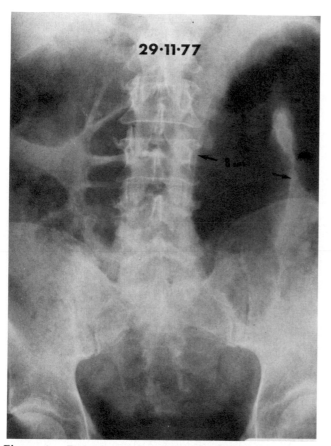

Figure 6a Redundant sigmoid loop dilated to 8 cm.

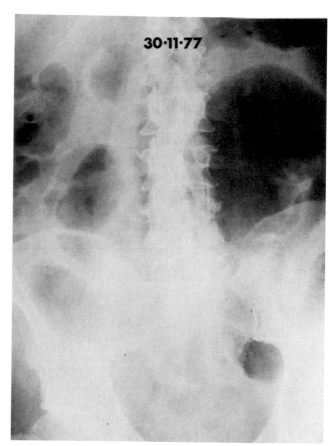

Figure 6b Next day it is 10 cm wide with mucosal islands visible.

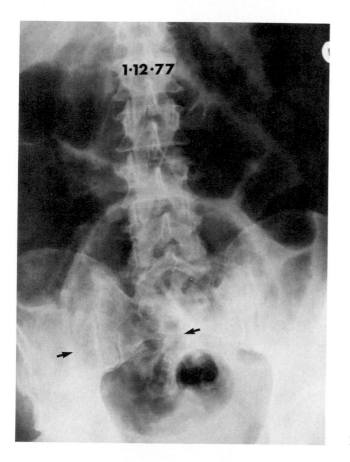

Figure 6c Twelve centimeters the day after (arrows).

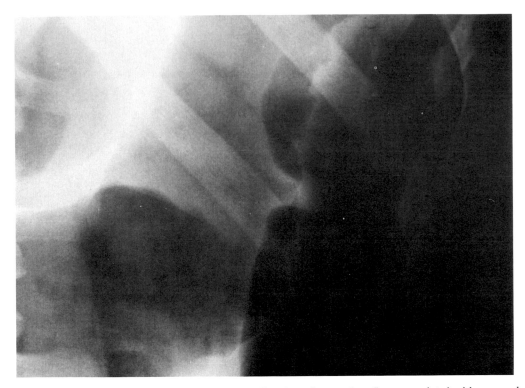

Figure 7 Early changes of toxic megacolon—dilatation of more than 5 cm associated with mucosal ulceration.

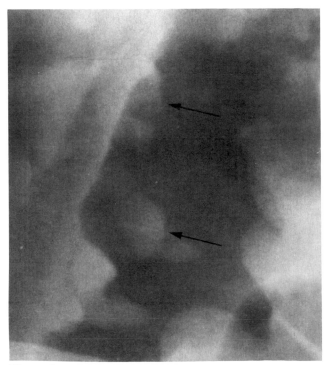

Figure 8 Mucosal islands (arrows).

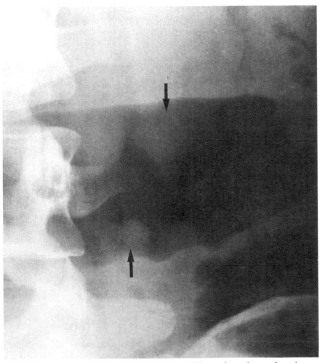

Figure 9 Mucosal islands (arrows). Note that the colon is not dilated.

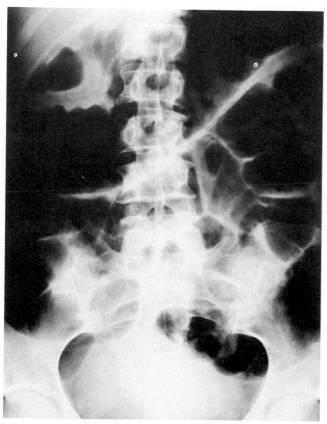

Figure 10 Mucosal islands are visible only at the edge of the bowel. In the center of the bowel the volume of gas has caused too much blackening for the mucosal islands to be visualized.

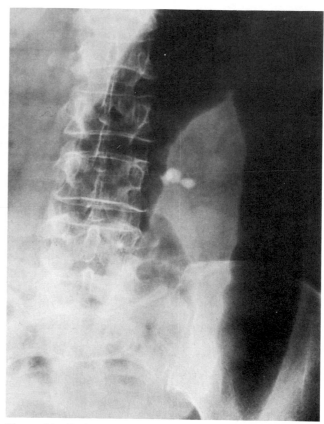

Figure 11 Early toxic megacolon but no mucosal islands visible. This was due to very extensive ulceration completely denuding the mucosa, leaving a relatively smooth surface.

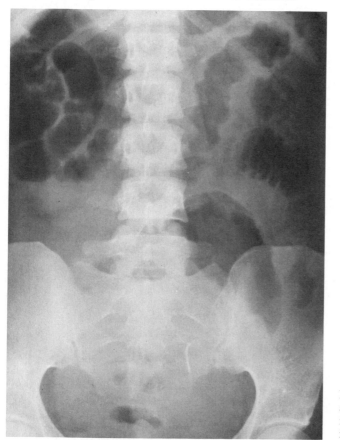

Figure 12 Gas shows an irregular edge in the transverse colon and sigmoid. Acute ulceration was present in the sigmoid, but not in the transverse colon, where the irregularity was due to inflammatory polyps.

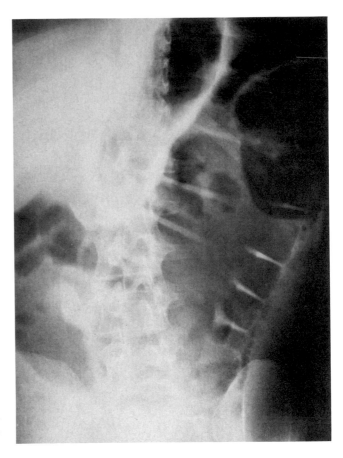

Figure 13 Gross gaseous distension of the transverse colon in a patient with idiopathic megacolon. Note the normal mucosal edge and haustration.

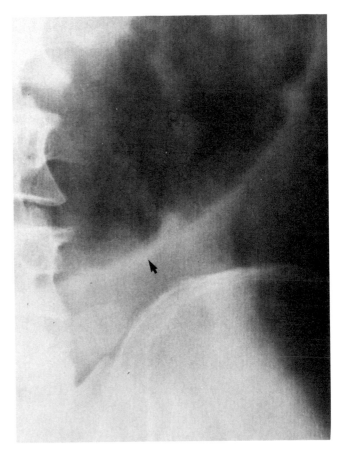

Figure 14 Bowel wall thickening of 6 mm in toxic megacolon. Serosal edge shown by arrow.

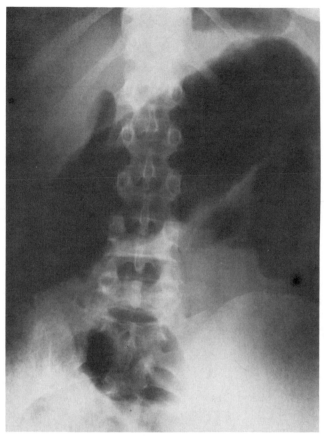

Figure 15a Toxic megacolon. The patient recovered on medical treatment.

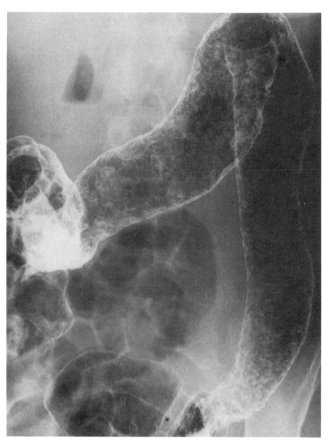

Figure 15b A double-contrast barium enema 6 months later shows extensive inflammatory polyps. The colon remains slightly dilated, perhaps reflecting neuronal damage.

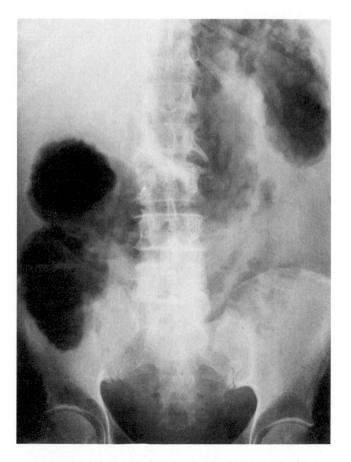

Figure 16 There is marked dilatation of the transverse and ascending colon with a mucosal appearance suggesting mucosal islands. This was due to a postoperative ileus with retained fecal residue.

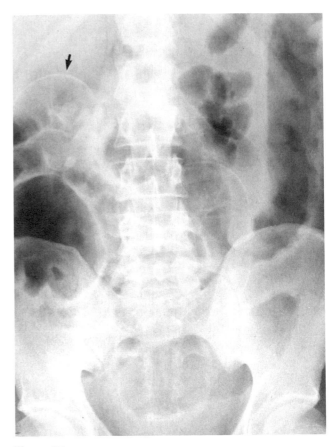

Figure 17

Figure 17 Perforation with free intraperitoneal air. Note the white line (arrow) due to air either side of the bowel wall. Active disease with ulceration is seen in the sigmoid and transverse colon, but the perforation had occurred in the sigmoid, which is also slightly dilated.

Figure 18a Active colitis with a granular mucosa extending into the transverse colon.

Figure 18b Perforation 11 days later. Note the retention of barium in the proximal colon. This is always on ominous sign of severe distal disease. Air is seen tracking around the bowel wall in the lower descending colon, indicating an extraperitoneal component to the free perforation.

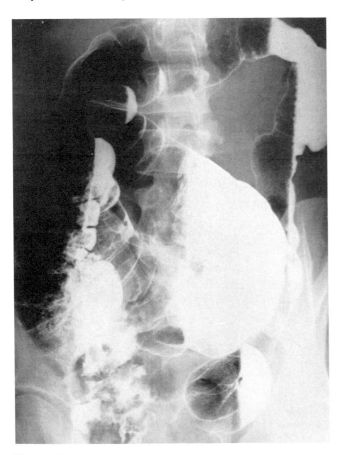

Figure 18a

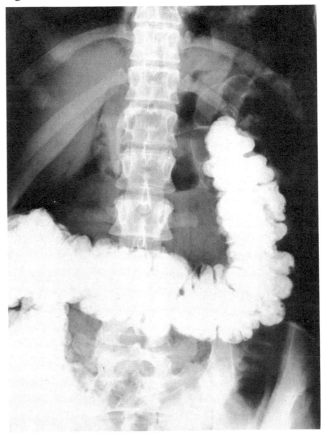

Figure 18b

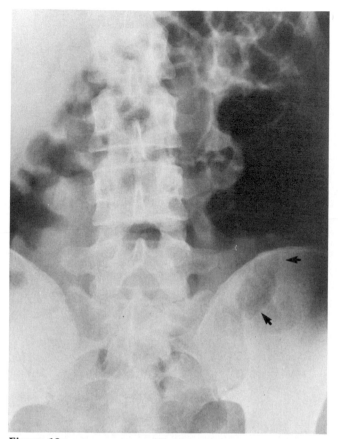

Figure 19a

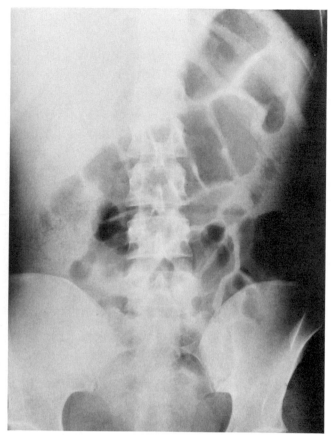

Figure 19b

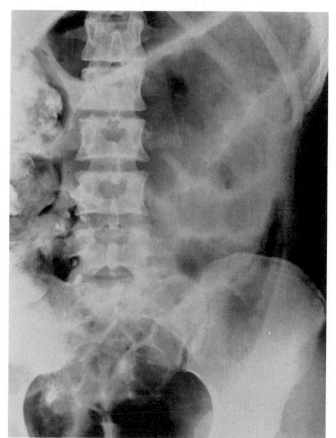

Figure 20

Figure 19a Localized acute disease without dilatation is just visible in the lower descending colon (arrows).

Figure 19b Sealed perforation 8 days later. Note the distension of the normal transverse colon. A small bowel ileus is present in the left iliac fossa. The loops are separated by some free fluid which supports the diagnosis of peritonitis.

Figure 20 Linear streaks of gas in the descending colon (arrow) due to deep ulceration and probably extraperitoneal perforation. Free intraperitoneal air was present within 24 hr. Note the retention of barium in the proximal colon following an instant enema some days before, the dilatation of the transverse colon, and gaseous distension of the small bowel—all signs indicating severe distal colitis. (From Ref. 28.)

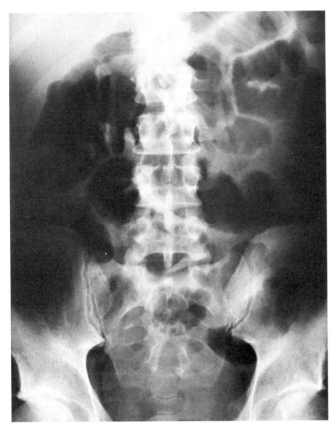

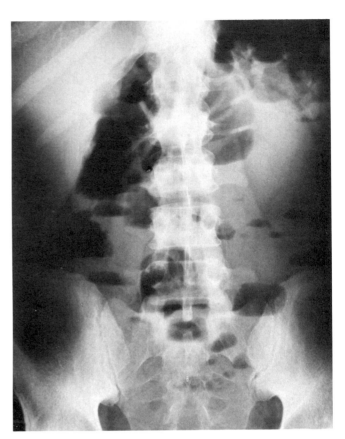

Figure 21 Severe distal colitis, with ulceration and early dilatation of the sigmoid colon. Proximal distension of relatively normal transverse colon and gaseous distension of small bowel are supportive signs of severe distal colitis.

Figure 22 Erect view of Figure 21. Free air is just visible under the liver edge. At operation a sigmoid perforation and large abscess in the right iliac fossa were found.

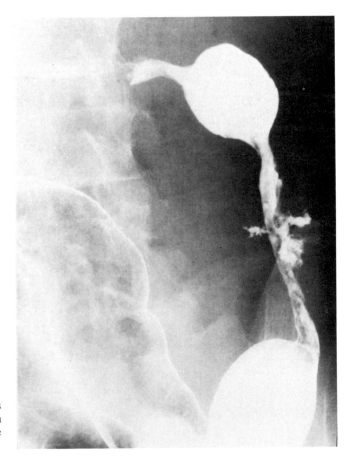

Figure 23 A patient with long-standing ulcerative colitis presented with a mass in the left iliac fossa. An instant barium enema shows several deep perforating tracks extending into the abscess.

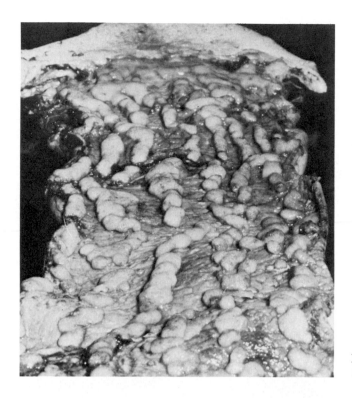

Figure 24 "Pseudopolypoid" mucosa resulting from extensive undermining ulceration.

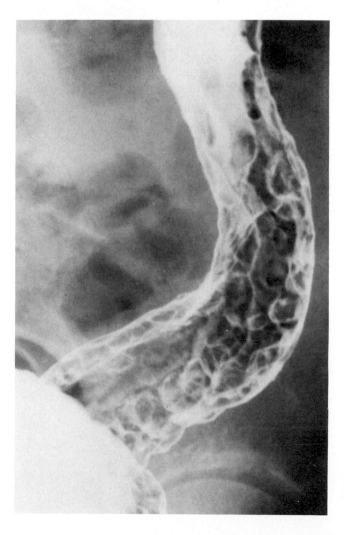

Figure 25 The mucosa appears polypoid and there is no irregularity of the mucosal line to suggest ulceration. This is an unusual case where there has been very extensive linear ulceration, leaving mucosal pseudopolyps set against a smooth background of exposed muscle.

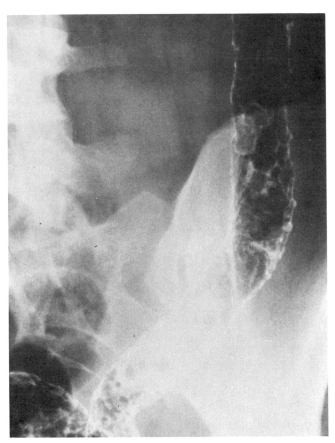

Figure 26a Instant enema performed during the recovery stage from an acute attack of colitis. Some ulceration remains and a number of polypoid lesions due to granulation tissue are present.

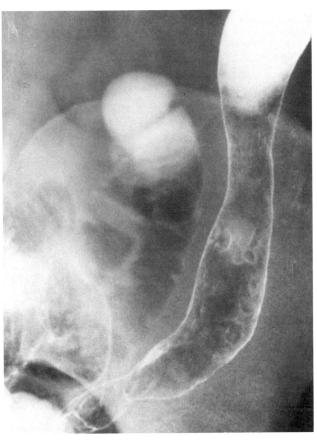

Figure 26b Several years later the colitis is relatively inactive. Several small postinflammatory polyps are visible.

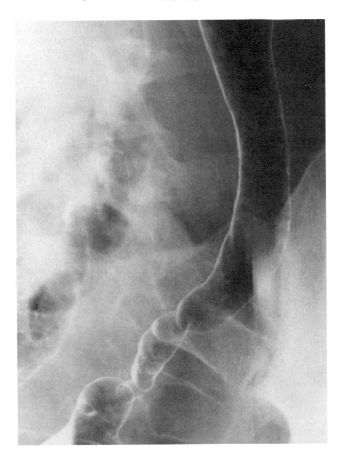

Figure 26c About 10 years after (a) the inflammatory polyps have disappeared. The sigmoid strictures are more pronounced.

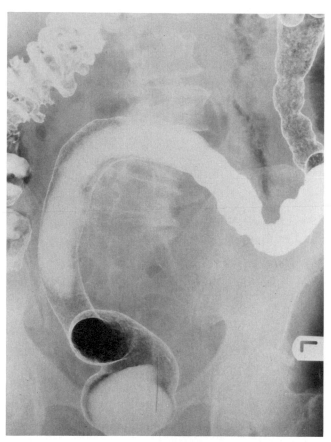

Figure 27a Active colitis to the splenic flexure.

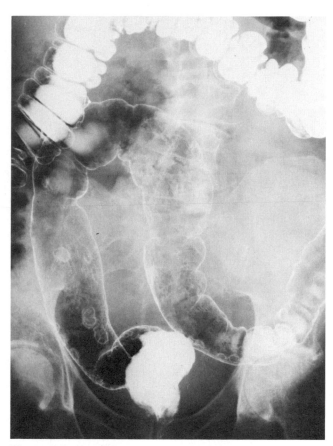

Figure 27b Several years later the colitis has become inactive; a number of sessile inflammatory polyps remain in the sigmoid colon. (From Ref. 34.)

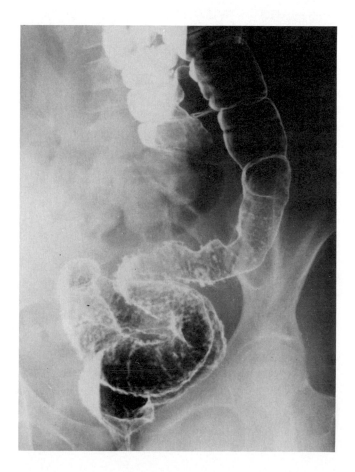

Figure 28 Ulceration in acute colitis causing disruption of the mucosal line.

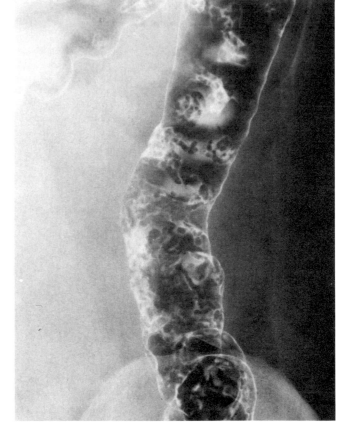

Figure 29

Figure 29 Numerous small inflammatory polyps may make the en face view of the mucosa rather irregular, but the mucosal line is smooth and intact.

Figure 30a Polypoid mucosal surface with some irregularity of the mucosal line. (From Ref. 28.)

Figure 30b Close-up view of the resected specimen showing a mass of regenerative nodules in between lines of residual ulceration.

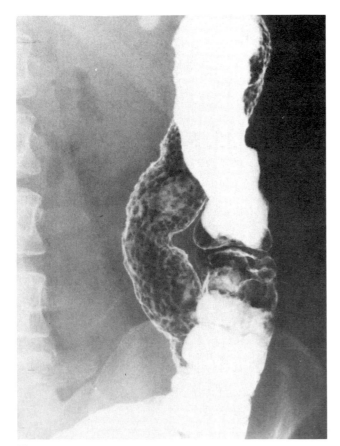

Figure 30a

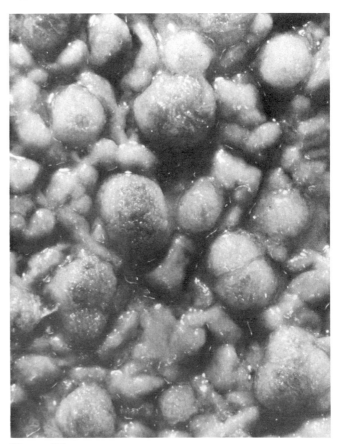

Figure 30b

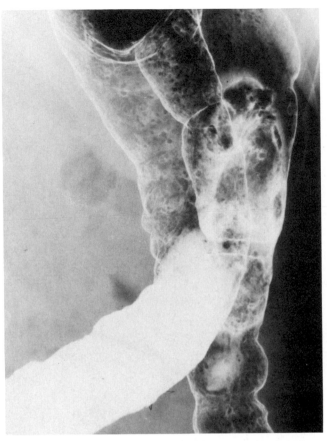

Figure 31a Numerous small inflammatory polyps. Background mucosa and mucosal line normal.

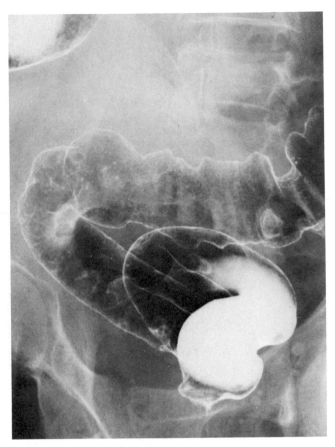

Figure 32 Inflammatory polyps composed of granulation tissue. A number of sessile polyps are present in the sigmoid. The surface of the polyps is granular, in keeping with the background mucosa. (From Ref. 34.)

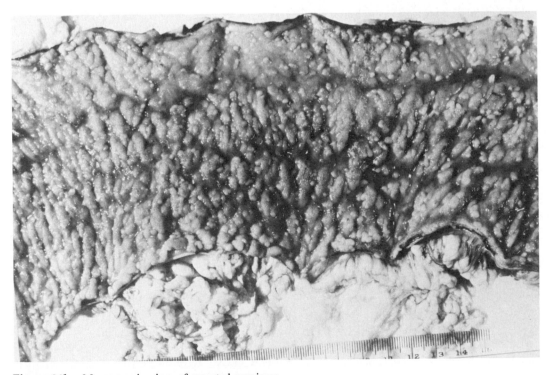

Figure 31b Macroscopic view of resected specimen.

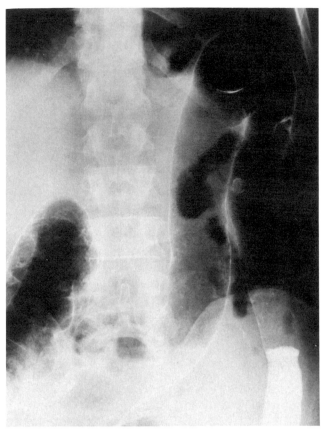

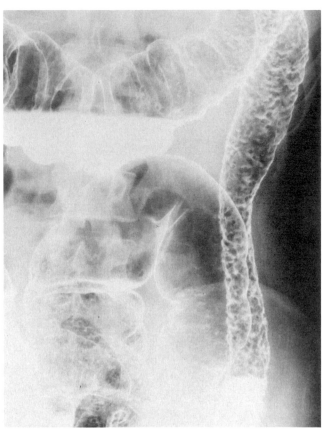

Figure 33 Two sessile polyps in the proximal descending colon. The surface of these polyps is smooth. Radiologically, it is impossible to suggest their nature. Endoscopic biopsy confirmed that they were both inflammatory polyps composed mainly of granulation tissue.

Figure 34 Inflammatory polyps in Crohn's disease. A mixture of sessile and short filiform polyps are present in the descending colon. (From Ref. 34.)

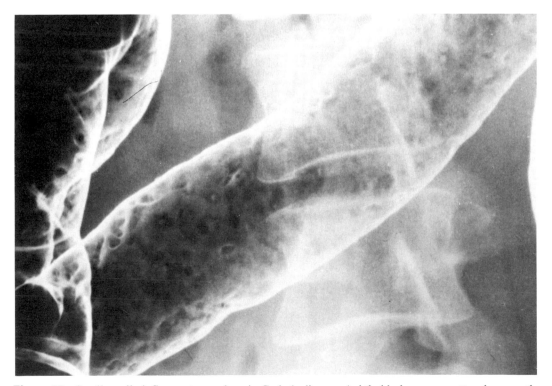

Figure 35 Small sessile inflammatory polyps in Crohn's disease. Aphthoid ulcers are scattered among the polyps.

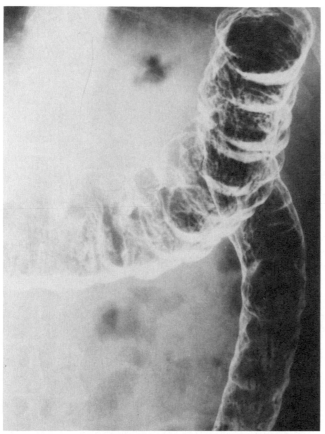

Figure 36 Extensive filiform polyps. The background mucosa is normal, as the colitis was in complete remission. (From Ref. 83.)

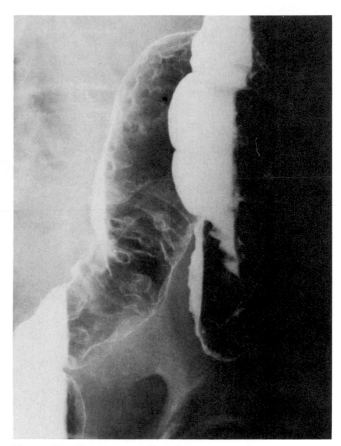

Figure 37 Numerous sessile inflammatory polyps.

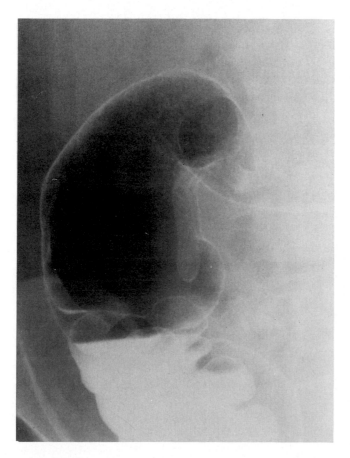

Figure 38 Unusually long filiform polyp arising from the hepatic flexure. It is not truly pedunculated, as it cannot be differentiated into a head or stalk.

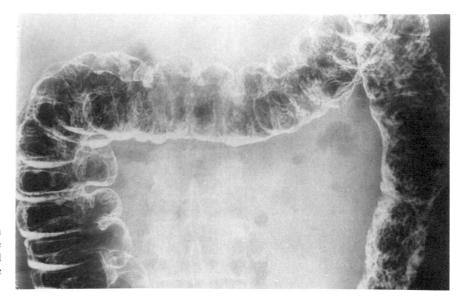

Figure 39 Numerous fine filiform polyps are present, giving the appearance of seaweed. The background mucosa and configuration of the colon is normal. The colitis was in complete remission.

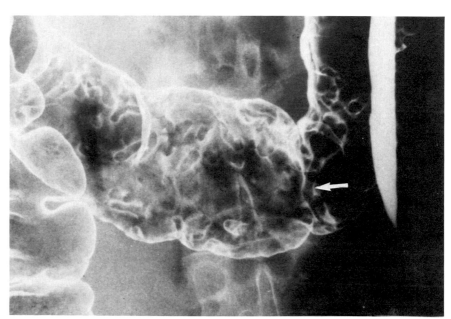

Figure 40 Filiform polyps in a patient with healed Crohn's colitis. A number of the polyps are adherent and one (arrow) bridges the lumen.

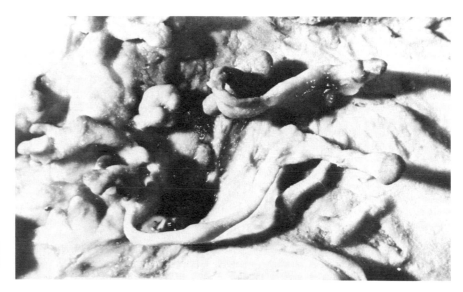

Figure 41 Close-up view of a resected colon with long filiform polyps that would bridge the lumen.

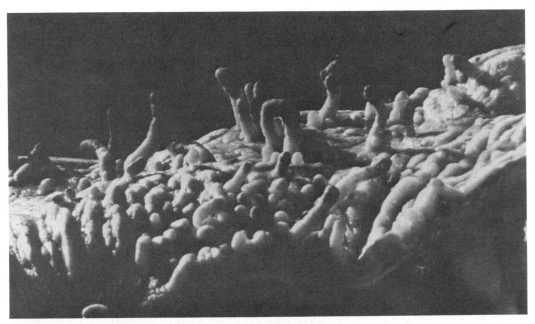

Figure 42 Macroscopic view of filiform polyps. In the center two polyps are adherent, fused at their tips. (From B.C. Morson, *The Pathogenesis of Colorectal Cancer*, 1978. W.B. Saunders, Philadelphia.)

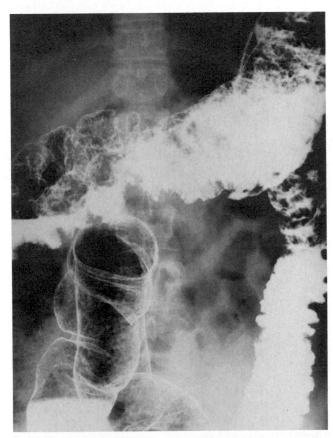

Figure 43 This patient presented with ankle edema, secondary to protein losing enteropathy, which resulted when active colitis was sumperimposed on a mass of inflammatory polyps. These are responsible for the extensive irregular filling defects in the transverse and descending colon.

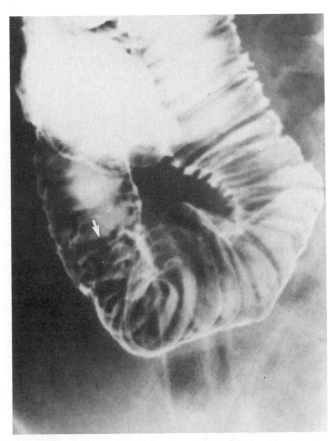

Figure 44 Crohn's disease with a few filiform polyps in the small bowel shown by double contrast (arrow).

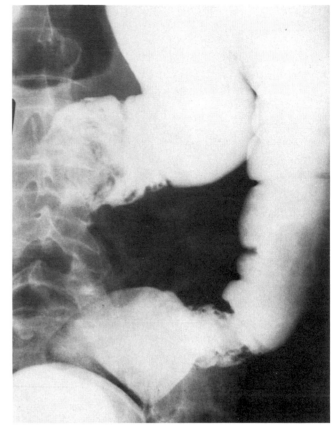

Figure 45 Localized mass of inflammatory polyps in the transverse colon preventing complete filling of the colon. Another short segment of inflammatory polyps is present in the proximal sigmoid. (From Ref. 34.)

Figure 46a The barium column is held up at the hepatic flexure.

Figure 46b After air insufflation the mass of filiform inflammatory polyps at the hepatic flexure, which were the cause of the obstruction, can be seen. Some smaller polyps are noted in the lower descending colon. (Courtesy of Professor Blum, Stadtspital Triemli, Zurich.)

Figure 45

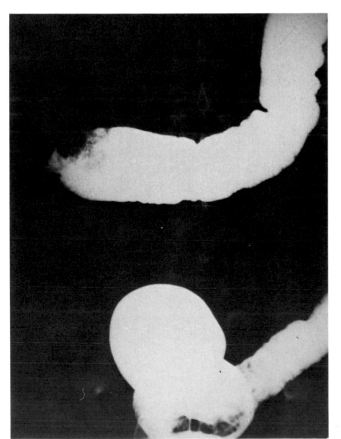

Figure 46a

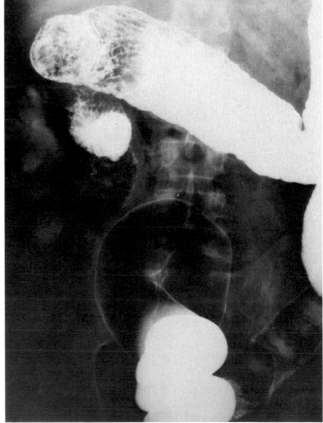

Figure 46b

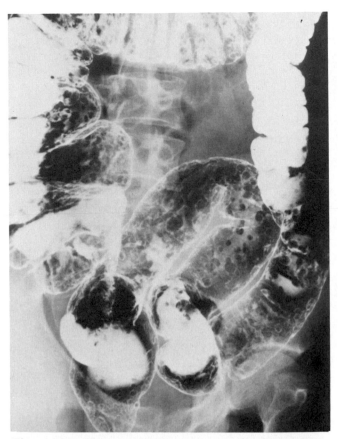

Figure 47

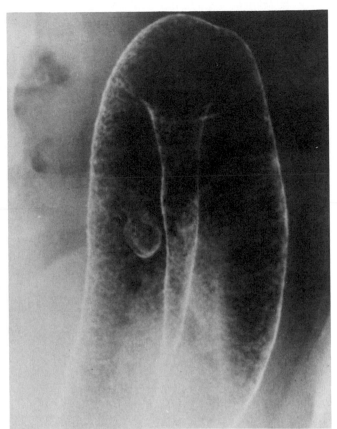

Figure 48

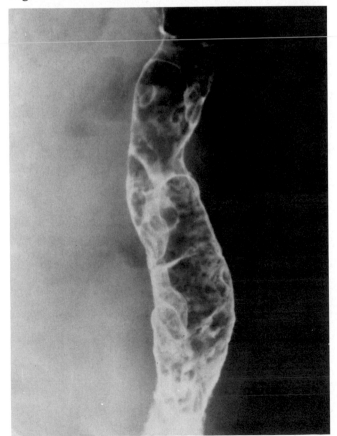

Figure 49

Figure 47 Typical case of familial adenomatous polyposis coli. There are a large number of small sessile polyps throughout the colon and rectum.

Figure 48 A 20-year-old patient with ulcerative colitis. The pedunculated polyp at the splenic flexure was a juvenile polyp.

Figure 49 Collection of pedunculated polyps in the descending colon of a 16-year-old patient with Crohn's disease. The polyps proved to be inflammatory in nature in spite of their pedunculation.

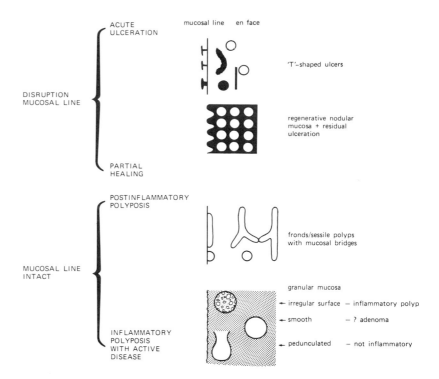

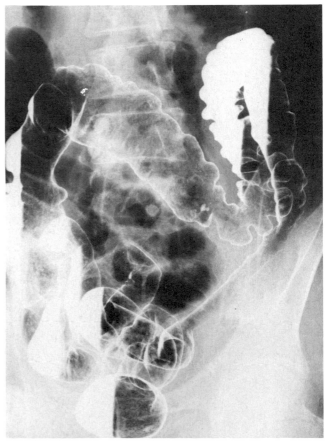

Figure 50 Diagrammatic representation of the causes of a polypoid mucosa in ulcerative colitis.

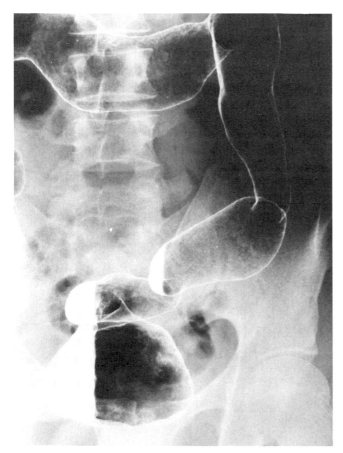

Figure 51 Two short strictures are present in the distal colon, in a patient with total ulcerative colitis and symptoms for 8 years. (From Ref. 28.)

Figure 52 Single long stricture in ulcerative colitis. (From Ref. 34.)

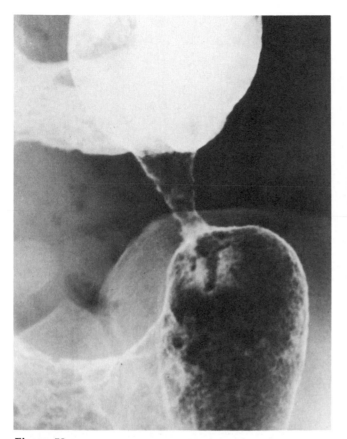

Figure 53

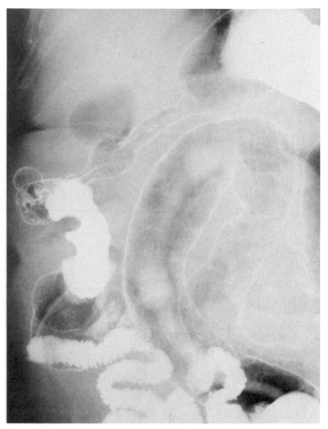

Figure 54

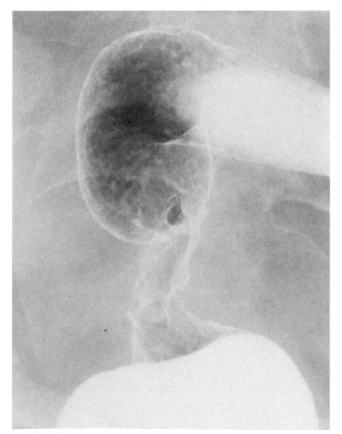

Figure 55

Figure 53   Short stricture in the descending colon. The mucosa on the medial side of the stricture is irregular. Endoscopic biopsy showed this to be due to severe dysplasia.

Figure 54   A stricture in the proximal colon in ulcerative colitis is unusual. This was benign but malignancy should always be considered.

Figure 55   Rectal stricture with an irregular lumen that was considered malignant radiologically but proved to be benign on biopsy. (From Ref. 34.)

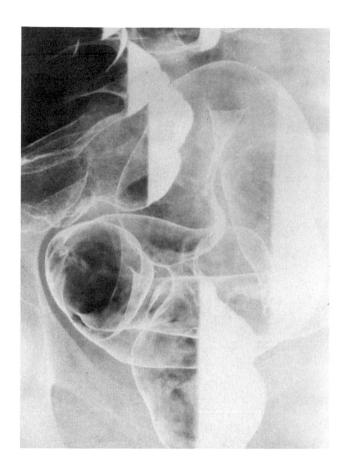

Figure 56a This patient had a 12-year history of colitis, which was in remission at the time of the examination. The rectal stricture appears relatively smooth and symmetrical. (From Ref. 34.)

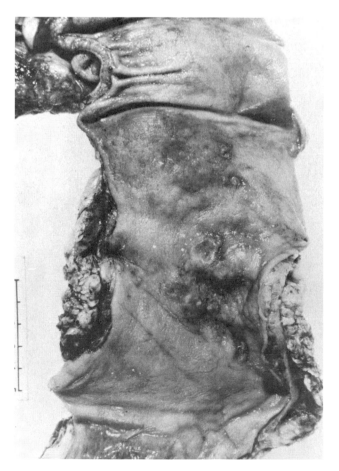

Figure 56b Resected specimen showing only minimal mucosal irregularity in an annular carcinoma where most of the tumor had spread submucosally.

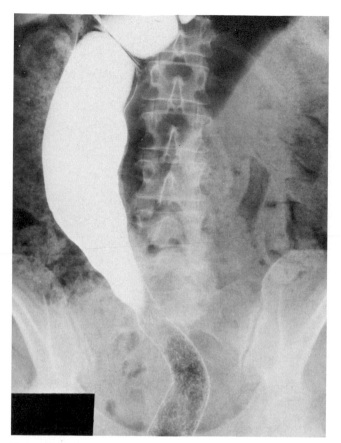

Figure 57a

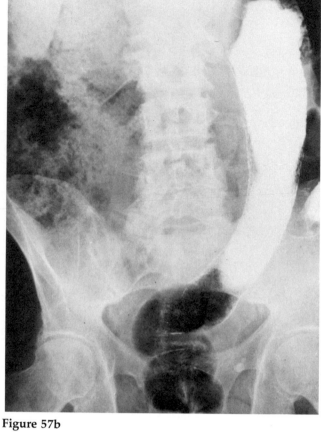

Figure 57b

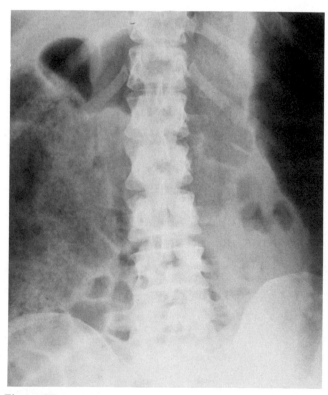

Figure 57 c

Figure 57 Three cases of fecal stasis in ulcerative colitis. Note the buildup of fecal residue in the proximal colon with active distal disease shown by instant enema in (a) and (b), and acute ulceration in the lower descending colon seen on a plain film in (c).

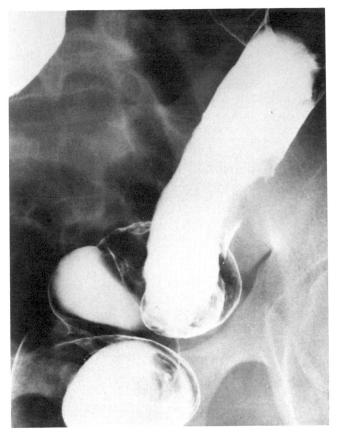

Figure 58a

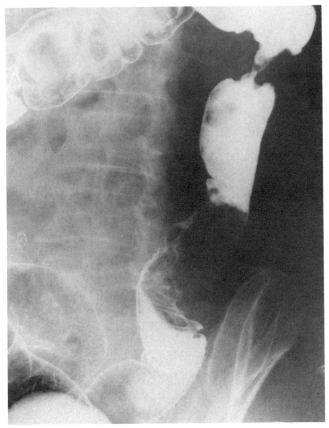

Figure 58b

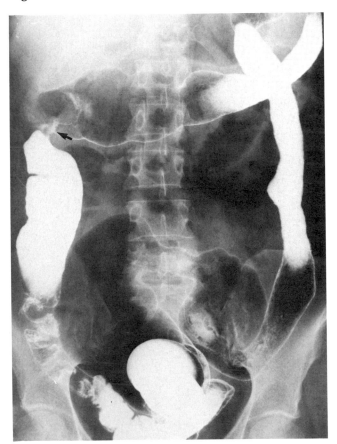

Figure 58c

Figure 58 Examples of carcinoma in ulcerative colitis. (a) An irregular plaquelike lesion in the lower descending colon. (b) Two carcinomas. (c) A plaquelike carcinoma at the hepatic flexure (arrow).

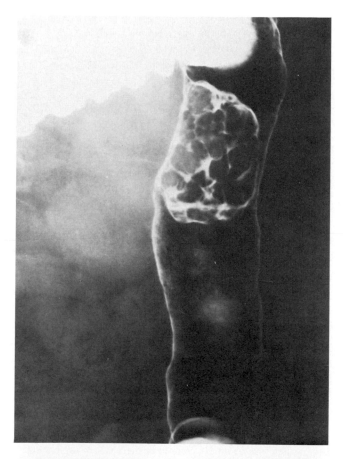

Figure 58d Unusual polypoid carcinoma in the descending colon. (From Ref. 34.)

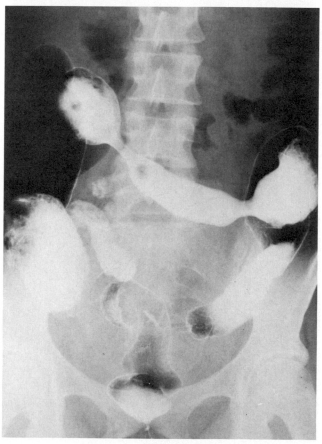

Figure 58e Annular tumor in the sigmoid. (From Ref. 34.)

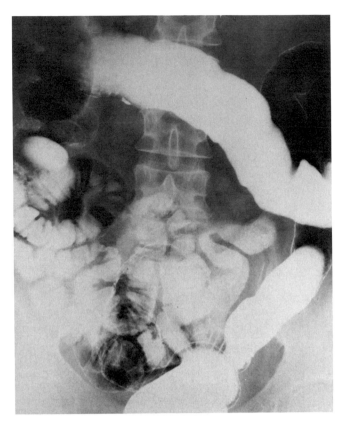

Figure 59a Total active ulcerative colitis.

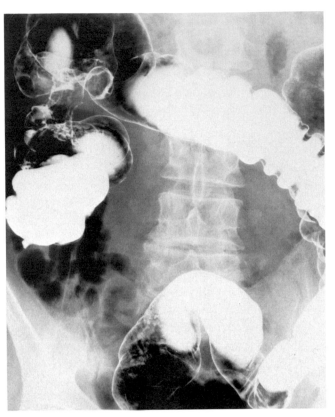

Figure 59b An annular carcinoma has developed 10 years later, which was about 20 years after the onset of the patient's symptoms.

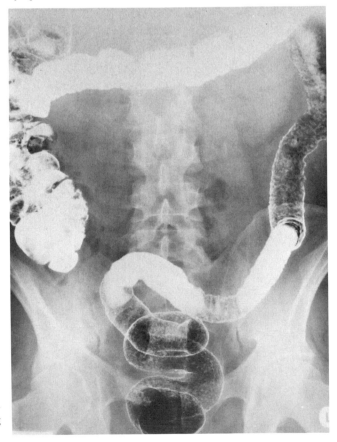

Figure 60 ''Extensive colitis''—by definition a colitis extending at least to the hepatic flexure on instant enema, and implying total histological involvement.

108

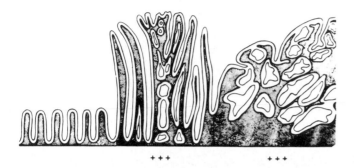

Figure 61 Diagramatic representation of dysplasia. A, normal mucosa; B, villous change; C, tubular budding. (+) represents mild and (+++) severe changes. (From Ref. 43.)

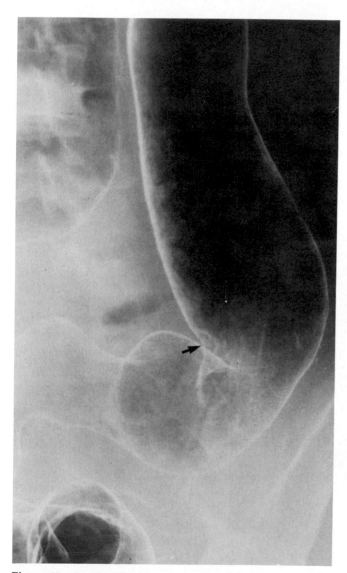

Figure 62 Small polypoid area of severe dysplasia (arrow). This patient had a carcinoma in the ascending colon.

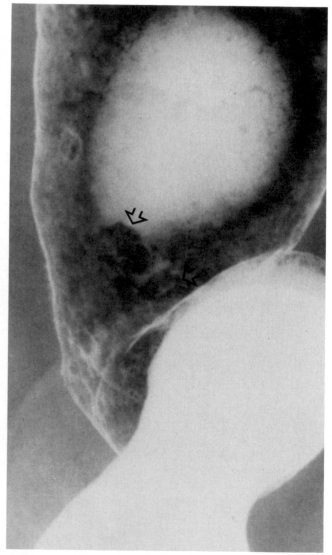

Figure 63 Area of mucosal irregularity due to severe dysplasia that is only slightly elevated (arrows).

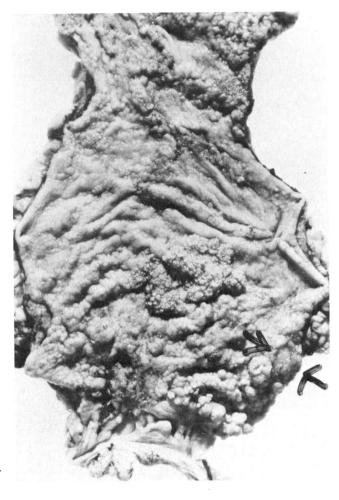

Figure 64 Severe dysplasia with scattered small villous lesions. An early carcinoma is present (arrows).

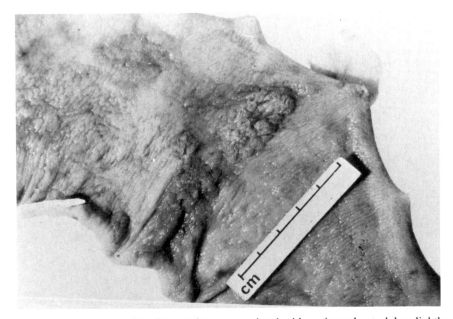

Figure 65 A small infiltrative carcinoma associated with an irregular nodular slightly elevated dysplastic lesion.

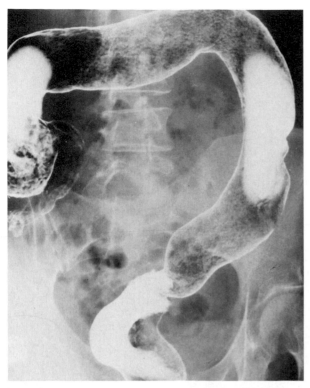

Figure 66a Instant enema showing total colitis with an irregular stricture in the sigmoid. (From Ref. 28.)

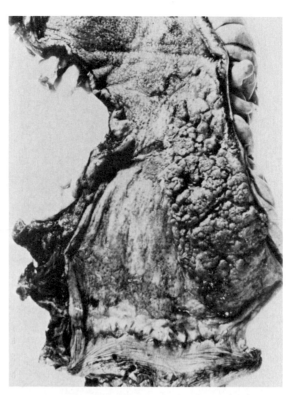

Figure 66b The resected specimen shows a villous tumor with a Dukes A carcinoma.

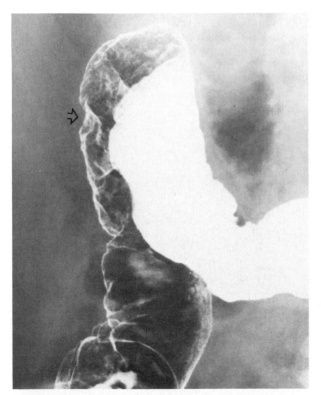

Figure 67a Early infiltrative carcinoma. Focal irregularity of the mucosa at the hepatic flexure is due to dysplasia. There is a localized area where the bowel wall is indrawn (arrow).

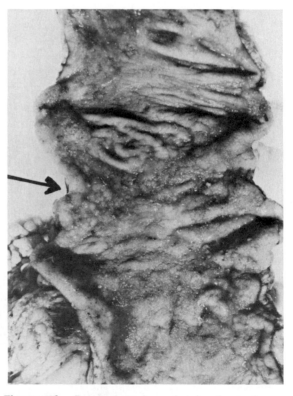

Figure 67b Resected specimen showing the carcinoma (arrow).

111

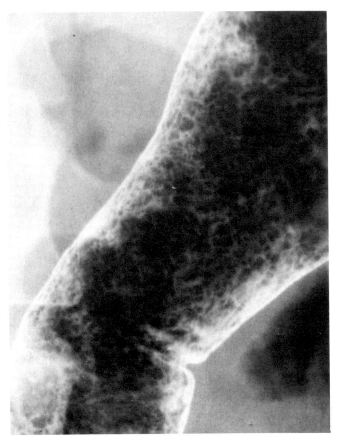

Figure 68 Dysplasia with flat polygonal surface.

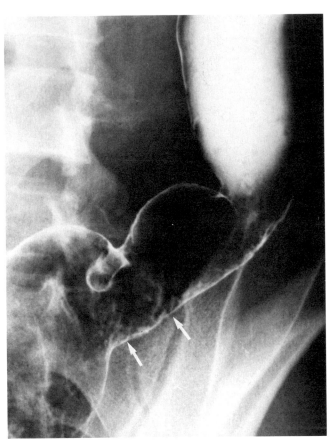

Figure 69 Inflammatory polyps associated with two short strictures. The larger polypoid lesion is an inflammatory polyp. Its base appears indrawn but this is due to the stricture. Just below this (arrows) are some smaller inflammatory polyps which are sessile and filiform. The sessile lesions produce a change that it is difficult to distinguish radiologically from dysplasia.

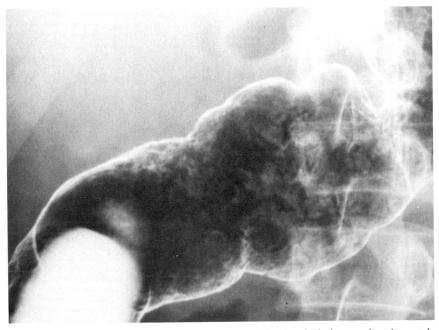

Figure 70 Dysplasia in a relatively flat mucosa. The dysplasia has produced a patchy nodular irregularity of the mucosa.

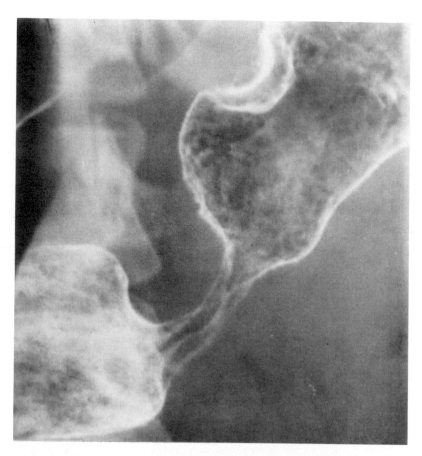

Figure 71 The polypoid lesion with an irregular indrawn base is a carcinoma. It is just proximal to a benign stricture.

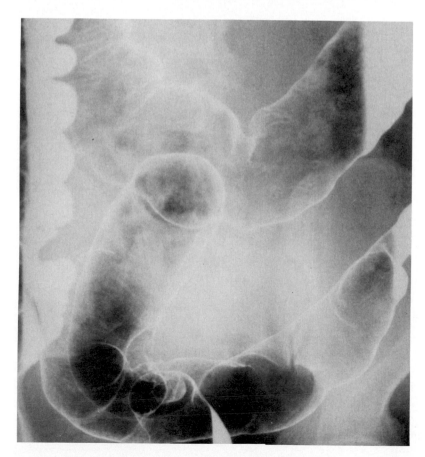

Figure 72 A pedunculated adenoma is present in the sigmoid, with a few filiform inflammatory polyps in the transverse colon in a patient with a long history of ulcerative colitis.

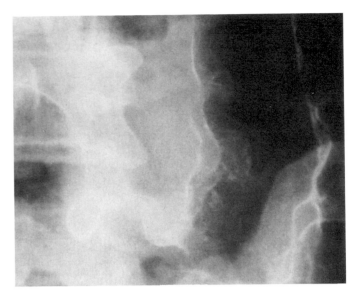

Figure 73a

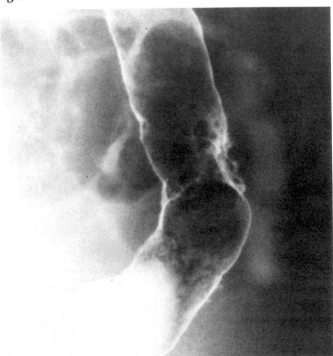

Figure 73b

Figure 73a – c Examples of early carcinoma in ulcerative colitis. All show two features in common; there is a polypoid lesion present with irregular indrawing of the base of the polyp—typical features of a malignant polyp.

114

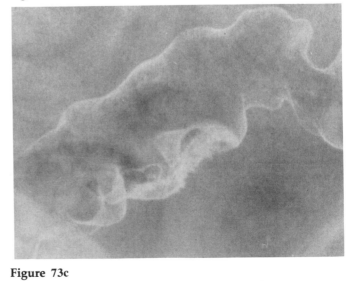

Figure 73c

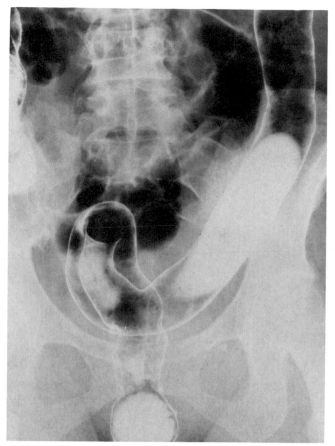

Figure 74a There is irregular narrowing of the rectum in a patient with a total colitis, which was of long standing and relatively inactive.

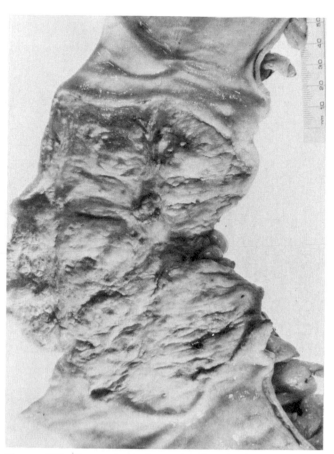

Figure 74b Resected specimen showing the irregular partly ulcerated surface of the malignant lymphoma in the rectum.

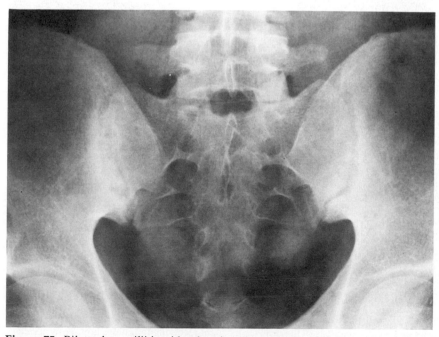

Figure 75 Bilateral sacroiliitis with sclerosis and erosions leading to irregular widening of both joint margins.

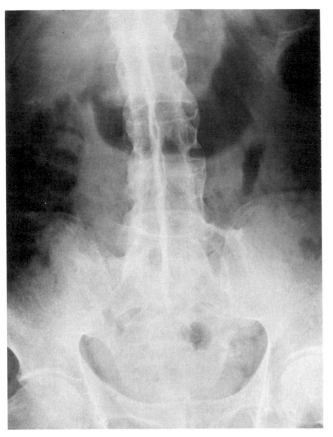

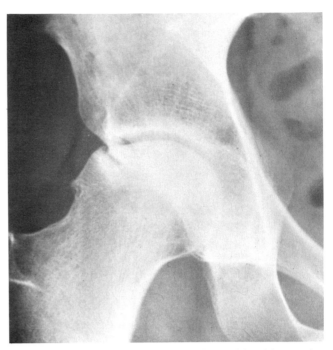

Figure 77 Avascular necrosis of the femoral head in a patient receiving a high dose of steroids for colitis. A typical lesion is present in the superior segment of the femoral head.

Figure 76 Advanced ankylosing spondylitis in a patient with distal ulcerative colitis.

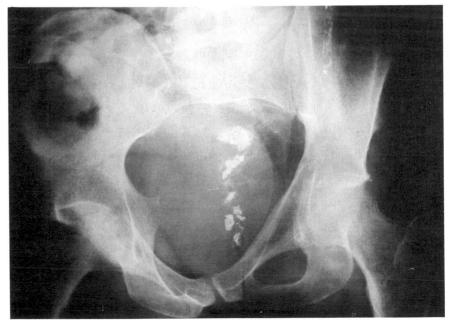

Figure 78 Bilateral chronic avascular necrosis of the femoral heads with loss of joint space and patchy sclerosis of the heads in a patient receiving long-term high-dose steroids.

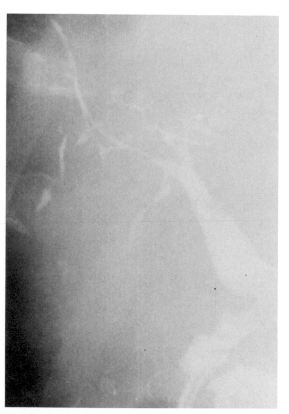

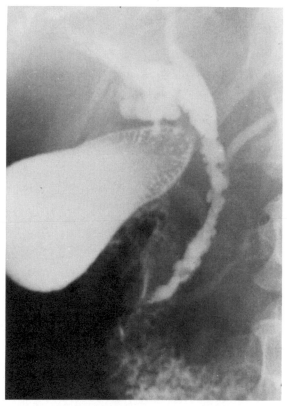

Figure 79 Sclerosing cholangitis with extrahepatic involvement. Note that the gall bladder is entirely normal.

Figure 80 Sclerosing cholangitis with intrahepatic involvement.

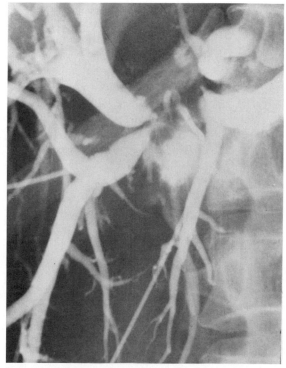

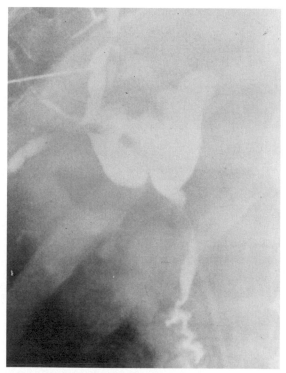

Figure 81 Occlusion of the main hepatic ducts due to a centrally placed cholangiocarcinoma producing the ''carrot sign.'' (Courtesy of Dr. R. Dick, Royal Free Hospital, London.)

Figure 82 Smooth stricture in the bile duct due to a cholangiocarcinoma. (Courtesy of Dr. R. Dick, Royal Free Hospital, London.)

4

Crohn's Disease

Crohn's disease is a chronic inflammatory condition in which the inflammation is transmural and characterized by the presence of noncaseating granulomas with fissuring like ulcers. The disease is often patchy in distribution and may affect any part of the gastrointestinal tract. Its cause is unknown and as yet there is no effective treatment.

The onset of Crohn's disease is commonest between the second and fourth decades, but may develop at any age. Several studies have shown a second peak incidence in the elderly (1,2). The possibility that this is due to the inclusion of cases with ischemic colitis has been suggested (1), but in practice proven cases of Crohn's disease presenting late in life are common.

Typical clinical features of the disease are diarrhea, abdominal pain, weight loss, and fever. The presence of rectal bleeding and perianal disease suggests colonic involvement. The National Cooperative Crohn's Disease study records a mean of 35 months from onset of symptoms until final diagnosis (Fig. 1) (3). Spontaneous remissions are a natural phenomenon. Thirty-two percent of randomized patients placed on placebo therapy went into remission by week 17 (3), and 53% of these were still in remission after 2 years. The age of onset did not affect the prognosis, as has been suggested previously (4).

Once the disease has presented there may be no change in its distribution, but slow progression of the mucosal lesions, with ulcerated areas developing into strictures (Fig. 2). However, relatively advanced lesions may resolve (5) with associated clinical improvement (Fig. 3). The converse is not always true, as only 18% of patients in symptomatic remission showed radiological evidence of improvement (3). Colonic disease appears to be subject to more fluctuation. Progression of left-sided disease, sometimes with regression on the right side or alternation of the segments involved has been reported (6). Distal ileal disease has been considered relatively static (7,8), but proximal extension in the small bowel as well as spread into the colon have been documented (9,10). Our radiological appreciation of the fluctuation in Crohn's disease is incomplete, as patients are not usually examined when in remission. The suggestion that the disease is more variable in certain parts of the gastrointestinal tract, may reflect the ability of contrast examinations to show early changes in that part, rather than any inherent difference.

Radiology does not provide a definitive diagnosis of Crohn's disease, so the probability that the patient is suffering from this disease must take into account all the clinical and histological features. However, it has an important role in establishing the diagnosis, and the demonstration or exclusion of Crohn's disease is a common reason for requesting a barium study. If disease is found in one part of the gastrointestinal tract, the remainder should be examined to assess the full extent of involvement. Further examination is required only if there has been a deterioration in the patient's condition, to show if there has been any gross change in the extent of disease, or to assess the development of a complication such as a fistula. If surgical excision is considered, a preoperative assessment of the entire gastrointestinal tract will also be needed.

RADIO-LOGICAL PATHOLOGY

The early changes of Crohn's disease involve hyperplasia of the lymphoid tissue with an obstructive lymphedema. The submucosa is widened, which causes the typical fold pattern thickening in the small bowel. Superficial ulceration of lymphoid follicles, or focal areas of lymphocytic infiltration, results in aphthoid-type ulcers, which may be superimposed on a mucosa with a normal or abnormal fold pattern (Figs.4–6). This very shallow ulceration may progress to deeper discrete ulcers (Fig. 7), or a linear or serpiginous configuration of more confluent ulceration (Figs.8–10). The distribution of the lesions is typically discontinous and asymmetric, so that there is normal bowel between abnormal segments along the length of the bowel, and patches of normal bowel amid ulcers running transversely across the lumen (Fig. 11). Cobblestoning is a classic feature of Crohn's disease in the small bowel. It is due to a combination of linear ulceration with fissuring ulcers forming transverse clefts between edematous mucosal remnants (Figs. 12 and 13). Fissuring is another typical feature of Crohn's disease and is seen as narrow crevices penetrating deeply into the wall.

Thickening of the bowel wall is due to a combination of submucosal edema, transmural inflammation, and adhesions, with fibrosis of the serosal surface. Large fleshy lymph nodes may be seen in the mesentery (Fig. 14). The combination of serosal inflammation and deep ulceration leads to fistula formation (Fig. 15). Healing following ulceration may lead to the formation of inflammatory polyps (Fig. 16).

ESOPHAGUS

Clinical examination of the oropharynx may show mucosal lesions in some 6–20% of patients who have overt Crohn's disease in part of the gastrointestinal tract. Esophageal involvement is by comparison very uncommon, and only a few cases have been reported radiologically. Ulceration, nodular thickening of the folds, and stricturing have been described (12–17) (Fig. 17). In one case an esophagobronchial fistula developed (14).

Double-contrast studies of the esophagus (14a) are needed to show the very early changes of Crohn's disease, such as superficial or apthoid ulceration (Figs. 18 and 19). Any patient with Crohn's disease complaining of dysphagia should be examined carefully for such lesions. Viral and monilial esophagitis can present with small nodular or longitudinal plaquelike lesions, or ulceration (Fig. 20). Radiologically, the differential diagnosis is difficult. Reflux esophagitis is usually localized to a short segment in the distal esophagus, usually just above a hiatus hernia. The esophagus is invariably narrowed at the site of ulceration, whereas there may be no narrowing with superficial ulceration in Crohn's disease.

STOMACH AND DUODENUM

Gastroduodenal disease is present in 0.5–7% of cases (see Table 1). Involvement of the antrum, pylorus, and first part of the duodenum appears to be a common combination and may lead to the ''ram's-horn'' sign (24), where there is a tubular narrowing of the gastric outlet simulating a Bilroth 1 gastrectomy or scirrhous carcinoma (25). The duodenal loop may show a range of changes, starting with blunted folds (Fig. 21) progressing to ulceration, cobblestoning, and stricturing (Figs. 22 and 23) (19). Strictures may cause gastric outlet obstruction (Fig. 24), which is an important complication of gastroduodenal involvement (19,24). Other parts of the bowel are often involved, so the entire gastrointestinal tract must be examined.

Aphthoid ulcers in the stomach have been demonstrated on double-contrast studies (26,27). The lesions are radiologically similar to chronic gastric erosions (Fig. 25), so histological confirmation is needed for their differentiation, and in only a few cases has endoscopic biopsy proved positive (26,27). Thickened gastric folds and discrete ulcers have been reported in up to 40% of patients with advanced Crohn's disease elsewhere in the gastrointestinal tract (28). The significance of these changes is uncertain, as advanced changes are rare by comparison.

If a patient has had a resection of 60 cm or more of small bowel, this will lead to an increased output of gastric acid (29) and is probably the cause of the higher incidence of peptic ulceration in Crohn's disease. This could explain some of the changes noted above, such as thickened folds, which are a feature of increased acid secretion (30), but not the presence of aphthoid ulcers, as no relationship between increased gastric acid and chronic gastric erosions has been proved.

Deformity of the duodenal cap may be due to peptic ulceration or Crohn's disease. These may be difficult to distinguish. Endoscopic examination suggests that Crohn's involvement of the duodenum is more common than was suspected, so that it is prudent never to rule out Crohn's disease, and to favor peptic ulceration only when the changes are absolutely typical.

SMALL BOWEL

Crohn's disease is known to involve the entire gastrointestinal tract, but the terminal ileum is affected in 55%, and remains the commonest site to be involved. Unfortunately, this is not the easiest part of the bowel in which to visualize radiologically the fine mucosal detail. Double-contrast studies can be employed (Fig. 26), but not with the same ease as for the stomach or colon. The endoscopist can examine only a limited part of the small bowel — the duodenum and distal terminal ileum — so that the overall examination of the small bowel remains the province of the radiologist.

Table 1 Incidence of Gastroduodenal Involvement in Crohn's Disease

Number of patients with gastroduodenal involvement	Total	Percent[a]	Series
12	300	4	Fielding et al., 1970 (18)
23	312	7	Thompson et al., 1975 (19)
7	383	1.8	Legge et al., 1970 (20)
4	750	0.5	Marshak and Wolf, 1955 (21)
3	600	0.5	Darrance, 1962 (22)
8	500	1.6	Jones et al., 1966 (23)

[a]Mean 2.6%.

The pathology of Crohn's disease is the same whatever part of the bowel is involved, but its radiological manifestations may vary, due to differences in methods of examination and gross structure of various parts of the bowel. Lymphedema and aphthoid ulceration are recognized as early changes in Crohn's disease (31–34). Aphthoid ulcers can be seen throughout the gastrointestinal tract, but edema tends to be recognized radiologically only in the small bowel. Edematous folds have been reported as the commonest superficial lesion of Crohn's disease in the small bowel (31). Fold changes and ulceration may occur together, or separately, so that three permutations are possible:

1. There is uniform thickening of the valvulae conniventes, which become rounded, so that barium is compressed between the swollen folds and appears spiky (Fig. 27). This is the least common change and not a specific radiological feature (Fig. 28). Ischemia in particular can mimic this appearance. Radiation enteritis must also be considered. Coeliac disease and edema from any cause can produce a thickened fold pattern, but are associated with dilatation (35), which is not a feature of Crohn's disease. Minor alterations of fold pattern are frequent in the irritable bowel syndrome (36). A high incidence of observer variation has been recorded in the assessment of fold pattern changes (37), so this is a difficult sign to assess. Screening of suspicious loops and compression views often help to confirm the presence of an abnormality.

2. Nodular defects distorting a relatively normal fold pattern. These are due to aphthoid ulcers. The area immediately around the ulcer is slightly elevated. This may appear round when en face, or as a crescentic filling defect when seen in profile (Fig. 29). The ulcer is not always apparent unless compressed to obtain a direct en face view when an irregular central ulcer crater about 1–3 mm in diameter with a surrounding halo will be seen (Fig. 30). Double contrast with air insufflation into the small bowel gives the most detailed view of aphthoid ulcers (Fig. 26), but they have been demonstrated by compression in 52.5% (33), and by an infusion technique in 43% of patients with Crohn's disease (38) (see Table 2).

There are a number of other causes of nodular filling defects in the small bowel, the commonest being lymphoid nodular hyperplasia of the terminal ileum. With compression views alone it may be difficult to distinguish this from Crohn's disease. Air insufflation is very useful to show the small regular 2-mm nodules against a normal mucosal background that are characteristic of lymphoid nodular hyperplasia (Fig. 31) and should be used whenever there is any doubt as to the state of the terminal ileum. Multiple submucosal

Table 2 Small Bowel Crohn's Disease: Frequency of Radiological Features

Feature	Series (with % frequency)		
	Goldberg et al. (49)	Nolan and Gourtsoyiannis (38)	Dyer et al. (37)
Narrowing	57		64
Aphthoid ulcers		43	
Fissuring	54	33	60
Longitudinal ulcers	49		
Cobblestoning	60	43	34
Thick folds	28	47	
Separation			
Loops	46	31	
Skip lesions	12	10	18
Strictures	21	46	32
Fistula	12		2
Pseudopolyps		1	

deposits from lymphoma, melanoma, or carcinoma are much larger than aphthoid ulcers, and if umbilicated the depression is central, often smaller, and more clear cut than the ragged superficial aphthoid ulcer.

3.   A mixed pattern, with nodular deformity and swollen folds, is probably the commonest presentation of the early changes in Crohn's disease (Figs. 32–34).

More advanced changes follow a pattern that is typical for Crohn's disease throughout the gastrointestinal tract. Ulceration may be transverse and fissure-like, or linear and longitudinal (Figs. 35 and 36). A secondary effect of ulceration is muscle spasm, which narrows the bowel (Fig. 37). The ''string sign'' describes a long, very narrow segment of diseased bowel (39). To some extent this appearance is due to underfilling, as infusion techniques will show intermittent distension of such segments (40). If during a small bowel examination a persistently narrowed or underfilled segment of small bowel is seen, this should be regarded as a warning sign of disease and an indication for careful screening of that segment.

A cobblestone pattern is common (Fig. 38) and is due to a mixture of longitudinal linear ulceration and transverse fissuring, with edematous intervening mucosa producing the raised cobbled appearance. The affected bowel is often narrowed and thick walled. The ulceration is asymmetric in distribution. Longitudinally, this results in skip lesions. Fibrosis affecting all the layers of the bowel wall is a common association with ulceration in chronic disease. Asymmetric involvement across the bowel leads to contraction of the abnormal side with ballooning out of the normal side. This is the mechanism for pseudodiverticular formation which is a common finding in advanced disease of the small bowel (Figs. 39–41).

Stricture formation is also common and their number and length variable. Multiple short strictures may be seen (Fig. 42). Careful examination often shows a transverse fissure at the site of the stricture (Figs. 43 and 44). The serosa and mesentery are also involved in Crohn's disease. Bowel wall thickening causes increased separation between loops, which tends to highlight diseased segments during a small bowel examination. The increased wall thickness can also be demonstrated ultrasonographically (Fig. 45) (42). The mesentery also contracts, rotating the bowel slightly, so that ulceration on the mesenteric border is seen en face (41).

Deep ulceration of the fissuring type may be contained within the thickened bowel wall, but its presence should lead to a careful search for tracts outside the bowel wall, which indicate abscess formation (Fig. 46). Frequently, another structure has become adherent to the diseased segment, so that penetration of an ulcer through the bowel wall leads to a fistula instead of an abscess.

Inflammatory polyps are uncommon in the small bowel in Crohn's disease, but have been reported (Fig. 47) (38).

The optimum examination technique to demonstrate Crohn's disease in the small bowel is the subject of some controversy. The suspected or known presence of Crohn's disease is considered by many to be an indication for a small bowel infusion (38,43–45), but there are only a few studies where direct comparisons between an infusion technique and standard examination have been made (46–48). One of the chief difficulties in evaluating such studies is that the protagonist for the new technique is always more highly motivated than the radiologist performing a routine examination which may not be his or her particular interest. Small bowel examinations seem particularly liable to fall prey to lack of enthusiasm. My personal experience of reviewing small bowel examinations referred to specialized gastrointestinal units is rather depressing, the majority of small bowel examinations being inadequate for one or other of the following reasons:

1.   Inadequate volume of barium given.
2.   Stasis of barium, usually in ileal loops, which is due to the above and/or that no accelerating agent was given.
3.   No compression views.

Such faults appear to be widespread, as in a National Cooperative Crohn's Disease Study (49), the panel of radiologists reviewing the examinations were forced to conclude that "the nature and extent of Crohn's disease in these patients must be interpreted with caution [as] many of the small bowel examinations were performed with inadequate amounts of barium or barium that precipitated." Inadequate examinations yield inadequate diagnoses. In a study of 161 patients with Crohn's disease, the mean delay in diagnosis was 4.3 years, due mainly to the failure to perform a small bowel examination (50), but also in this series 10 patients had to be excluded who had been referred with a diagnosis of Crohn's disease which was proved to be incorrect. Whatever method of examination, it must be done properly if the maximum information from that style of examination is to be realized. Granted an adequate examination technique, it is important to establish whether or not there is an innate diagnostic superiority for one form of examination, bearing in mind whether such additional information will be relevant to the patient's management.

The prevailing opinion is that duodenal intubation with the infusion of a large volume of barium is more accurate and reliable in the diagnosis of both early and advanced lesions of Crohn's disease (38,43–45). Saunders and Ho (46) compared 150 intubation studies with 26 conventional small bowel examinations and found 2 patients with Crohn's disease and 2 fistulas that were not shown by the conventional study. Ekberg (47), compared 43 small bowel enemas to 43 conventional studies. Sixty percent were performed within a year of each other, with a maximum separation of 4½ years. Lesions demonstrated by small bowel enema but not by conventional study included minor ulceration in 6, transmural ulceration in 8, cobblestoning in 2, strictures in 4, and mucosal edema in 16 patients. Transmural ulceration, strictures, and edema were more clearly shown in each case. Vallance (48) reported 16 patients who had been examined by both techniques. No detail of the pathological findings was given, but only 25% of the conventional studies were abnormal compared to 62.5% of the enemas, and no enema was equivocal, whereas 25% of the conventional examinations were. Hildell et al. (51), in a review of the accuracy of radiological methods in Crohn's disease, had performed both examinations in nine patients, and concluded that the small bowel enema was better for showing the early changes of aphthoid ulceration and mucosal edema.

In many cases the technical performance of the conventional studies was below par, with too little barium given and compression studies limited to the terminal ileum (48). Nevertheless, the small bowel enema is definitely superior in certain areas. Strictures are more clearly defined by the infusion of a large volume of dilute barium. This distends the bowel, which highlights any small strictures (38), The difference in distension between a conventional and intubation study is obvious when one considers that the upper limit for the jejunum is 27 mm for a follow-through, and up to 40 mm during small bowel enema. However, such a large volume of fluid may be a hindrance in demonstrating a fistula. Filling of the bowel is very rapid, so that the fistula can be difficult to localize. To overcome this, small infusion volumes have been recommended (47).

Aphthoid ulcers and mucosal edema appear to be demonstrated more clearly by small bowel enema. This is also due to the greater distension of the bowel. As it dilates the secondary folds of the valvulae conniventes are lost, and only the primary folds remain (52). The variations in fold pattern that are so common in conventional studies do not occur. Any alteration in the fold is easier to assess. However, it is interesting to note that the highest reported incidence of aphthoid ulceration was found in conventional studies (33). As a general rule in barium work, once a diagnostic skill has been developed using a technique that readily demonstrates the pathology, it is often possible to apply this diagnostic ability to other examinations where it is harder to show the lesion, and still achieve a similar degree of accuracy. Many radiologists are not familiar with the appearance of aphthoid ulceration in the small bowel. These can be shown on the standard follow-through, but this may be easier once the appearance of the lesion has been appreciated from a small bowel enema. The same applies to mucosal edema.

The clinician's main concern, when requesting a small bowel examination in a patient suspected clinically of having Crohn's disease, is to be told if the small bowel is normal or abnormal. If abnormal, a description of the approximate extent of the disease and the nature of the mucosal changes is useful in broad terms, but only a few specific details affect management directly. For example, the presence of a fistula is important, as this is an indication for surgery. Multiple strictures usually indicate that little response to medical treatment is likely, and surgery will be needed at some stage. It is often difficult to correlate the radiological appearance of the bowel with the patient's general condition. Some patients with gross changes may seem relatively healthy, whereas those with a short ulcerated segment may have marked symptoms. Generally, ulceration is associated with acute inflammation, which causes systemic changes, whereas strictures represent a fibrotic stage of the disease and lead to mechanical problems usually of an obstructive nature.

Surgeons may like a detailed view of the small bowel preoperatively, and a small bowel enema has been recommended for this (38). Unfortunately, it is difficult to transcribe the radiological appearance of the small bowel to the surgical findings during operation. Only rough comparisons can be made. It is helpful for the surgeon to know that there is no proximal skip lesion from the main segment of disease. Some overall assessment of how much bowel needs to be resected can be made, but precise measurements are impossible. The need for this is also debatable. The histological changes of Crohn's disease are much more extensive than the macroscopical lesions, so it is impossible to show the full extent of the disease radiologically. Resection through active overt disease may lead to problems with anastomotic breakdown, but whether resection through an aphthoid ulcer is any different to resection through an apparently normal mucosa is uncertain.

The description of every minute mucosal lesion is not important, but the ability to show such lesions is, as it is then possible to give a definite radiological opinion as to whether the small bowel is normal or abnormal. A routine examination needs to be able to fulfill this criterion. Given expertize and a good technique, the standard follow-through examination is comparable to the small bowel enema. It has many advantages; the patient does not have to endure intubation; several examinations can be performed at the same time without completely blocking a room or utilizing all the radiologist's time, and it may be supplemented by air insufflation to give double-contrast views of the terminal ileum in difficult cases. Which examination is used is subject to personal preference, but the small bowel enema may be recommended for problem cases and preoperative assessment of Crohn's disease.

COLON   The earliest macroscopic abnormality in Crohn's disease that pathologists recognize is aphthoid ulceration (53,54). These are very superficial lesions that were not recognized clearly on single-contrast examinations (Fig. 48). Marshak (55) described small nodular defects with ulceration that probably represented aphthoid ulcers, but the radiological appearances of apthoid ulceration were not fully appreciated until changes on double-contrast enemas were compared with the findings at endoscopy (56,57). En face the ulcer crater is about 1–3 mm in diameter. It is filled with barium which is dense and of rather a coarse texture. This is probably due to flocculation of barium on the slough covering the surface of the ulcer. The crater is surrounded by a halo, which is due to the mucosa around the ulcer being slightly elevated from edema and inflammatory changes. Otherwise, the adjacent mucosa is normal (Fig. 49).

Aphthoid ulcers are found in 44–72% of patients with Crohn's colitis (57–59). They may be the only abnormalities and scattered throughout an otherwise normal colon (Fig. 50), or they be present at the edge of more advanced lesions (Fig. 51). This type of ulceration may also occur in yersinial enterocolitis, ischemic colitis, Behçet's disease, and amebiasis (57,60,61). It is therefore not pathognomonic of Crohn's disease, although in Western countries aphthoid ulceration is most unlikely to be due to any other cause, and represents an important radiological feature of Crohn's disease.

Small reddened areas with an intact mucosa may be seen endoscopically in the very early stages of Crohn's disease (62). These have been termed erythematous plaques and are not visible radiologically, as there is no mucosal defect. Two radiological abnormalities that have been suggested as being early changes of Crohn's disease are fine nodularity and prominence of the innominate groove pattern.

A fine nodular mucosa may be due to lymphoid follicular hyperplasia. This is a common finding in children and has been reported in 13% of double-contrast barium enemas in adults (62a), where small nodules about 2–4 mm in diameter were seen mainly over a short segment in the proximal colon. Follicular hyperplasia has been considered an early stage of Crohn's disease (63) (Fig. 52), prior to the breakdown of the mucosa and formation of aphthoid ulceration. The validity of this is uncertain, although the size of the follicles does seem to be significant. In a recent study (63a) 73% of follicles more than 4 mm in diameter were associated with inflammatory bowel disease, whereas inflammatory bowel disease was not present in patients with follicles less than 3 mm in size. Larger follicles are a normal finding in the rectosigmoid (Fig. 53), so the same importance cannot be attached to their size; but generally follicles more than 4 mm in diameter should be regarded with suspicion and warrant further investigation.

Prominence of the innominate groove pattern (Chap. 1) has been suggested as an early manifestation of Crohn's disease (51). This could be due to mucosal edema, but unlike the small bowel this is not in my experience seen either radiologically or endoscopically in the large bowel. Purgatives may effect the grove pattern (64), so causes other than Crohn's disease should be considered on the rare occasions that a prominent groove pattern is visible.

Mucosal edema may be responsible for another sign that has been reported as pathognomonic of Crohn's disease—transverse stripes (65). These are deep transverse grooves, more than 1 cm long, which run parallel to each other across the bowel wall (Fig. 54). Comparisons to resected specimens has suggested that transverse stripes are due to fissure-like ulcers with intervening swollen mucosal folds (65). Personal experience suggests that this sign is also uncommon. It is hardly ever seen in resected specimens that have been fixed. It may be that the appearances reported were due to muscular contraction of the colon immediately following resection.

A transverse linear component has been reported in 42% of Crohn's colitis (59). This may be due to several factors. Residual parts of the haustral clefts will cause a transverse line (Fig. 55). Aphthoid ulceration often has a transverse orientation (Fig. 56), or may be associated with some mucosal edema accentuating the transverse line (Fig. 58). Transverse stripes as the sole abnormality must be very rare, and should lead to the consideration of tuberculosis where transverse ulceration is typical.

Aphthoid ulcers are so superficial that there is often no evidence of any projection from the mucosal line. Deeper ulcers with well-defined punched-out craters usually undercut the mucosal edge, forming collar-stud-shaped projections from the mucosal line (Fig. 57). En face the configuration of the ulcer may be rounded, serpiginous, or longitudinal (Fig. 59). Discrete ulcers are separated from other lesions by flat mucosa. Confluent ulcers are so close that no normal intervening mucosa can be identified (Fig. 57). Discrete ulcers are often identified at the periphery of confluent ulceration (Fig. 57). Thorn-shaped ulcers (66) represent fissures (Fig. 60 and 61). When these are combined with a linear ulceration, a cobblestone mucosa results (Fig. 62). This is found in about 25% of patients with advanced Crohn's colitis (55).

A diffuse granular mucosa has been reported in Crohn's colitis (Chap. 6). This may be a more common feature of Crohn's disease than has been appreciated. In one study (67) a granular mucosa in part of the colon was present in 25% and was the sole abnormality in 7% of the patients thought to have Crohn's disease (Fig. 63).

Deformity due to fibrosis is a prominent feature of Crohn's disease. Fibrosis is associated with ulceration (Fig. 64) and if this is asymmetric, so is the deformity. Strictures are seldom symmetric as in ulcerative colitis, and are usually pulled toward one side, a "purse string" deformity (Fig. 65) (55,66). Pseudodiverticula are common, usually on the antimesenteric border (Fig. 67). Their development is comparable to the deformity of the duodenal cap from peptic ulceration. Pseudodiverticula are often associated with ulceration, but remain when the ulcers have healed, so that they may be seen in a colon that appears otherwise normal (Fig. 66). These must then be differentiated from the sacculations of systemic sclerosis (68). These are square-shaped with wide mouths and not pulled in slightly at their necks as are the pseudodiverticula of Crohn's disease. If there is any doubt, a mouthful of barium will show complete loss of esophageal peristalsis in systemic sclerosis.

The asymmetry of Crohn's colitis is one of its most distinguishing features. It is present both longitudinally and transversely. A skip lesion refers to an abnormal segment of bowel which is separated from one or more other such segments by normal bowel (69) and reflects the longitudinal asymmetry of the disease (Fig. 68). Transversely, this is seen as marked alteration of the mucosa when one side of the bowel wall is compared to the other. For example, deep ulceration may be present on one side when the other is normal (Fig. 69).

Rectal sparing is another facet of the asymmetry of Crohn's disease. The rectum appears normal radiologically and sigmoidoscopically in about 50% of patients with Crohn's colitis (70).

Involvement of the distal ileum is often apparent on barium enema. The ileocecal valve is thickened and may contain several fistulous tracts (Fig. 70). Thickening of the wall of the terminal ileum may cause an extrinsic impression on the medial wall of the cecum (71). Crohn's disease may involve the appendix and sometimes the lumen can be seen to be ulcerated. This may be complicated by abscess formation (72).

ANAL LESIONS   Chronic anal disease due to to Crohn's involvement presents with a red discoloration to the skin, multiple fissures, and skin tags. The fissures are really longitudinal ulcers in the anal canal (Fig. 71). These may extend up to the anorectal ring and lead to perianal or ischiorectal abscess formation (73) (Figs.72 and 73). Spontaneous discharge of these abscesses leads to fistula formation. The anal canal and distal rectum may be grossly deformed. It is best to use a soft rubber catheter when performing a barium enema. This may have to be inserted high into the rectum if a fistula opens above the sphincter and is causing incontinence (Fig. 75).

About 36% of patients with Crohn's disease have anal disease (74). The incidence is only about 25% if the small bowel is involved, rising to 67% with colonic disease (75) (Fig. 74). If the rectum is involved, almost all patients will show some clinical anal abnormality.

Anal Crohn's disease in an important clinical stigma of the disease. Its presence warrants radiological investigation of the entire gastrointestinal tract. About 24% of patients will not have intestinal symptoms, as the anal lesions may precede overt intestinal disease by a mean of 4 years (76). If the anal disease is severe, full bowel preparation would be most uncomfortable for the patient, and the instant enema is recommended as the initial examination (Fig. 76). If this does not show much of the colon and surgery is considered, a full double-contrast barium enema is indicated.

ASSOCIATED DIVER-TICULAR DISEASE

The incidence of Crohn's disease shows a small second peak in the elderly. When the disease develops in patients of this age there is a tendency for it to involve the distal colon, and it is therefore likely to be superimposed on preexisting diverticular disease, which is very common in the elderly. This combination is clinically significant, as there is a higher incidence of pericolic abscess formation (77), and if resection is considered it is important for the surgeon to be aware of the presence of Crohn's disease as a complicating factor.

There are two problems with these diseases for the radiologist. One is to distinguish them; the other is to diagnose their presence together. The following features should be considered:

1. Small intramural diverticula should not be confused with aphthoid ulcers. The pool of barium in the diverticulum is clearly defined, round, and dense. There is no surrounding halo. A plication deformity of the mucosa is often associated with these diverticula (Fig. 77).

2. Deep fissuring ulcers in the sigmoid are unlike the smooth interdigitating muscle clefts of diverticular disease (78). The muscle abnormality may be present without diverticula, but in most cases diverticula are seen arising from the apices of the clefts, so there is no problem in establishing the presence of diverticular disease.

3. The diagnosis of Crohn's disease superimposed on diverticular disease depends on recognizing several changes:
   a. The typical changes of Crohn's disease in the mucosa of the lumen (Fig. 78), either within or adjacent to the diverticular disease.
   b. The way that Crohn's disease will alter the general configuration of diverticular disease (Figs. 78 and 79). A number of the diverticula may not fill and the muscle change becomes less pronounced, not so regular or obliterated.
   c. Crohn's disease affecting the diverticulum. As this contains the mucosa, it may be affected directly and so become ulcerated (Figs. 80,81). This muscle layer of the bowel wall forms a natural barrier to perforation following ulceration. The domes of the diverticula project through this layer, and without its protective benefit ulceration more commonly leads to perforation, which explains the higher incidence of pericolic abscess formation (77). The abscesses tend to track longitudinally and may join up with other diverticula (Fig. 82) or communicate with the lumen (Fig. 83). A long track of 10 cm or more is highly suggestive of Crohn's disease (79), although cases have been found where tracks of this length were present in uncomplicated diverticular disease (80,81).

REFERENCES

1. Kyle, J., (1971)., An epidemiological study of Crohn's disease in north-east Scotland. Gastroenterology 61; 826.
2. Norlen, B.J., Krause, U., Bergman, L. (1970). Epidemiological study of Crohn's disease. Scand. J. Gastroenterol. 5; 385.
3. Mekhjian, H.S., Switz, M., Melnyk, C.S., et al. (1979). Clinical features and natural history of Crohn's disease. Gastroenterology 77; 898.
4. Korelitz, B.L., Gribetz, D., Kopel, F.B. (1968). Granulomatous colitis in children: a study of 25 cases and comparisons with ulcerative colitis. Paediatrics 42; 446.
5. Hywel-Jones, J., Lennard-Jones, J.E. (1969). Reversibility of radiological appearances during clinical improvement in colonic Crohn's disease. Gut 10; 738.
6. Hildell, J., Lindstrom, C., Wenckert, A. (1979). Radiographic appearances in Crohn's disease. 11. The course as reflected at repeat radiography. Acta Radiol. Diagn. 20; 933.

7. Marshak, R.H., Lindner, A.E., (1970). Granulomatous colitis and ileocolitis with emphasis on the radiological features. Prog. Gastroenterol. 1; 357.

8. Nelson, J.A., Margulis, A.R., Goldberg, H.I., Lawson, T.L. (1973). Granulomatous colitis: significance of involvement of the terminal ileum. Gastroenterology 64; 1071.

9. Schofield, P.F. (1965). The natural history and treatment of Crohn's disease. Ann. Coll. Surg. Engl. 36; 258.

10. Truelove, S.C., Pena, S. (1976). Course and prognosis of Crohn's disease. Gut 17; 192.

11. Basu, M.K., Asquith, P. (1980). Oral manifestations of inflammatory bowel disease. Clin. Gastroenterol. 92; 307.

12. Legge, D.A., Coulson, H.C., Judd, E.S. (1970). Roentgen features of regional enteritis of the upper gastrointestinal tract. Am. J. Roentgenol. 110; 355.

13. Dyer, N.M., Cook, P.L., Kemp Harper, R.A., (1969). Oesophageal strictures associated with Crohn's disease. Gut 10; 549.

14. Lynn, W.S., Caon, H.K., Gureghian, P.A., et al. (1975). Crohn's disease of the oesophagus. Amer. J. Roentgenol. 125; 359.

14a. Laufer, L. (1976). The esophagus. In *Double Contrast Gastrointestinal Radiology,* Laufer, I. Saunders, Philadelphia, p. 92.

15. Hellemon, E.W., Kepkay, P.H. (1954). Segmental esophagitis, gastritis and enteritis. Gastroenterology 26; 83.

16. Gelfand, M.D., Krone, C.L. (1968). Dysphagia and oesophageal ulceration in Crohn's disease. Gastroenterology 55; 510

17. Haggitt, R.C., Meissner W.A. (1973). Crohn's disease of upper gastrointestinal tract. Am. J. Clin. Pathol. 59; 613.

18. Fielding, J.F., Toye, D.K.M., Benton D.C. (1970). Crohn's disease of the stomach and duodenum. Gut 11; 1001.

19. Thompson, W.M., Cockrill, H., Rice R.P. (1975). Regional enteritis of the duodenum. Am. J. Roentgenol. 123; 252.

20. Legge, D.A., Carlson, H.C., Judd, E.S. (1970). Roentgenologic features of regional enteritis of upper gastrointestinal tract. Am. J. Roentgenol. 110; 355.

21. Marshak, R.H., Wolf, B.S. (1955). Roentgenologic findings in regional enteritis. Am. J. Roentgenol. 74; 1000.

22. Darrance, F.Y. (1962). Regional enteritis of the duodenum. Am. J. Roentgenol. 88; 658.

23. Jones, G.W., Dooley, M.R., Schoenefield, L.J. (1966). Regional enteritis with involvement of the duodenum. Gastroenterology 51; 1018.

24. Farman, J., Fuengenbuerg, D., Dallemand, S., Clark-Kuo, C. (1975). Crohn's disease of the stomach. The ''Ram's horn'' sign. Am. J. Roentgenol. 123; 242.

25. Nelson, S.W. (1969). Some interesting and unusual manifestation of Crohn's disease of the stomach, duodenum and small intestine. Am. J. Roentgenol. 107; 86.

26. Laufer, I., Trueman, T., DeSa, D. (1976). Multiple superficial gastric erosions due to Crohn's disease of the stomach—radiologic and endoscopic diagnosis. Br. J. Radiol. 49; 726.

27. Ariyama, J., Webhin, L., Lindstrom, C.G., Nerkert, A., Roberts, G.M. (1980). Gastroduodenal erosions in Crohn's disease. Gastrointest. Radiol. 5; 121.

28. Stevenson, G.W., Laufer, I. (1979). Crohn's disease of the duodenum. In *Double Contrast Gastrointestinal Radiology,* Laufer, I. Saunders, Philadelphia, p. 357.

29. Fielding, J.F., Cooke, W.T. (1970). Peptic ulceration in Crohn's disease. Gut 11; 998.

30. Rhodes, J., Evans, K.T., Lawrie, J.H., Forrest, A.P.M. (1968). Coarse mucosal folds in the duodenum. Q. J. Med. 61; 151.

31. Ekberg, O., Lindstrom, C. (1979). Superficial lesions in Crohn's disease of the small bowel. Gastrointest. Radiol. 4; 389.

32. Sellink, J.L. (1976). *Radiological Atlas of Common Diseases of the Small Bowel.* Stenfert Kroese, Leiden, p. 70.

33. Engelholm, L., Maingnet, P., Potuliege, P. (1976). Radiology in early Crohn's disease of the small intestine. In *The Management of Crohn's Disease.* Excerpta Medica, Leiden, p. 73.

34. Hildell, J., Lindstrom, C., Wenckert, A. (1979). Radiographic appearances in Crohn's disease. 1. Accuracy of radiographic methods. Acta Radiol. Diagn. 20; 609.

35. Farthing, M.J.G., McLean, A.M., Bartram, C.I., et al. (1981). Radiologic features of the jejunum in hypoalbuminemia. Am. J. Roentgenol. 136; 883.

36. Kumar, P., Bartram, C.I. (1979). Relevance of the barium follow-through examination in the diagnosis of adult coeliac disease. Gastrointest. Radiol. 4; 285.

37. Dyer, N.H., Rutherford, C., Visick, J.H., Dawson, A.M. (1970). The incidence and reliability of individual radiographic signs in the small intestine in Crohn's disease. Br. J. Radio. 43; 401.

38. Nolan, D.J., Gourtsoyiannis, N.C. (1980). Crohn's disease of the small intestine: a review of the radiological appearances in 100 consecutive patients examined by a barium infusion technique. Clin. Radiol. 31; 597.

39. Kantor, J.L. (1934). Regional (terminal) ileitis: its roentgen diagnosis. JAMA 103; 2016.

40. Nolan, D.J., Piris, J. (1980). Crohn's disease of the small intestine; a comparative study of the radiological and pathological appearances. Clin. Radiol. 31; 591.

41. Tsukasa, S., Tokudome, K., Irisa, T., et al. (1978). Roentgenographic diagnosis of Crohn's disease of the small intestine. Stomach Intest. 13; 335.

42. Flischer, A.C., Muhletaker, C.A., James, A.E. (1981). Sonographic assessment of the bowel wall. Am. J. Roentgenol. 136; 887.

43. Herlinger, H. (1978). A modified technique for double contrast small bowel enema. Gastrointest. Radiol. 3; 201.

44. Fleckenstein, P., Pedersen, G. (1975). The value of the duodenal intubation method (Sellink modification) for the radiological visualization of the small bowel. Scand. J. Gastroenterol. 10; 423.

45. Dyet, J.F., Pratt, A.E., Flouty, G. (1976). The small bowel enema; description and experience of a technique. Br. J. Radiol. 49; 1039.

46. Saunders, D.F., Ho, C.S. (1976). The small bowel enema; experience with 150 examinations. Am. J. Roentgenol. 127; 743.

47. Ekberg, O. (1977). Crohn's disease of the small bowel examined by double contrast technique; a comparison with the oral technique. Gastrointest. Radiol. 1; 355.

48. Vallance, R. (1980). An evaluation of the small bowel enema based on an analysis of 350 consecutive examinations. Clin. Radiol. 31; 227.

49. Goldberg, H.I., Caruthers, S.B., Nelson, J.A., Singleton, J.W. (1979). Radiographic findings of the National Cooperative Crohn's Disease Study. Gastroenterology 77; 925.

50. Dyer, N.H., Dawson, A.M. (1970). Diagnosis of Crohn's disease. A continuing source of error. Br. Med. J. 1; 735.

51. Hildell, J., Lindstrom, C., Wenckert, A. (1979). Radiographic appearances in Crohn's disease. 1. Accuracy of radiographic methods. Acta Radiol. Diagn. 20; 609.

52. Sloan, R.D. (1957). The mucosal pattern of the mesenteric small intestine —an anatomic study. Am. J. Roentgenol. 77; 651.

53. Brooke, B.N. (1953). What is ulcerative colitis? Lancet 1; 1220.

54. Lockhart-Mummery, H.E., Morson, B.C. (1960). Crohn's disease (regional enteritis) of the large intestine and its distinction from ulcerative colitis. Gut 1; 87.

55. Marshak, R.H. (1975). Granulomatous disease of the intestinal tract (Crohn's disease). Radiology 114; 3.

56. Laufer, I., Mullens, J.E., Hamilton, J. (1976). Correlation of endoscopy and double-contrast radiography in the early stages of ulcerative and granulomatous colitis. Radiology 118; 1.

57. Simpkins, K.C. (1977). Aphthoid ulcers in Crohn's colitis. Clin. Radiol. 28; 601.

58. Brahme, F. (1967). Granulomatous colitis. Roentgen appearances and course of the lesions. Am. J. Roentgenol. 99; 35.

59. Kelvin, F.M., Oddson, T.A., Rice, R.P., et al. (1978). The double contrast barium enema in Crohn's colitis and ulcerative colitis. Am. J. Roentgenol. 131; 207.

60. Vantrappen, G., Agg, H.O., Ponetee, E., et al. (1977). Yersinia enteritis and enterocolitis: gastroenterological aspects. Gastroenterology 72; 220.

61. Weinfield, A. (1966). The roentgen appearance of intestinal amebiasis. Am. J. Roentgenol. 96; 311.

62. Watier, A., Devroede, G., Perey, B. (1980). Small erythematous mucosal plaques: an endoscopic sign of Crohn's disease. Gut 21; 835.

62a. Kelvin, F.R., Max, R.J., Norton, G.A., et al. (1979). Lymphoid follicular pattern of the colon in adults. Am. J. Roentgenol. 133; 821.

63. Laufer, I. (1977). Air contrast studies of the colon in inflammatory bowel disease. CRC Crit. Rev. Diagn. Imaging 9; 421.

63a. Kenney, P.J., Koehler, R.E., Shackleford, G.D. (1982). The clinical significance of large lymphoid follicles of the colon. Radiology 142; 41.

64. Ansell, G. (1969). Radiological manifestations of drug induced disease. Clin. Radiol. 20; 133.

65. Welin, S., Welin, G. (1973). A pathognomonic roentgenologic sign of regional ileitis (Crohn's disease). Dis. Colon Rectum 16; 473.

66. Young, A.C. (1969). *Inflammatory Disease of the Colon—A Textbook of X-ray Diagnosis,* Vol. IV, Shanks, S.C., Kerley, P. (Eds.). H.K. Lewis, London, 6th ed., p. 454.

67. Donoghue, D., Dawson, A.M., Bartram, C.I., et al. (1982). Differentiating features between ulcerative and Crohn's colitis. In preparation.

68. Brunton, F.J., Guyer, P.B. (1979). Diverticulum formation in Crohn's disease of the colon. Clin. Radiol. 30; 39.

69. Schacter, W. (1975). Definitions of inflammatory bowel disease of unknown etiology. Gastroenterology 68; 591.

70. Lennard-Jones, J.E., Lockhart-Mummery, H.E., Morson, B.C. (1968). Clinical and pathological differentiation of Crohn's disease and proctocolitis. Gastroenterology 54; 1162.

71. Berridge, F.R. (1971). Two unusual radiological signs of Crohn's disease of the colon. Clin. Radiol. 32; 443.

72. Cohen, W.N., Denbeston, L. (1970). Crohn's disease with predominant involvement of the appendix. Am. J. Roentgenol. 110; 361.

73. Lockhart-Mummery, H.E. (1975). Crohn's disease: anal lesions. Dis. Colon Rectum 18; 200.

74. Rankin, G.B., Watts, D., Melnyk, C.S., et al. (1979). National Cooperative Crohn's Disease Study; extraintestinal manifestations and perianal complications. Gastroenterology 77; 914.

75. McGovern, V.J., Goulston, S.J.M. (1968). Crohn's disease of the colon. Gut 9; 164.

76. Baker, W.N., Milton-Thompson, G.J. (1971). The anal lesion as the sole presenting symptom of intestinal Crohn's disease. Gut 12; 865.

77. Meyers, M.A., Alonso, D.R., Morson, B.C., et al. (1978). Pathogenesis of diverticulitis complicating granulomatous colitis. Gastroenterology 74; 24.

78. Schmidt, G.T., Lennard-Jones, J.E., Morson, B.C., et al. (1968). Crohn's disease of the colon and its distinction from diverticulitis. Gut 9; 7.

79. Marshak, R.H., Janowitz, H.D., Present, D.H. (1970). Granulomatous colitis in association with diverticula. N. Engl. J. Med. 283; 1080.

80. Loeb, P.M., Berk, R.N., Saltzstein, S.L. (1974). Longitudinal fistula of the colon in diverticulitis. Gastroenterology 67; 720.

81. Ferrucci, J.T., Ragsdale, B.D., Barrett, P.J. (1976). Double tracking in the sigmoid colon. Radiology 120; 307.

FIGURES 1 THROUGH 84

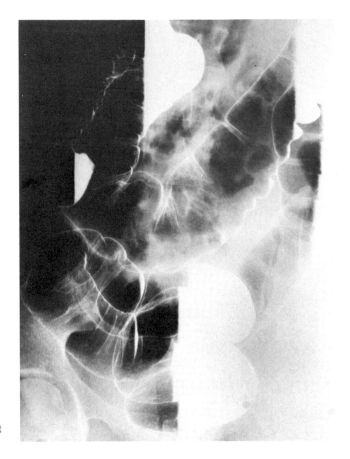

Figure 1a Patient presenting with diarrhea. Double-contrast barium enema did not show any significant abnormality.

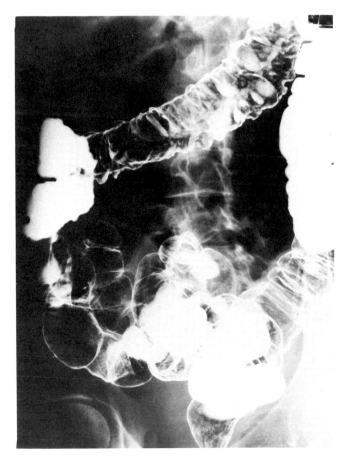

Figure 1b One month later, advanced changes of Crohn's disease.

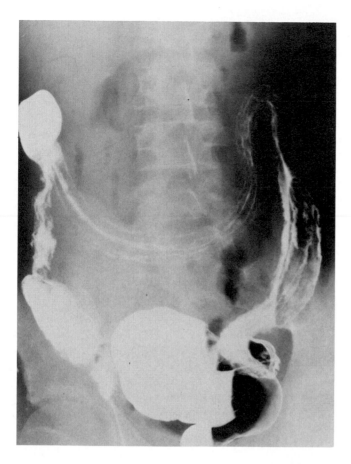

Figure 2a The progression of Crohn's disease over 12 years. (a) At presentation, extensive deep linear ulceration.

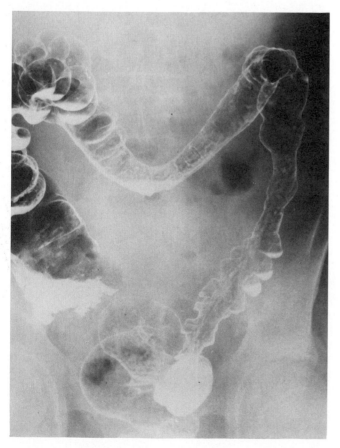

Figure 2b One year later this has largely healed. Some patchy ulceration remains and the left hemicolon is narrowed with pseudodiverticula formation.

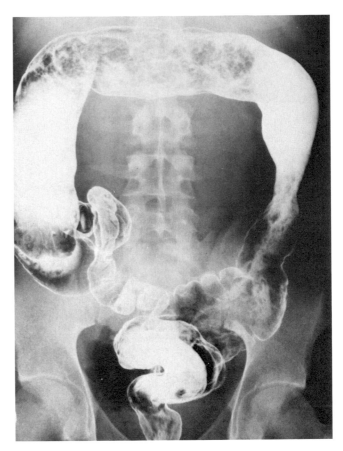

Figure 2c Six years later the colitis is at a burned out stage. The bowel is tubular but there is no active ulceration or pseudodiverticula.

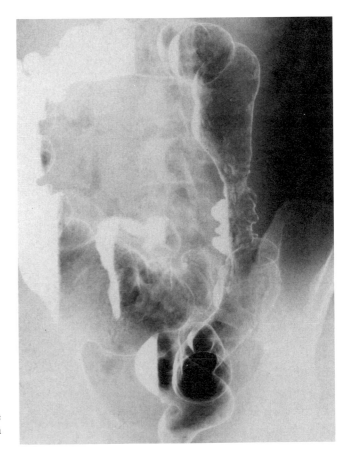

Figure 2d Twelve years after the onset of the colitis, some active disease has returned and ulceration with pseudodiverticula are again seen in the descending colon.

136

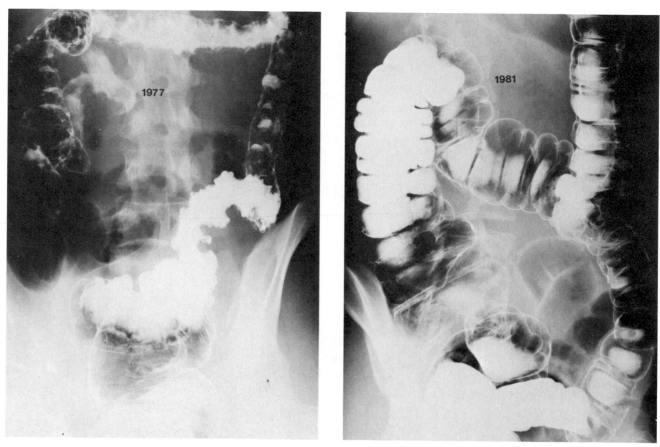

Figure 3 Healing of advanced Crohn's disease in 4 years with medical treatment.

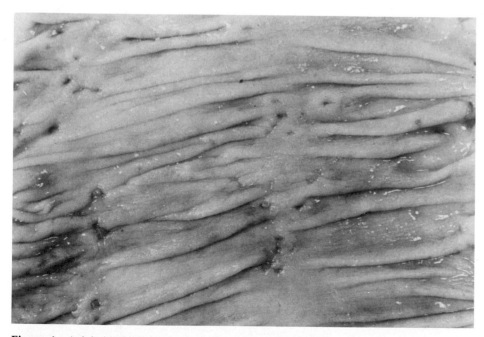

Figure 4 Aphthoid ulceration in the colon. Normal fold pattern.

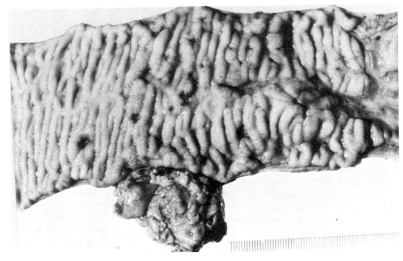

Figure 5 Aphthoid ulceration in the small bowel with thickened folds.

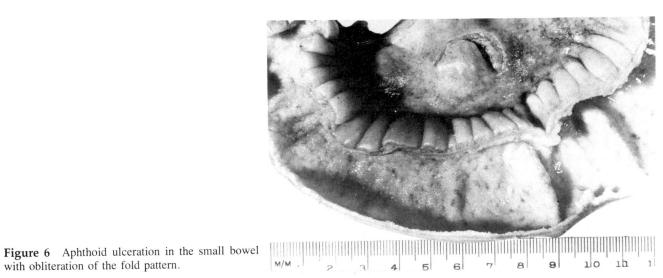

Figure 6 Aphthoid ulceration in the small bowel with obliteration of the fold pattern.

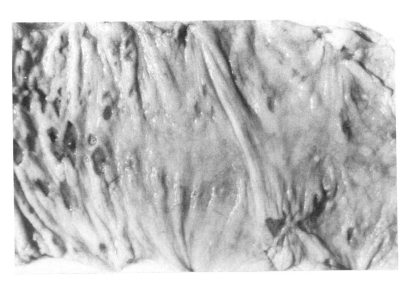

Figure 7 Mixture of aphthoid and larger discrete ulcers. Note the normal background mucosa.

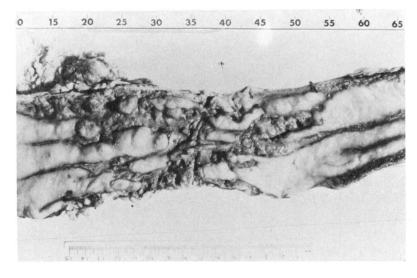

Figure 8 Deep linear ulceration.

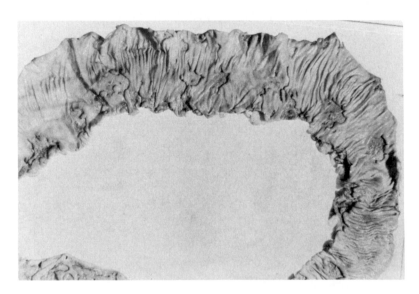

Figure 9 Large discrete ulcers with an irregular outline.

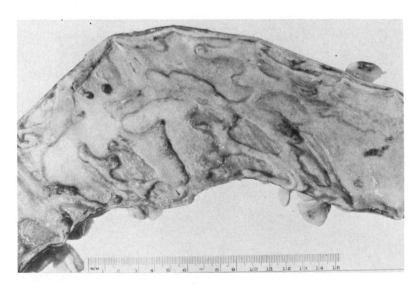

Figure 10 Extensive serpiginous ulceration.

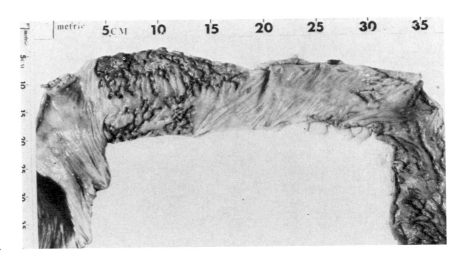

Figure 11 Skip lesions.

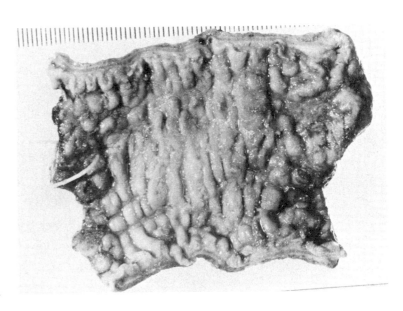

Figure 12 Cobblestoning in the small bowel.

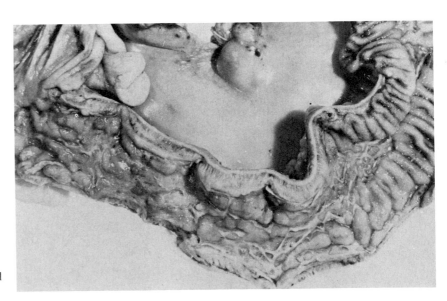

Figure 13 Cobblestoning in the terminal ileum.

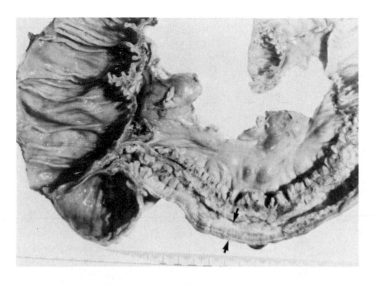

Figure 14 Thickening of the bowel wall in Crohn's disease of the terminal ileum (arrows).

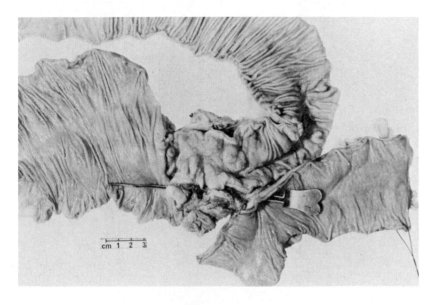

Figure 15 Ileosigmoid fistula.

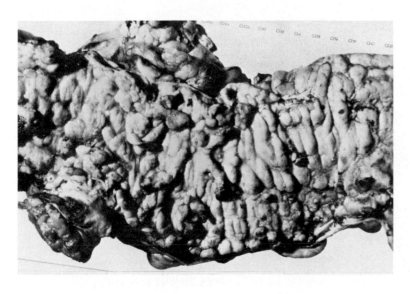

Figure 16 Filiform inflammatory polyps with some cobblestoning of the background mucosa.

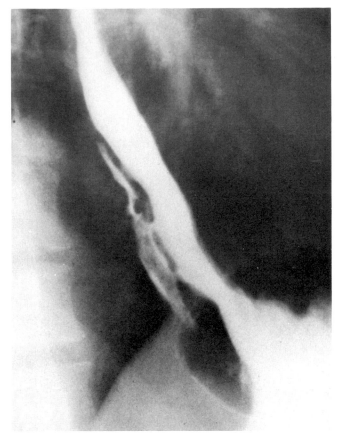

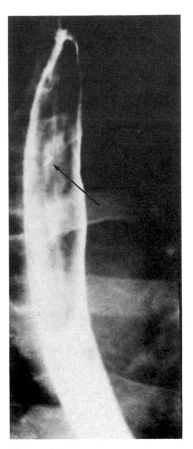

Figure 17 Deep linear ulcer with thickened folds in the lower esophagus. (From Ref. 13.)

Figure 18a

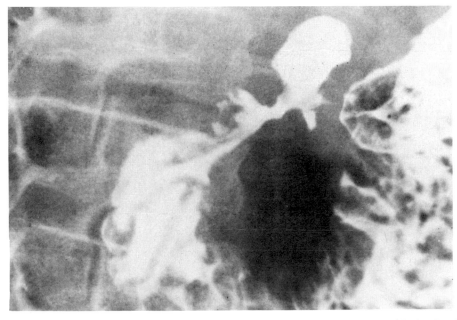

Figure 18b (a) A small superficial ulcer is present (arrow) in a patient with duodenal Crohn's disease (b).

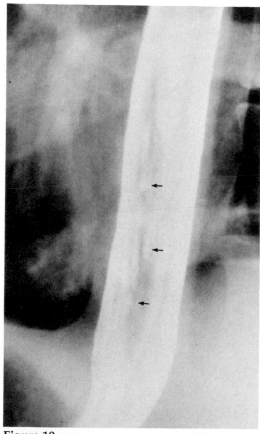

Figure 19

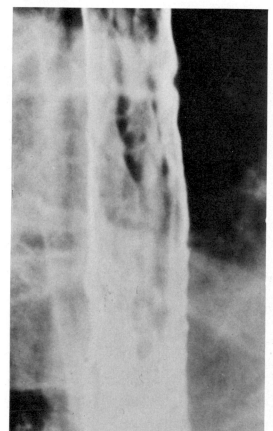

Figure 20

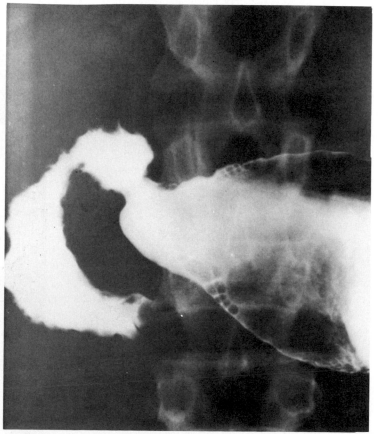

Figure 21

Figure 19 Double-contrast esophagogram showing aphthoid ulcers (arrows). (Courtesy of Dr. H. Kressel, University Hospital of Pennsylvania, Philadelphia.)

Figure 20 Narrowing of the first part of the duodenum with ulceration. The folds in the second part of the loop are effaced. The pylorus was involved and remained open.

Figure 21 Linear plaquelike lesions in a patient with moniliasis.

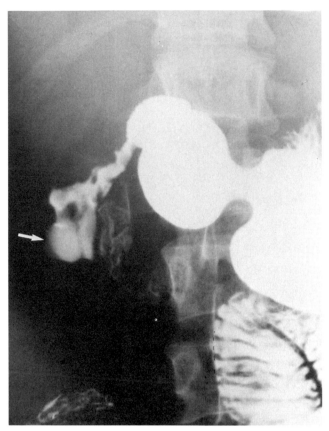

Figure 22 Stricturing in the proximal part of the duodenum with the formation of a large pseudodiverticulum (arrow).

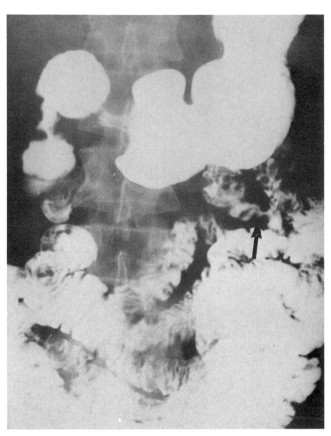

Figure 23 Ulceration and stricturing in the duodenum and proximal jejunum (arrow).

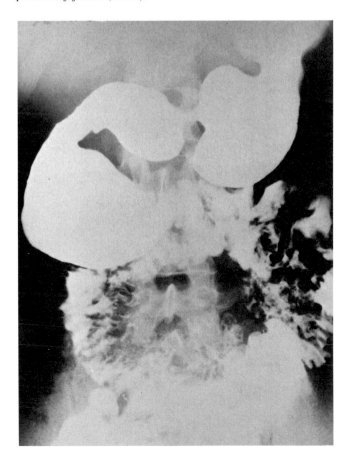

Figure 24 Stenosis of the third part of the duodenal loop. The patient presented with gastric outlet obstruction.

144

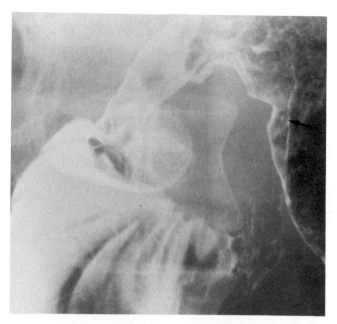

Figure 25 Gastroduodenal disease with aphthoid ulceration in the antrum (arrow).

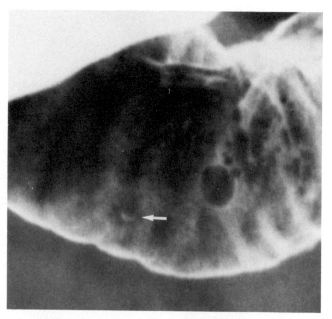

Figure 26 Double-contrast view of the small bowel showing an aphthoid ulcer (arrow).

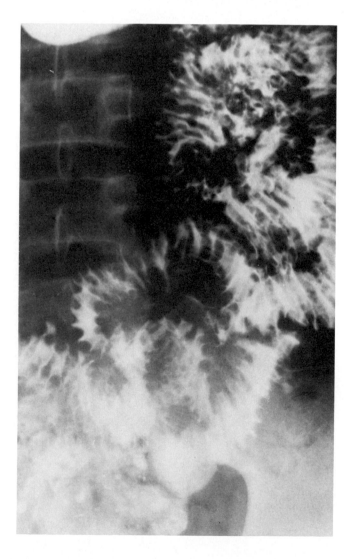

Figure 27 Lymphedema of the valvulae conniventes. Barium is compressed between the thickened folds, producing a spiky pattern.

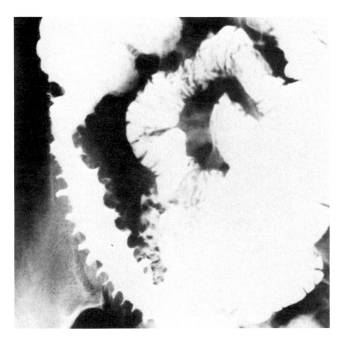

Figure 28 Thickened folds with some ulceration developing in the distal small bowel shortly after a right hemicolectomy. Ischemia might be a cause of this, but endoscopy confirmed recurrent Crohn's disease.

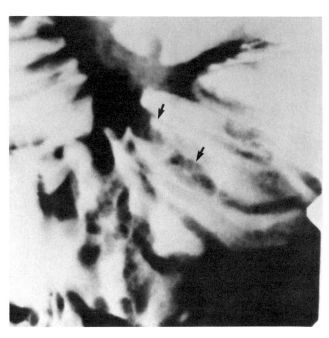

Figure 29 Tangential and en face views of aphthoid ulcers (arrows). Note the way edema around the ulcer expands the fold, causing a nodular filling defect.

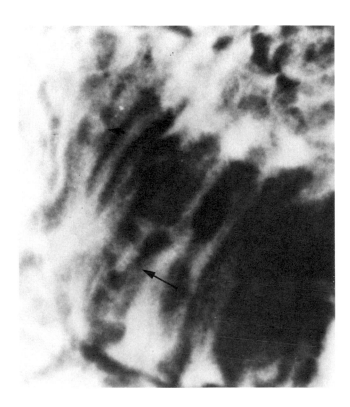

Figure 30 Compression views demonstrating aphthoid ulceration (arrows).

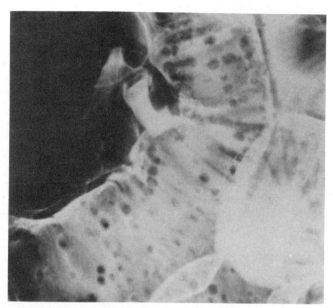

Figure 31 Double-contrast view of the terminal ileum showing numerous 2-mm filling defects set against a normal mucosal surface—a typical appearance of follicular lymphoid hyperplasia. (From Igor Laufer, *Double Contrast Gastrointestinal Radiology*, 1979. W.B. Saunders and Co.)

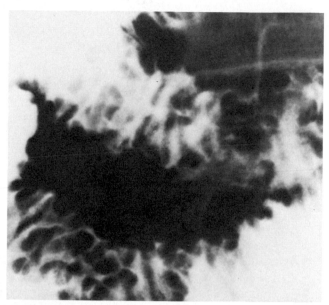

Figure 32 Mixed pattern of superficial ulceration and fold thickening.

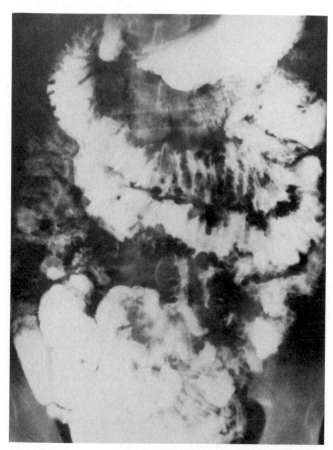

Figure 33 Extensive Crohn's disease throughout the jejunum. There is irregular thickening of the folds due to the superimposition of diffuse superficial ulceration.

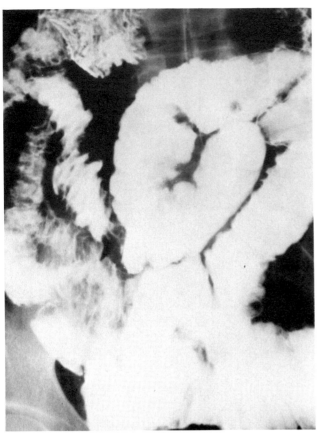

Figure 34 There is irregular thickening of the folds in part of the jejunum, with slight dilatation and effacement of the fold pattern in the rest. This is probably in response to marked submucosal edema with superficial ulceration causing the irregularity of the mucosal edge.

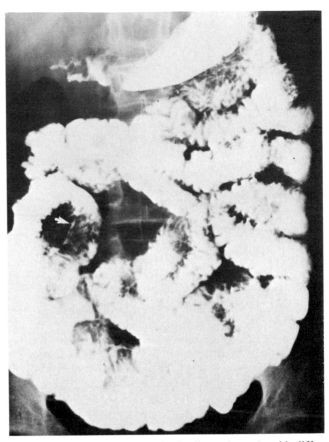

Figure 35 Short linear ulcer in the ileum (arrow), with diffuse early disease in the jejunum.

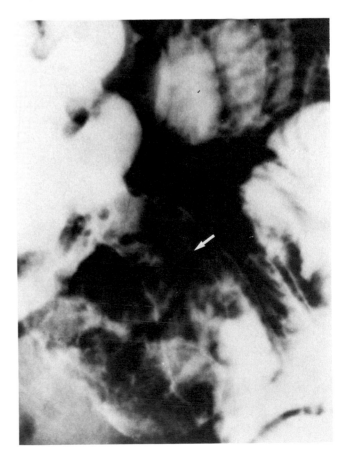

Figure 36 Linear ulceration in the terminal ileum shown on double contrast (arrow).

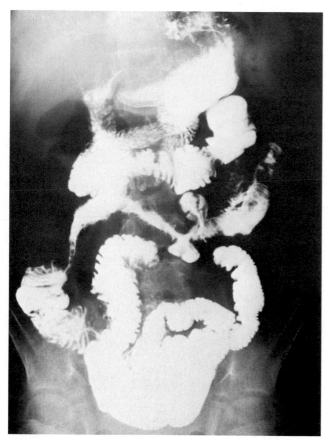

Figure 37a Narrowing and ulceration in a segment of the jejunum.

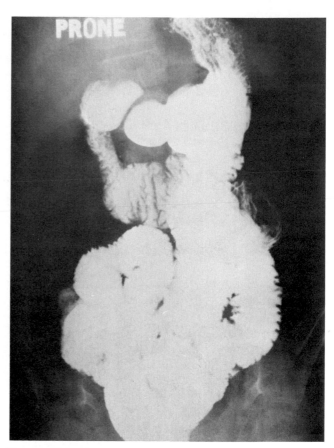

Figure 37b After 2 months of medical treatment the ulceration has healed and the bowel has returned to normal configuration.

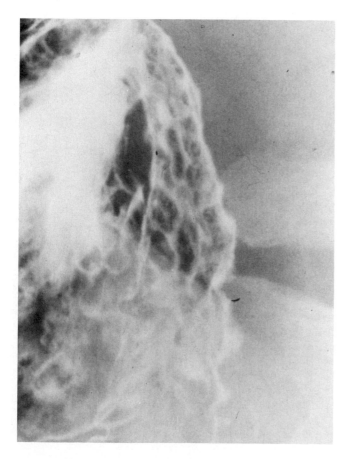

Figure 38 Cobblestoning in the terminal ileum shown on double contrast.

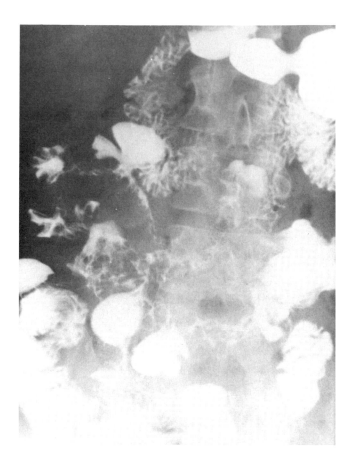

Figure 39 Extensive pseudodiverticular formation.

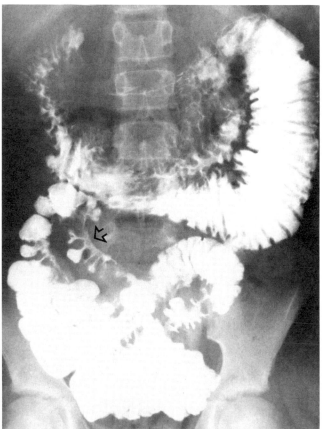

Figure 40 Typical case of advanced disease in the small bowel. The jejunum is slightly dilated before it narrows into a long linear ulcer (arrow) with pseudodiverticula. There is then a normal skip segment before another stricture.

150

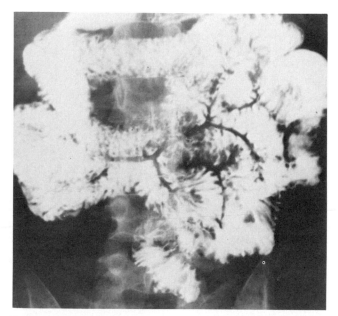

Figure 41a

Figure 41 (a) Early changes of Crohn's disease in the midjejunum. (b) Seven years later advance changes are present with narrowing and deep ulceration. Small areas of bowel not involved have ballooned out, forming large pseudodiverticula. The residual fold pattern in these is deformed, radiating to the base of the pseudodiverticulum, creating the "shell sign."

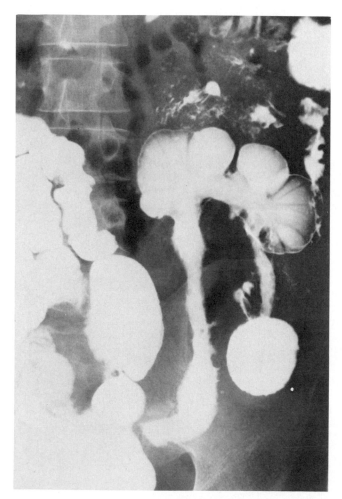

Figure 41b

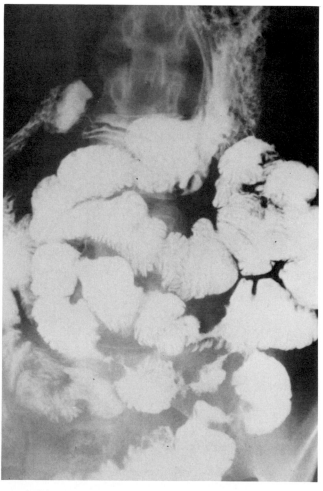

Figure 42   Multiple short strictures.

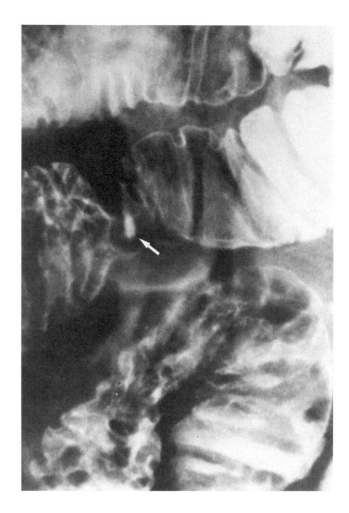

Figure 43 A small fissure is present (arrow) at the site of a short stricture.

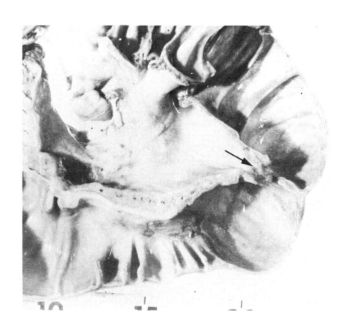

Figure 44 Resected terminal ileum showing ulceration (arrow) at the site of a short stricutre. Just distal to this is some patchy ulceration and thickening of the bowel wall on the mesenteric side. Note how the other side of the bowel is not involved—the transverse asymmetry of Crohn's disease.

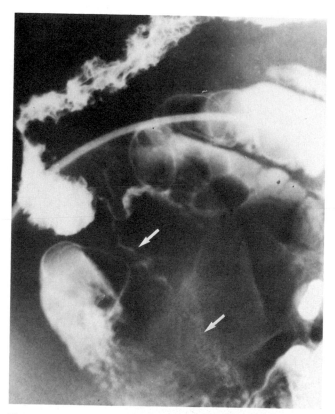

Figure 45a Crohn's disease of the terminal ileum (arrows).

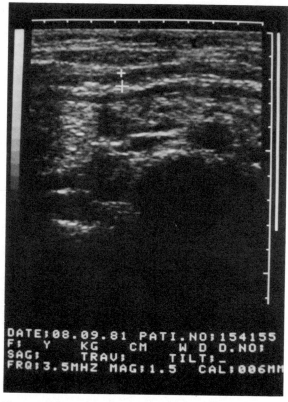

Figure 45b Ultrasonograph along plane of terminal ileum showing bowel wall thickening of 6 mm.

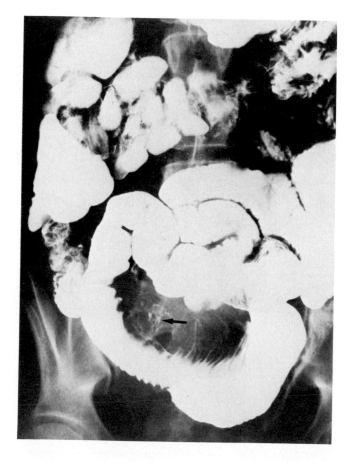

Figure 46 Barium is seen tracking into an abscess cavity (arrow). The abscess mass is causing extrinsic compression of surrounding small bowel.

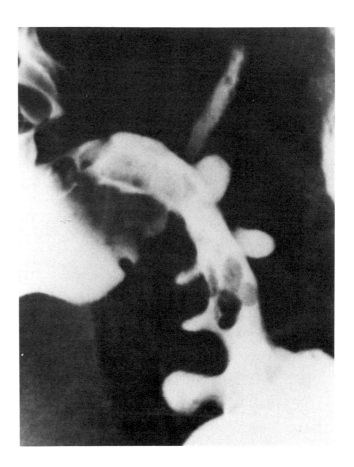

Figure 47 Stenotic terminal ileum with pseudodiverticula and several filling defects due to inflammatory polyps.

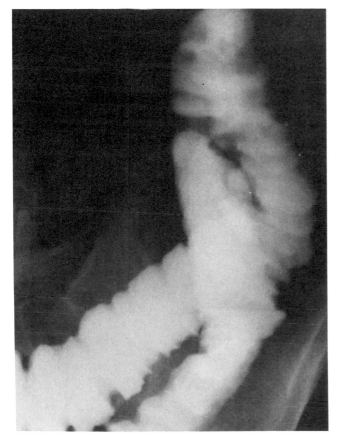

Figure 48a Single-contrast barium enema. The fold pattern appears thickened but there is no evidence of ulceration.

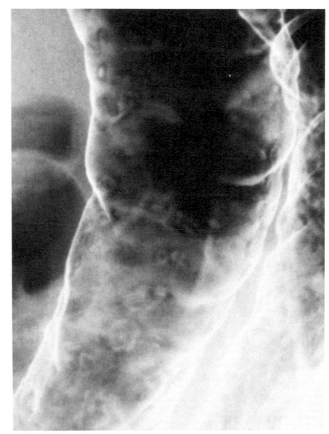

Figure 48b A double-contrast barium enema performed within a few days shows multiple aphthoid ulcers.

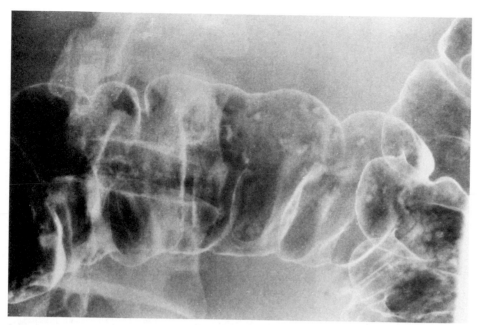

Figure 49a

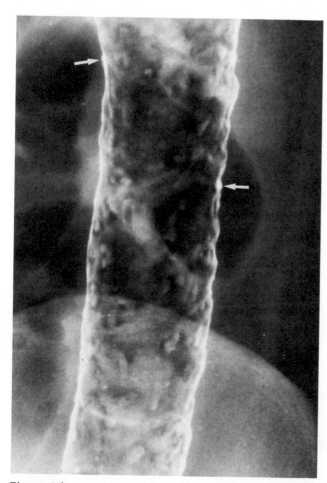

Figure 49b

Figure 49a–d Examples of aphthoid ulceration in Crohn's disease. The ulcers are of variable size and tend to be rounded or oval about 1–4 mm in diameter. The halo around the ulcer is due to its edematous elevated border. The background mucosa is normal, so the mucosal line is intact, except where an ulcer is caught tangentially (arrows). The haustration may be normal or slightly deformed.

155

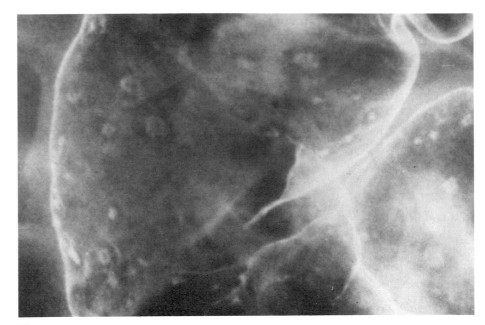

Figure 49c

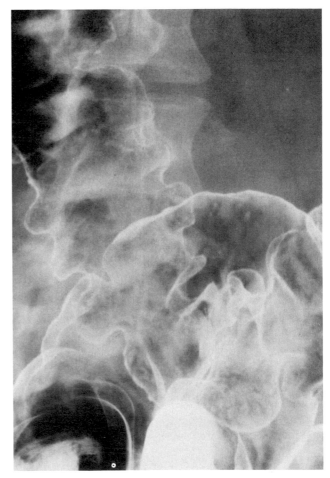

Figure 49d

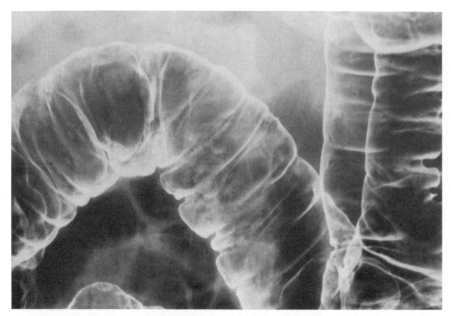

Figure 50 Scattered aphthoid ulcers in an otherwise normal-looking colon.

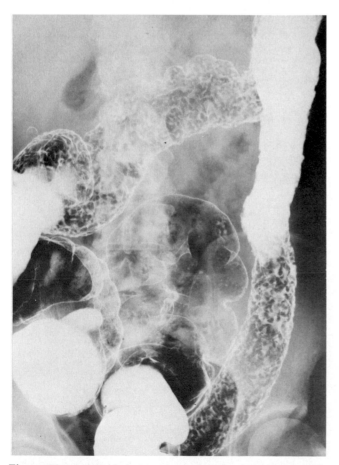

Figure 51 Aphthoid ulcers are present in the sigmoid colon. The transverse and descending colons are covered by a mass of inflammatory polyps.

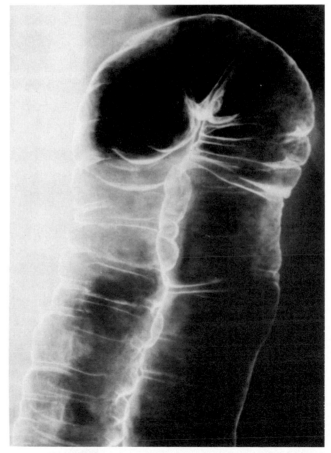

Figure 52 A fine nodular pattern, compatible with follicular lymphoid hyperplasia, is just visible at the splenic flexure. No ulceration was seen radiologically, but endoscopically small erythematous plaques were visible and biopsy confirmed Crohn's disease.

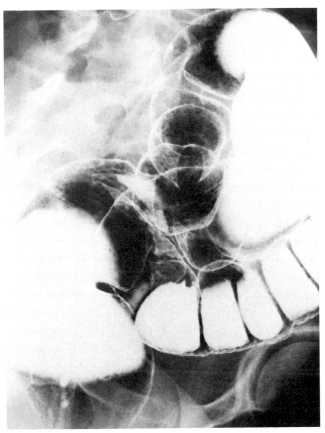

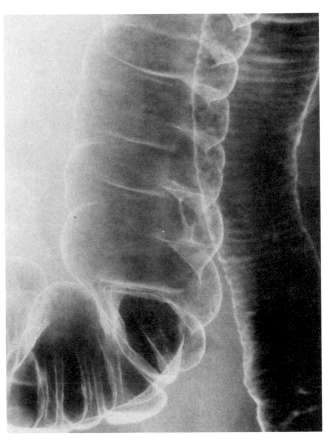

Figure 53 Follicular lymphoid hyperplasia in the rectosigmoid. Note the larger follicles in the rectum. No evidence of inflammatory bowel disease.

Figure 54 Transverse stripes in the descending colon.

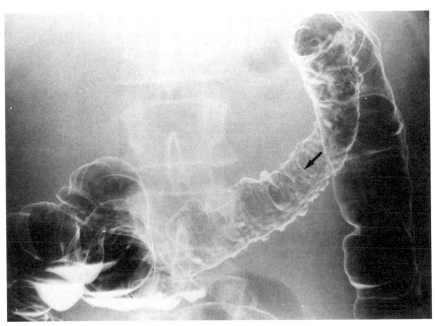

Figure 55 Residual haustration in the transverse colon causing some transverse lines (arrow).

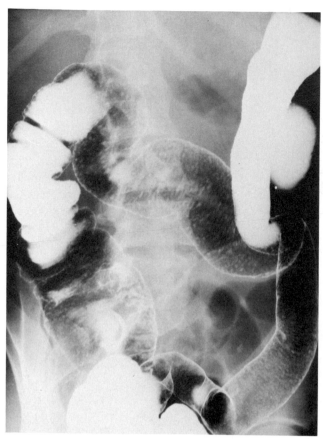

Figure 56 Extensive aphthoid ulceration with a transverse orientation.

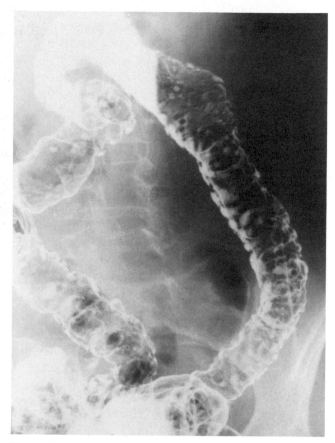

Figure 57 Discrete to confluent rounded ulceration with typical collar-stud projections from the mucosal line.

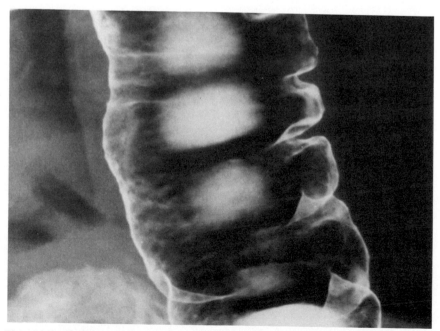

Figure 58 Small aphthoid ulcers with some mucosal edema accentuating the transverse linear pattern.

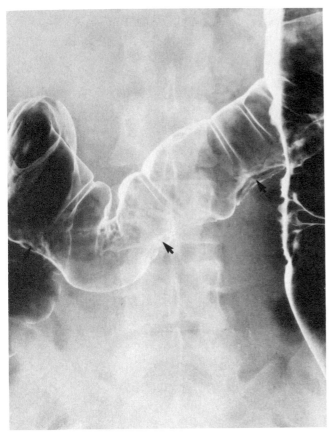

Figure 59   Linear ulceration on the antimesenteric border of the transverse colon (arrows).

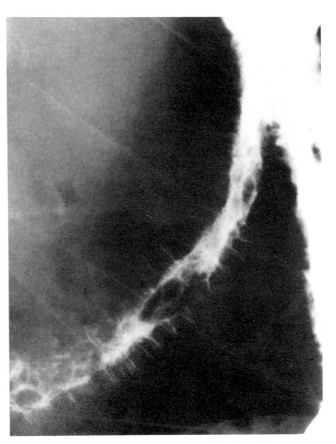

Figure 60   Mass of deep thorn-shaped fissuring ulcers.

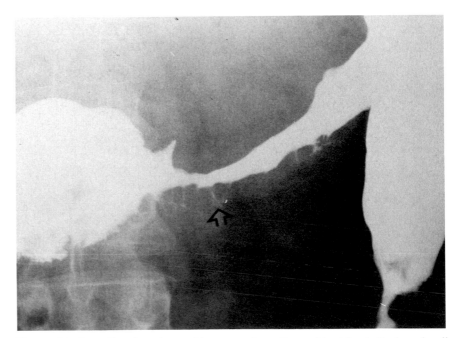

Figure 61   Deep fissuring ulcers with some undercutting and tracking in the bowel wall (arrow).

160

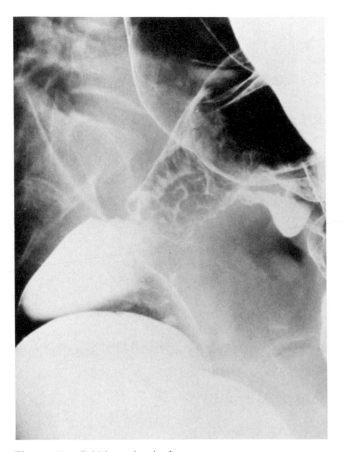

Figure 62 Cobblestoning in the rectum.

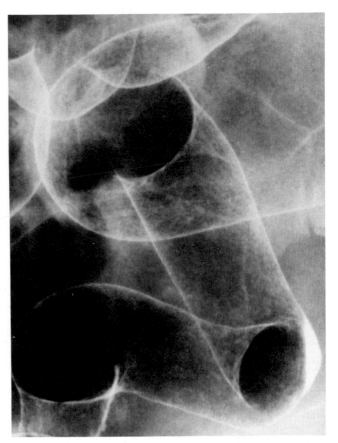

Figure 63 Distal granular colitis in a patient with Crohn's disease.

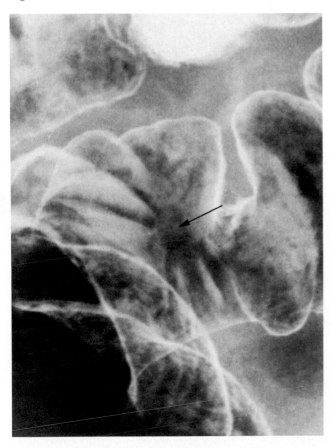

Figure 64 Radiating folds caused by fibrosis around an ulcer (arrow).

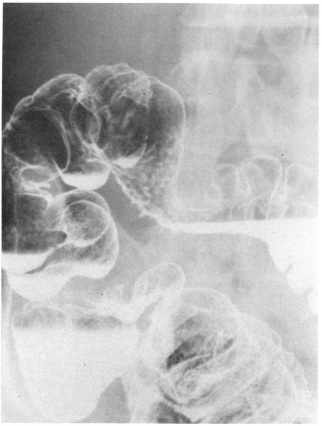

Figure 65 Ulceration on the antimesenteric border, leading to a "purse string" deformity.

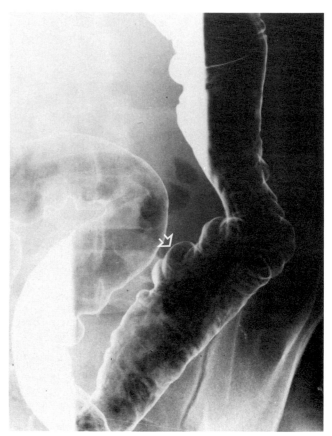

Figure 66 Pseudodiverticula (arrow). No active ulceration visible.

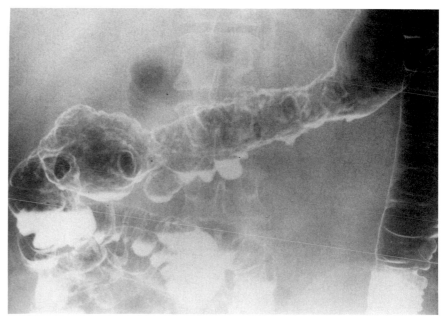

Figure 67 Pseudodiverticula on the antimesenteric border of the transverse colon associated with active ulceration of a mixed pattern.

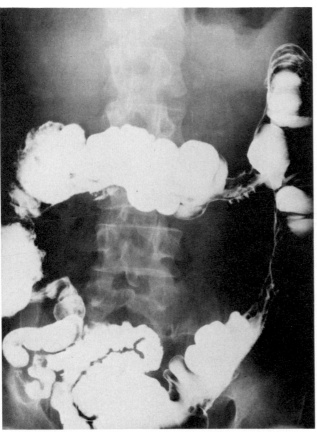

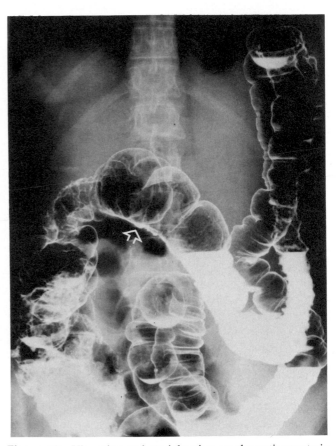

Figure 68 Normal skip segments in the midtransverse colon and splenic flexure—longitudinal asymmetry.

Figure 69 Ulceration and straightening on the antimesenteric border of the proximal colon (arrow) when the other side of the bowel wall is normal—transverse asymmetry.

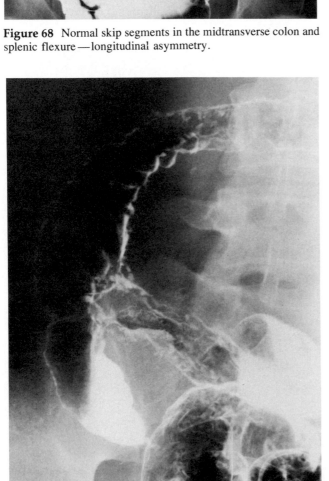

Figure 70 The ileocecal valve is thickened and irregular with several fistulous tracks into the terminal ileum.

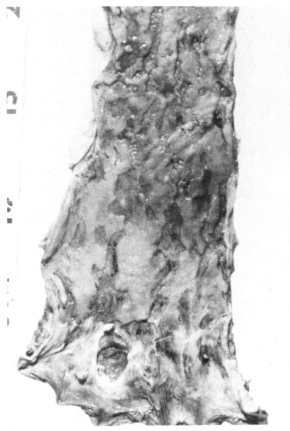

Figure 71

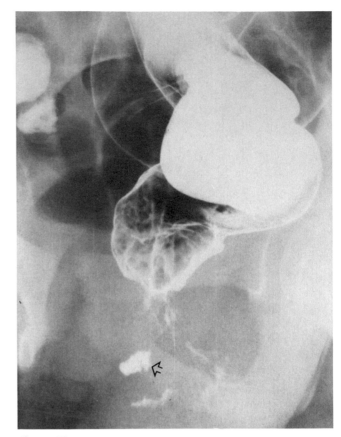

Figure 72

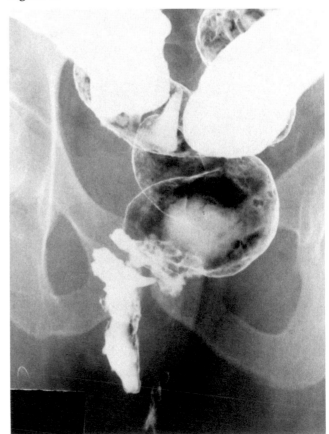

Figure 73

Figure 71   Gross stricturing and deformity of the anorectal region with a track leading into a perianal abscess (arrow).

Figure 72   Linear ulceration in the rectum extending down into the anal canal.

Figure 73   Ischiorectal abscess secondary to anal Crohn's disease.

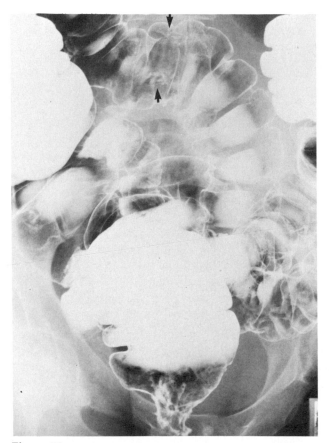

Figure 74

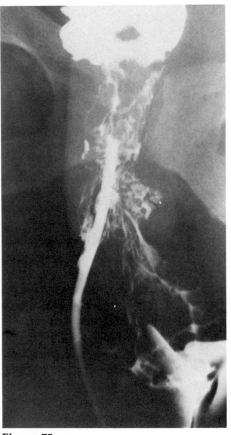

Figure 75

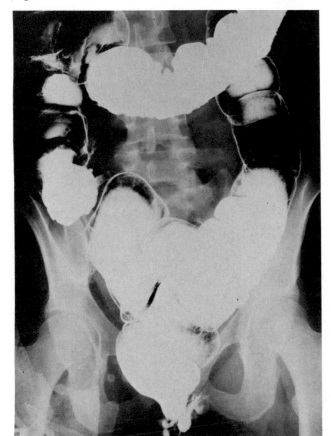

Figure 76

Figure 74 Prominent anal Crohn's disease with patchy involvement of the transverse colon (arrows).

Figure 75 Severe anorectal disease with extensive fistulas on the left side leading to incontinence. The soft rubber catheter had to be inserted high into the rectum to overcome this.

Figure 76 Instant enema in a patient with anal Crohn's disease. The entire colon has been demonstrated. Patchy disease in the ascending and transverse colons is visible.

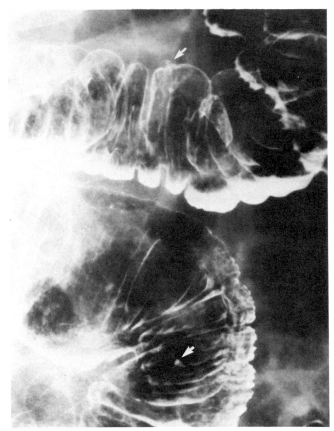

Figure 77

Figure 77 Intramural diverticula (arrows) with a typical plication deformity of the mucosa.

Figure 78 (a) Diverticular disease only. (b) Two years later Crohn's disease superimposed on diverticular disease. Discrete ulceration is present in the lumen, and several of the diverticula in the descending colon have not filled.

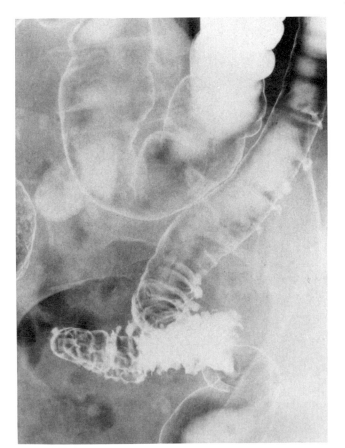

Figure 78a

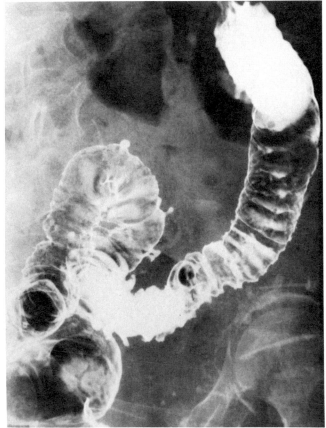

Figure 78b

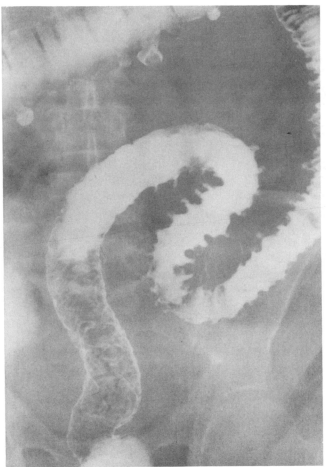

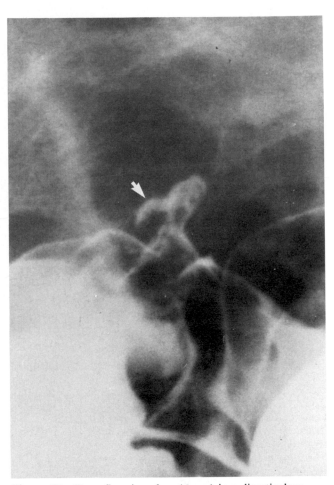

Figure 79 Linear ulceration is present in the rectosigmoid. A number of the diverticula are ulcerated and the muscle clefts are irregular.

Figure 80 Deep fissuring ulcer (arrow) in a diverticulum. (From Ref. 77)

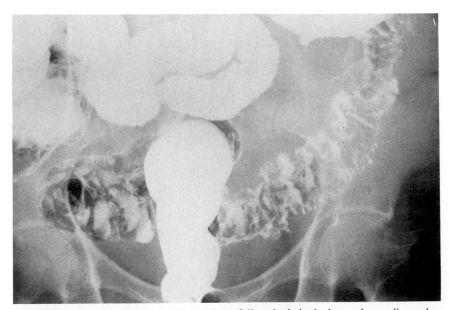

Figure 81 Irregular ulceration of a number of diverticula in the lower descending colon.

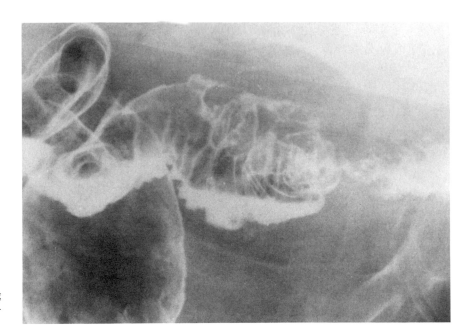

Figure 82 Dissecting abscess linkng several diverticula. Crohn's disease confirmed on resection. (From Ref. 77.)

Figure 83 Diagrammatic representation of the possible fistulous communications that can result from deep fissuring ulceration. (1) Ulceration in dome of diverticulum; (2) formation of small pericolic abscess following perforation due to ulceration; (3) longitudinal tracking from pericolic abscess; (4) fissuring ulcer creating a track into the diverticulum; (5) deep fissuring ulcer leading into a longitudinal track; (6) and (7) linking up with another ulcerated diverticulum. (From Ref. 77.)

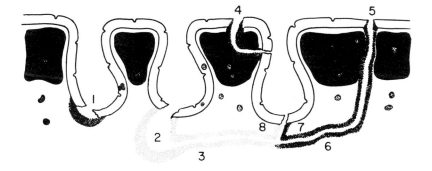

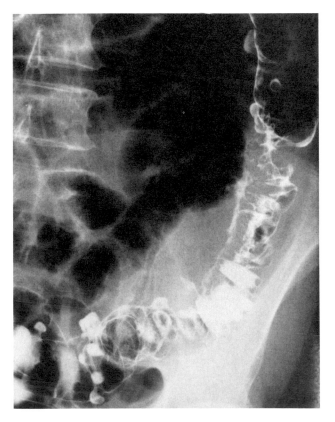

Figure 84 Long track in Crohn's disease outlining a dissecting abscess that links up with several diverticula to communicate with the lumen at either side. (Courtesy of Dr. R. Mason, Middlesex Hospital, London.)

5
Complications of Crohn's Disease

There is some overlap between the complications of Crohn's disease and ulcerative colitis. Toxic megacolon and post inflammatory polyps may be seen in both but are less common in Crohn's disease, as severe attacks of colitis are less frequent. These and other complications, such as the arthropathies and hepatic abnormalities that are common to ulcerative colitis, were discussed in Chapter 3.

Complications specific to Crohn's disease are related to the underlying pathology of the disease. The characteristic deep fissuring ulceration may penetrate the bowel wall. This might be expected to result in perforation with free intraperitoneal air and a generalized peritonitis, but this is unusual, as the transmural inflammation, which is another characteristic feature of the disease, produces adhesions between the serosa of affected bowel and neighboring structures. Any leak tends therefore to be contained by these adhesions and results in the formation of an abscess. If a structure is closely adherent to the bowel, it may also be penetrated by the ulcer, causing a fistula. Both are common and important complications of Crohn's disease.

Colonic strictures may be seen in Crohn's disease and ulcerative colitis, but seldom cause any problems. The same cannot be said for small bowel strictures in Crohn's disease. These often lead to obstruction, and are a common reason for surgery.

The urinary tract may be involved quite frequently, either from inflamed bowel, or indirectly from mesenteric thickening and abscess formation, or rarely by amyloid deposition. In practice such lesions are seldom a major problem in management.

PERFORATION As Crohn et al. (1) observed: "Deep fissures leading to perforation occur slowly enough to permit walling off by adhesions to a neighbouring viscus, to the parietal peritoneum, or to the omentum.'' For this reason, abscess or fistula formation is the more usual result of perforation of the bowel wall (2). However perforation with free intraperitoneal air is seen in 2–3% of cases (3,4). This may be due to direct penetration of the bowel wall from ulceration, fissuring, or necrosis, or to the rupture of a chronic intraabdominal abscess (Fig. 1). The commonest site for perforation is the ileum (5). This appears to be most likely to happen during an acute exacerbation of disease, where there is also an element of distal obstruction. The dilated bowel proximal to the stricture may be the site of perforation. The volume of free air is small, and less than that seen in a perforated duodenum. Perforation of the colon is very rare (Fig. 2) , except where toxic megacolon has developed (Fig. 3) (6), and then multiple sealed or free perforations may be present (Fig. 4).

INTRA-ABDOMINAL ABSCESSES

Abscesses may form spontaneously in 9–28% of patients (7–9). The presenting features are fever, abdominal pain, and a palpable mass. It left untreated the abscess may either perforate into a related adherent structure, creating a fistula, or rupture into the peritoneal cavity, causing generalized peritonitis. The development of an abscess not only produces systemic effects, but places the patient further at risk, as the abscess may lead to more complications.

Abscesses are also a common postoperative complication. Their location may differ from the spontaneous variety, as spillage into the abdominal cavity during operation or afterwards from anastomotic leakage usually results in pelvic or subphrenic collections, whereas a spontaneous abscess is related to the site of disease, so is commonest within the small bowel. Large collections may have one surface in contact with the parietal peritoneum; the majority are surrounded by loops of small bowel, which are bound together by dense adhesions (7). Rarely an abscess may develop within the leaves of the mesentery.

Plain films are not much help in detecting abscesses related to the small bowel (Fig. 5). A barium study of the small bowel will show the presence of a mass, but it can be difficult, as it is clinically, to distinguish a mass of inflamed bowel loops from an abscess. Both cause separation of bowel loops. In an abscess this will be localized and may affect only one side (Fig. 6), whereas bowel wall thickening will displace adjacent bowel on either side roughly in parallel with the diseased segment (Fig. 7). The mass effect of the abscess will compress any normal folds, and the diagnosis is confirmed if a track of barium is seen extending into or towards the mass (Fig. 6).

A psoas abscess is now much more likely to be due to Crohn's disease than to tuberculosis (10). This may present with hip flexion or a lump in the groin. A plain film may show bulging of the psoas outline or air within the sheath, but the exact extent of the abscess is most accurately defined by computerized tomography (Fig. 8). Most cases are due to ileal disease, so that a small bowel meal should be performed.

Ultrasonography is an extremely useful method for screening patients with suspected abscesses. Localization is possible with about 90% accuracy (11). The majority are cystic in appearance, but may contain some echoes. A lot of gas within the abscess will prevent penetration, but small amounts may produce either dense echoes without shadowing, or shadowing without echoes, allowing the abscess to be defined ultrasonically (12). The ''microbubble'' theory has been proposed to explain why a number of abscesses are strongly echogenic (12,13). Abscesses must be distinguished from bowel wall thickening due to Crohn's disease. This causes a sonolucent zone 5 mm or more in thickness around the lumen of the bowel (Fig. 9), the contents of which usually produce quite strong echoes. Abscesses have poorly defined walls and are often oval in shape (Figs. 10 and 11), but it may be possible to trace extensions between loops of bowel, or its shape is governed by the contour of an adjacent organ (e.g., the liver) (Fig. 12). The distinction from other fluid-filled collections can be difficult (14). Ascites is echo-free and bowel loops are clearly defined floating within the fluid. Small volumes can be displaced with gravity. Hematomas may separate out into a cystic and solid component as the clot retracts, but hematomas can be similar to abscesses depending on their state of development (15).

Fluid collections in the subphrenic spaces and abscesses within the liver (16) should be sought. Once a possible abscess is localized, the diagnosis may be confirmed, and its bacteriological content established, by fine needle aspiration biopsy. Treatment of the abscess by catheter drainage should then be considered (17). This is a rapidly expanding field, and readers are referred to Ferrucci and Wittenberg's excellent book on this subject (17a).

Computerized tomography (CT) is more accurate than ultrasound for the detection of intraabdominal abscesses (18) and will define the extent of the abscess more clearly. This is particularly true with retroperitoneal lesions, and CT is the method of choice in a suspected psoas abscess.

FISTULA A fistula is an abnormal communication between two epithelial surfaces. The spontaneous development of a fistula may be internal to bowel, bladder, or other structure, or external to the abdominal wall or vagina. The development of a fistula is due to transmural inflammation and deep fissuring ulceration leading to perforation of an adherent structure (1,5) (Fig. 13).

Spontaneous internal fistula have been reported in 6–33% of patients (3,8,19–25) (see Table 1). The incidence of fistula formation relates to the severity of the disease and the length of bowel involved (9). Fistulas are more common in patients with ileocolitis than in those with small bowel disease only (24). When the terminal ileum is involved, the ileocecal valve is often abnormal and short fistulous tracts are seen in about 7% of cases (26). Other common terminations for small bowel fistula are to the cecum, to other ileal loops, or to the sigmoid. Any of the viscera may be involved (Figs. 14 and 15). Gastrocolic, coloduodenal, and ileoduodenal fistulas have been reported (27–29), and even involvement of the superior mesenteric venous system, with portal pyemia and barium entering the mesenteric veins during small bowel meal (30).

The presence of an internal fistula is accepted as an indication for surgery, so their radiological demonstration is important. An ileocolic fistula is usually demonstrated by premature filling of the distal colon during a small bowel examination (Fig. 16). Absence of this sign does not exclude a fistula (31). In some cases this may be due to a poor technique of examination, with too long an interval between films, so that early filling of the distal colon

Table 1 Incidence of Internal Fistula Due to Crohn's Disease

Series	Reported % incidence
Crohen and Yarnis, 1958 (19)	17.5
Colcock, 1964 (20)	18
Atwell et al., 1965 (21)	14
Schofield, 1965 (22)	12
Gjone et al., 1966 (23)	10
Edwards, 1969 (9)	12
Kemp Harper, 1971 (3)	10
Steinberg et al., 1973 (8)	6
Rankin et al., 1979 (24)	16.3
Brahme, 1980 (25)	33

[a]Mean 14.9%

is overlooked because the entire colon has filled. Probably some fistulas open and close spontaneously, so it may depend on the timing of the examination in relation to this. In some cases the pressure gradient across the fistula may be inadequate for the passage of contrast (Fig. 17). One might expect all colonic fistulas to show up on barium enema, but this is not always the case (Fig. 18). It is probably better to look for fistula along the physiological pathway (e.g., an ileocolic fistula) by a small bowel examination first, and then examine the distal side of the fistula by a barium enema. This combination should confirm the presence of the fistula, show its exact site, and indicate the extent of bowel involvement on either side, which will be useful information for the surgeon planning resection. With ileocolic fistulas the disease in the small bowel is usually extensive, but the colonic involvement may be quite limited, often to just a small area around the fistula (Fig. 15b), or the mucosa may appear normal and just tacked on the the fistula (Fig. 13). A prefistula formation stage may be seen when diseased small bowel has become adherent to part of the colon and invaded the bowel wall, causing deformity and irregularity of the mucosa without breaking through to form a fistula (Fig. 19).

Fistulas between loops of small bowel may be single or multiple. Single fistulas are easy to miss and often require careful compression studies to be demonstrated. Multiple fistulas are obvious and often arranged in a stellate fashion, with diseased bowel in the center feeding into a number of fistulas, which lead out like spokes from a hub to communicate with other parts of the bowel at the periphery (Fig. 20).

Spontaneous external fistulas are uncommon. Indeed, Crohn originally did not think that these occurred, but a number of cases have been reported, almost all associated with small bowel disease (8). Most fistulas to the anterior abdominal wall complicate laparotomy. Following anastomotic breakdown a horrific number of fistulas may develop, which drain out feculent fluid through the incisional sites, including stab wounds for drains. A further complication is dehiscence of the laparotomy wound. In such patients it is important to catheterize each site, inject water-soluble contrast, and establish if the opening leads into just a short blind-ended track, into an abscess or is intercommunicating with other tracks. If a fistula is present, which part of the bowel it communicates with must be established. Barium studies may then be helpful to show how much normal bowel is left and to confirm the levels of the fistulas.

STRICTURE FORMATION

Inflammatory changes within the bowel wall lead to a change in tone in the muscularis, which results in narrowing of the bowel and loss of its normal fold pattern. Ulceration is therefore associated with narrowing of the lumen. An extreme sign of this is the "string sign" of Kantor. Underfilling of the bowel tends to exaggerate the degree of narrowing, as when sufficient pressure is applied during a small bowel enema, some distensibility is visible in these narrowed segments. The lack of complete rigidity probably explains why the narrowing can appear so marked radiologically and yet the patient is not obstructed. If a stricture is defined as persistent fixed narrowing, the narrowing associated with diffuse ulceration is not really stricture formation and should be described simply as "narrowing."

True stricture formation is due to fibrosis within the bowel wall. Fibrosis is common in Crohn's disease and may be found in any layer of the wall. Strictures are therefore common in Crohn's disease and have been reported in the small bowel in 21%, and in the large bowel in 8% of cases (26). In the colon the strictures tend to be short and single. The strictured segment is often angulated, with ulceration on the antimesenteric border (Fig. 21). In the small bowel the strictures are more variable in length and frequently multiple. Compression views of short strictures may show a small ulcer at the site of the stricture. Pseudodiverticular change is a common accompaniment, reflecting the asymmetric distribution of the changes in

Crohn's disease. Strictures once formed tend to be slowly progressive. In the small bowel this invariably leads to obstruction and the need for surgical intervention. (Fig. 22).

INTESTINAL OBSTRUCTION

Overt intestinal obstruction is often preceded by several months or years of episodes of attacks of colicky abdominal pain, which may be associated with distension and vomiting. These attacks can be precipitated by the ingestion of certain foods. Peanuts seem particularly prone to cause problems.

Obstruction due to stricturing in the large bowel is rare (Fig. 23) and most cases are due to small bowel disease. Small bowel obstruction is a common problem in the stenotic phase of the disease. In the National Cooperative Crohn's Disease Survey (26), 13% had small bowel obstruction, which was the reason for surgery in 45.2% (32). Comparing these patients to those without obstruction showed that those with small bowel obstruction had more fistulas, linear ulceration, angulation, extrinsic masses, separation of loops, asymmetric disease, and abscesses. In patients with large bowel obstruction there was also an increased incidence of fistulas, rectal abscesses, extrinsic inflammatory masses, and more rectal disease than in those without obstruction. These findings reflect a general trend that patients with obstruction have have extensive severe disease with strictures often complicated by abscess or fistula formation.

Plain films may confirm the presence of small bowel obstruction in about 60% (33) (Fig. 24), but there may not be any gas in the fluid-filled loops, so that these are not visible (34). Real-time ultrasound can then show distended loops with increased peristalsis (35). Should there be any doubt as to the level or presence of obstruction, this can be accurately demonstrated by a barium infusion (Fig. 25) (36), which does not cause any complication with the obstruction or subsequent operation. Rarely, an enterolith or plum stone (37) can be seen causing a ball valve obstruction between two strictures (Fig. 26). Marked small bowel dilatation secondary to chronic obstruction is a more common feature of stenotic jejunal disease than of ileal disease, where the dominant abnormality tends to be just the diseased bowel (38) (Figs. 27 and 28).

Following operation, obstruction may develop in about 9% of cases (39) and is the second most common reason for reoperation (40). Ileus may be seen in the immediate postoperative phase, but later problems will be mechanical, due either to adhesions or recurrent disease with stricture formation. Distinguishing these radiologically requires careful examination with compression (41), ideally using a small bowel enema, although adhesions can still be accurately shown on a standard small bowel meal. Peristaltic contractions can be difficult to distinguish from strictures, and an intravenous relaxant is useful if this is proving to be a problem. If there is any doubt about the mucosa, air should be insufflated into the colon and refluxed into the small bowel. Narrowing at an ileocolic anastomosis is almost diagnostic of recurrent disease, and any abnormality in the distal 10 cm of small bowel should be regarded as being due to recurrent Crohn's disease unless there is exceptional good radiographic evidence to the contrary. Adhesions cause a fixed deformity, either between loops or to the parietal peritoneum. The bowel tends to be sharply angulated at the point of fixation, with fixed folds running toward that point. Compression is essential to demonstrate fixation (41,42). The absence of any mucosal abnormality excludes Crohn's disease (Figs. 29 and 30).

HEMORRHAGE

Low-grade blood loss is common in Crohn's disease and many patients become iron deficient. Rectal bleeding may be noted, and this tends to happen more often when the active disease is in the distal large bowel, but about 10% of patients with small bowel disease have been reported as having overt rectal bleeding (9,19). Blood loss is usually occult, and only rarely does massive hemorrhage occur (Fig. 20). Persistent bleeding is an indication for operation in less than 2% of cases (20).

If a patient continues to bleed despite supportive therapy, surgery may be considered. The problem then is to localize the site of hemorrhage if extensive disease is present. Plain films and barium studies are of no value, and the only investigation worth performing is angiography with selective superior and inferior mesenteric angiograms. Provided that hemorrhage is occurring at the rate of about 2 ml/min, the bleeding point will be revealed by extravasation of contrast into the lumen of the bowel. An infusion of pitressin (0.2 unit/min) can be used to provide temporary control of the hemorrhage (43).

If a diagnosis of Crohn's disease has not been established, it is possible to make the diagnosis angiographically from the following features: dilated vasa recta, often with terminal coiling, an intense but patchy parenchyma phase showing an increased wall thickness, and a positive zoning sign (44). To detect these changes requires good-quality angiograms and possibly subtraction films. These signs should be looked for if an angiogram is performed for hemorrhage where the cause is unknown.

PANCREATITIS

Pancreatitis should be considered if a patient presents with pain, which is atypical for abdominal Crohn's disease but is typical for pancreatitis and is associated with nausea and vomiting. The diagnosis is supported by an elevated serum amylase.

Pancreatitis has been associated with Crohn's disease where there is duodenal involvement, and following treatment with azathioprine. Disruption of the ampulla from ulceration or fistula formation is a possible mechanism for Crohn's disease to cause pancreatitis, and is supported by marked filling of the pancreatic duct during barium meals in some patients who have had pancreatitis (45). However, overt pancreatitis with duodenal involvement is rare. Of patients treated with azathioprine, 4.4% have been reported to develop pancreatitis (46). This is independent of duodenal involvement, and its development within 21 days of starting treatment suggests an immune response, but no definite cause has been established.

CARCINOMA

There are a number of reports of carcinoma associated with Crohn's disease (47–52), and a higher risk of intestinal cancer than the risk in the general population (48,51). Carcinoma tends to arise in areas affected by Crohn's disease, so is more common in the ileum and proximal colon (48,51,52). Bypassed loops and sites of fistulas are also high-risk areas (49,51).

Compared to ulcerative colitis, however, carcinoma is not such a major concern in the long-term management of Crohn's disease. This is fortunate, as the radiological features of a carcinoma can be difficult to differentiate from the disease process itself. As carcinomas are likely to occur in areas of chronic disease, malignancy can be overlooked. In one study the presence of a tumor was not suspected in 51% of cases (50). Radiological features typical of malignancy, such as a stricture with shouldering or a nodular mass with an indrawn base, should not be attributed automatically to Crohn's disease, and the possibility of a cancer must be borne in mind (Fig. 31).

URINARY TRACT INVOLVEMENT

Urinary tract abnormalities may be present in about 10% of patients with Crohn's disease (53). These are not all symptomatic, are usually overshadowed by the intestinal disease, and are rarely the main problem.

Hydronephrosis may be present in 6.6–9% of cases (54,55). This is due to ureteric obstruction secondary to inflammatory changes with retroperitoneal extension of an abscess.

As the right ureter is closely related to the terminal ileum, the right side is more often affected. The predominant symptom may be difficulty in walking, with inability to extend the right hip, and pain in the loin or flank. This reflects muscle spasm rather than renal involvement, and symptoms of urinary infection are uncommon. Intravenous urography or ultrasonography will demonstrate the hydronephrosis, with urography showing the level of obstruction with a conical tapering end to the ureter, compatible with periureteric fibrosis (53). If both ureters are involved, the most likely cause is a pelvic abscess.

The bladder is usually involved by contiguous ileal Crohn's disease, which produces either inflammatory changes in the bladder wall or a fistula into it. Ileovesicular fistulas have been reported in 2–7% of cases (55,56). These may present with pneumaturia, but are seldom shown on contrast examinations (Fig. 32) and are best detected by cystoscopy (56). Inflammatory changes in the bladder wall may interfere with bladder contraction and can lead to problems in micturition with an increased residual volume (57). Urography may show thickened edematous folds, a deformed dome to the bladder with a spiculated edge, which is usually on the right side due to involvement from the terminal ileum (Fig. 33). A pelvic abscess will cause extrinsic compression of the bladder. The soft tissue mass of the abscess may be apparent on plain films, but this is shown best by either ultrasonography or CT.

Renal tract stones may form in 3–10% of patients (3,55,58,59). Some of these may be uric acid stones, which are radiolucent. These may develop following colectomy, which leads to intestinal bicarbonate loss. If there is a high ileostomy output, the urine will become concentrated and of low pH, which are suitable conditions for urate stone formation (58). Most stones are radiopaque, being formed of calcium oxalate or phosphate. Dietary oxalate is normally bound to free calcium, forming an insoluble complex, but in patients with steatorrhea the free calcium is bound to the excess fatty acids, so that oxalate remains unbound and soluble. Provided that the colon is intact, this will then be absorbed (60). Hyperoxaluria may therefore occur in patients with ileal dysfunction. If this is then combined with a low urinary volume (e.g., from diarrhea), calcium oxalate may be precipitated in the kidneys.

Secondary amyloidosis is a rare complication of Crohn's disease (61), but can cause the nephrotic syndrome (62). This should be considered if the kidneys appear enlarged, and confirmed by demonstrating amyloid on rectal biopsy. A point to note here is that secondary amyloid from any cause involves the rectum, and may itself simulate a proctitis (63), so the presence of Crohn's disease should always be clearly documented before any association is made between the nephrotic syndrome and inflammatory bowel disease.

BILIARY TRACT ABNORMALITIES   The incidence of cholelithiasis is probably not increased in colonic disease, but there is an increased incidence of gallbladder disease in patients with ileostomies (64), and up to a third of patients with long-standing ileal disease or resection may have cholesterol stones (65–67). The reason for this is malabsorption of bile acids secondary to ileal dysfunction. This leads to a decrease in the concentration of bile acids, with a corresponding rise in biliary cholesterol, which then precipitates in the gallbladder. Most of these stones appear to be asymptomatic, as no increase in cholecystectomy has been reported.

REFERENCES

1. Crohn, B.B, Ginzburg, L., Oppenheimer, G.D. (1932). Regional ileitis. JAMA 99; 1325.
2. Waye, J.D., Lithgow, C. (1967). Small bowel perforation in regional enteritis. Gastroenterology 53; 625.
3. Kemp Harper, R.A. (1971). The radiological spectrum of Crohn's disease. Proc. R. Soc. Med. 64; 1181.

4. Kyle, J., Cardis, T., Dungan, T., Ewen, S.W.B. (1968). Free perforation in regional enteritis. Am. J. Dig. Dis. 13; 275.

5. Nasr, K., Morowitz, D.A., Anderson, J.G.D., Kirsner, J.B. (1969). Free perforation in regional enteritis. Gut 10; 206.

6. Javett, S.L., Brooke, B.N. (1970). Acute dilatation of colon in Crohn's disease. Lancet 2; 126.

7. Nagler, S.M., Poticha, S.M. (1979). Intra-abdominal abscess in regional enteritis. Am. J. Surg. 137; 350.

8. Steinberg, D.M., Cooke, W.T., Alexander-Williams, J. (1973). Abscess and fistula in Crohn's disease. Gut 14; 865.

9. Edwards, H. (1969). Crohn's disease, an enquiry into its nature and consequences. Ann. R. Coll. Surg. Engl. 44; 121.

10. Kyle, J. (1971). Psoas abscess in Crohn's disease. Gastroenterology 61; 149.

11. Taylor, K.J.W., Sullivan, D.C., Watson, J.F. McI., Rosenfield, H.T. (1979). Ultrasonography and gallium for the diagnosis of abdominal and pelvic abscesses. Gastrointest. Radiol. 3; 281.

12. Kressel, H.Y., Filly, R.A. (1978). Ultrasound appearance of gas-containing abscesses in the abdomen. Am. J. Roentgenol. 130; 71.

13. Yeh, H.C., Wolf, B.S. (1977). Ultrasonic study to identify stomach tap water micro-bubbles. J. Clin. Ultrasound 51: 170.

14. Doust, B.D., Quiroz, F., Stewart, J.M. (1977). Ultrasonic distinction of abscesses from other intra-abdominal fluid collections. Radiology 125; 213.

15. Wicks, J.D., Silver, T.M., Bree, R.L. (1978). Gray scale features of haematomas: an ultrasound spectrum. Am. J. Roentgenol. 131; 977.

16. Newlin, N., Silver, T.M., Stuck, K.J. (1981). Ultrasound features of pyogenic liver abscesses. Radiology 139; 155.

17. Gerzof, S.G., Robbins, A.H., Birkett, D.II., et al. (1979). Percutaneous catheter drainage of abdominal abscesses guided by ultrasound and computerized tomography. Am. J. Roentgenol. 133; 1.

17a. Ferrucci, J.T., Wittenberg, J. (1981). *Interventional Radiology of the Abdomen.* Williams & Wilkins, Baltimore.

18. Halbe, M.D., Daffner, R.H., Morgan, C.L. et al. (1979). Intra-abdominal abscess: current concepts in radiologic evaluation. Am. J. Roentgenol. 133; 9.

19. Crohn, B.B., Yarnis, H. (1958). *Fistula Formation in Regional Ileitis.* Grune & Stratton, New York, p. 52.

20. Colcock, B.P. (1964). Regional enteritis: a surgical enigma. Surg. Clin. N. Am. 44; 779.

21. Atwell, J.D., Duthie, H.L., Goligher, J.C. (1965). The outcome of Crohn's disease. Br. J. Surg. 52; 966.

22. Schofield, P.F. (1965). Natural history and treatment of Crohn's disease. Ann. R. Coll. Surg. Engl. 36; 258.

23. Gjone, E., Onung, G.M., Myren, J. (1966). Crohn's disease in Norway 1956-63. Gut 7; 372.

24. Rankin, G.B., Watts, D., Melynk, C.S., et al. (1979). National Cooperative Crohn's Disease Study: extraintestinal manifestations and perianal complications. Gastroenterology 77; 914.

25. Brahme, F. (1971). Roentgenology of Crohn's disease. In *Regional Enteritis.* International Symposium. Nordiska Bokhandeln, Stockholm, p. 81.

26. Goldberg, H.I., Caruthers, S.B., Nelson, J.A., et al. (1979). Radiographic findings of the National Cooperative Crohn's Disease Study. Gastroenterology 77; 925.

27. Metzger, W.H., Ranganath, K.A. (1976). Crohn's disease presenting as a gastrocolic fistula. Am. J. Gastroenterology 65; 258.

28. Korelitz, B.I. (1977). Colonic-duodenal fistula in Crohn's disease. Am. J. Dig. Dis. 22; 1040.

29. Van Patten, W.N., Bargen, J.A., Dockerty, M.B. et al. (1954). Regional enteritis. Gastroenterology 26; 347.

30. Reiner, L., Freed, A., Bloom, A. (1978). Enterovenous fistulization in Crohn's disease. JAMA 239; 130.

31. Fario, V.W., Wilk, P., Turnbull, R.B., et al. (1977). Ileosigmoidal fistula complicating Crohn's disease. Dis. Colon Rectum 20; 381.

32. Mekhjian, H.S., Switz, D.M., Watts, H.D., et al. (1979). National Cooperative Crohn's Disease Study: factors determining recurrence of Crohn's disease after surgery. Gastroenterology 77; 907.

33. Lo, A.M., Evans, W.E., Carey, L.C. (1966). Review of the small bowel obstruction at Milwaukee Country General Hospital. Am. J. Surg. 111; 884.

34. Gough, I.R. (1978). Strangulating adhesive small bowel obstruction with normal radiographs. Br. J. Surg. 65; 431.

35. Sheible, W., Goldberger, L.F. (1979). Diagnosis of small bowel obstruction: the contribution of diagnostic ultrasound. Am. J. Radiol. 133; 685.

36. Nolan, D.J., Marks, C.G. (1981). The barium infusion in small intestinal obstruction. Clin. Radiol. 32; 651.

37. Katz, I., Fischer, R.M. (1957). Enteroliths complicating regional enteritis. Am. J. Roentgenol. 78; 653.

38. Marshak, R.H., Wolf, B.S. (1953). Chronic ulcerative granulomatous jejunitis and ileo-jejuntitis. Am. J. Roentgenol. 70; 93.

39. Ritchie, J.K. (1971). Ileostomy and excisional surgery for chronic inflammatory disease of the colon: a survey of one hospital region. Gut 12; 528.

40. DeDombal, F.T., Barton, I., Goligher, J.C. (1971). The early and late results of surgical treatment of Crohn's disease. Br. J. Surg. 58; 805.

41. Bartram, C.I. (1980). The radiological demonstration of adhesions following surgery for inflammatory bowel disease. Br. J. Radiol. 53; 650.

42. Miller, R.E., Sellink, J.L. (1979). Enteroclysis: the small bowel enema. How to succeed and how to fail. Gastrointest. Radiol. 4; 269.

43. Podolny, G.A. (1978). Crohn's disease presenting with massive lower gastrointestinal haemorrhage. Am. J. Roentgenol. 130; 368.

44. Herlinger, H. (1972). Angiography of Crohn's disease. Clin. Gastroenterol. 1(2); 383.

45. Legge, D.A., Harry, M.B., Hoffman, N., et al. (1971). Pancreatitis as a complication of regional enteritis of the duodenum. Gastroenterology 61; 834.

46. Strudevant, R.A.L., Singleton, J.W., Deren, J.J., et al. (1979). Azothioprine related pancreatitis in patients with Crohn's disease. Gastroenterology 77; 983.

47. Hywel-Jones, J. (1969). Colonic cancer and Crohn's disease. Gut 10; 651.

48. Darke, S.G., Parks, A.G., Grognon, J.L., Pollock, D.J. (1973). Adenocarcinoma and Crohn's disease. Br. J. Surg. 60; 169.

49. Nesbit, R.R., Elbadansi, N.A., Morton, J.H., Cooper, R.A. (1976). Carcinoma of the small bowel — a complication of regional enteritis. Cancer 37; 2948.

50. Fleming, R.A., Pollock, A.C. (1975). A case of "Crohn's carcinoma." Gut 16; 533.

51. Weedon, D.D., Shorter, R.G., Ilstrup, D.M., et al. (1973). Crohn's disease and cancer. N. Engl. J. Med. 289; 1099.

52. Valdes-Dapena, A., Rudolph, I., Hidayat, A., et al (1973). Adenocarcinoma of the small bowel in association with regional enteritis. Cancer 37; 2938.

53. Bagby, R.J., Clements, J.L., Patrick, J.W., et al. (1973). Genito-urinary complications of granulomatous bowel disease. Am. J. Roentgenol. 117;297.

54. Present, D.H., Rabinowitz, J.G., Banks, P.A. (1969). Obstructive hydroenphrosis; frequent but seldom recognized complication of granulomatous disease of the bowel. N. Engl. J. Med. 280; 523.

55. Greenstein, A.J., Janowitz, H.D., Saclar, D.B. (1976). The extra-intestinal complications of Crohn's disease and ulcerative colitis. Medicine 55; 401.

56. Kyle, J., Murray, C.M. (1969). Ileovesical fistula in Crohn's disease. Surgery 66; 497.

57. Joffe, W. (1976). Roentgenologic abnormalities of the urinary bladder secondary to Crohn's disease. Am. J. Roentgenol. 127; 297.

58. Gelzayd, E.A., Breuer, R.I., Kirsner, J.B. (1968). Nephrolithiasis in inflammatory bowel disease. Am. J. Dig. Dis. 13; 1027.

59. Grossman, M.S., Nugent, F.W. (1967). Urolithiasis as a complication of chronic diarrhoeal disease. Am. J. Dig. Dis. 12; 491.

60. Chadwick, V.A., Nodha, K., Dowling, R.H. (1973). Mechanism for hyperoxaluria in patients with ileal dysfunction. N. Engl. J. Med. 289; 172.

61. Fansen, O., Nygaard, K., Elgio K. (1977). Amyloidosis and Crohn's disease. Scand. J. Gastroenterol. 12; 657.

62. Wallenstein, L., Serebro, H.A., Calle, S. (1966). Chronic regional enteritis complicated by nephrotic syndrome due to amyloidosis: antemortem clinical study. JAMA 198; 555.

63. Goldgraber, M.B., Kirsner, J.B. (1957). Specific diseases simulating ''non-specific'' ulcerative colitis (lymphogranuloma venereum, acute vasculitis, scleroderma and secondary amyloidosis). Ann. Int. Med. 47; 939.

64. Jones, M.R., Gregory, D., Evans, K.T., Rhodes, J. (1976). The prevalence of gall bladder disease in patients with ileostomy. Clin. Radiol. 27; 561.

65. Heaton, K.W., Read, A.E. (1969). Gallstones in patients with disorders of the terminal ileum and disturbed bile salt metabolism. Br. Med. J. 3; 494.

66. Baker, A.L., Kaplan, M.M., Norton, R.A. (1974). Gallstones in inflammatory bowel disease. Am. J. Dig. Dis. 19; 102.

67. Cohen, S., Kaplan, M., Gottlich, L. (1971). Liver disease and gallstones in regional enteritis. Gastroenterology 60; 237.

FIGURES 1 THROUGH 33

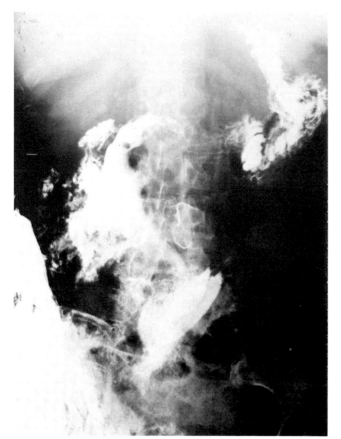

Figure 1

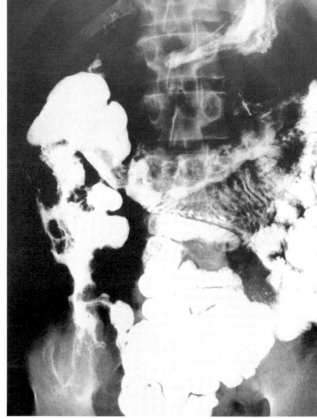

Figure 2

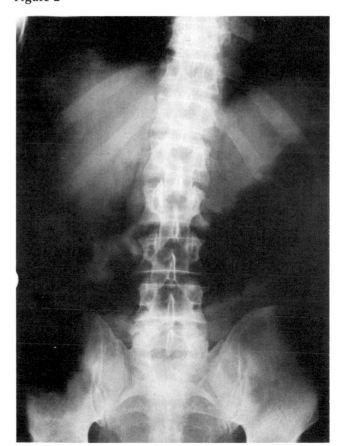

Figure 1 Duodenal Crohn's disease with abscess formation and rupture of the abscess leading to gross intra- and retroperitoneal contamination.

Figure 2 Perforation of the ascending colon leading to a paracolic abscess which tracked down into the pelvis. (From Ref. 68.)

Figure 3 Toxic megacolon in Crohn's disease with perforation. Free air is noted under the liver edge.

Figure 3

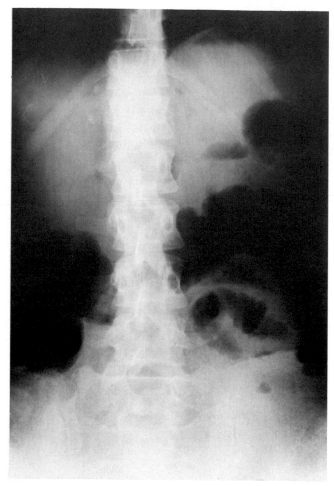

Figure 4a   Toxic megacolon in Crohn's disease.

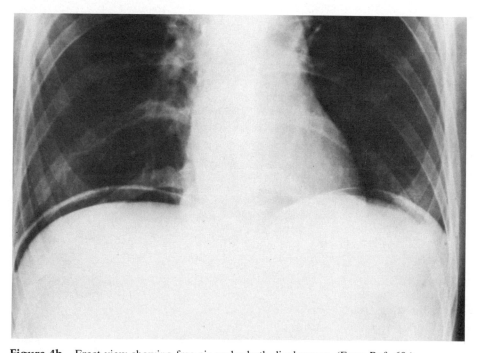

Figure 4b   Erect view showing free air under both diaphragms. (From Ref. 69.)

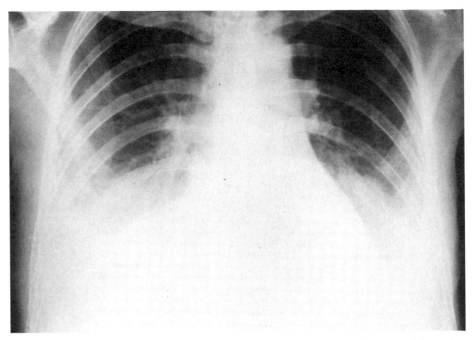

Figure 4c Basal effusions due to bilateral subphrenic abscesses developing several days after emergency colectomy. Multiple colonic perforations were present at operation.

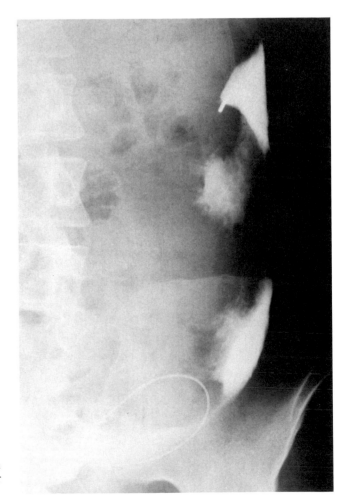

Figure 4d Extensive intraabdominal sepsis. A sinogram shows a pelvic collection extending into the left paracolic gutter space and superiorly to the left subphrenic cavity.

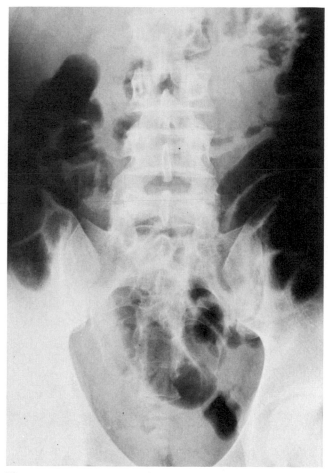

Figure 5a

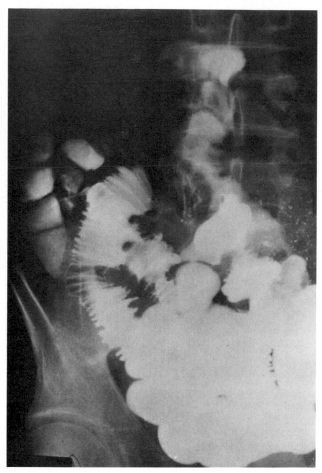

Figure 5b

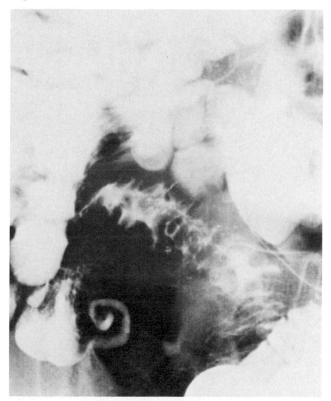

Figure 5c

Figure 5 (a) The patient was admitted with suspected appendicitis. The plain film shows some dilated small bowel and the suggestion of a soft tissue mass in the right iliac fossa, compatible with an appendix mass. (b) Edematous distal ileal loops. (c) Compression view showing a normal appendix and acute Crohn's disease of the terminal ileum. At operation an abscess was found surrounding the terminal ileum.

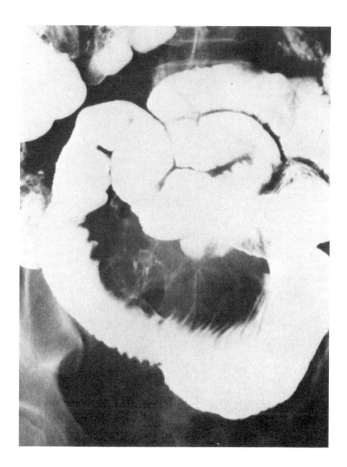

Figure 6 Terminal ileal disease with perforation and abscess formation causing displacement and extrinsic compression on one side of the bowel loop surrounding the abscess.

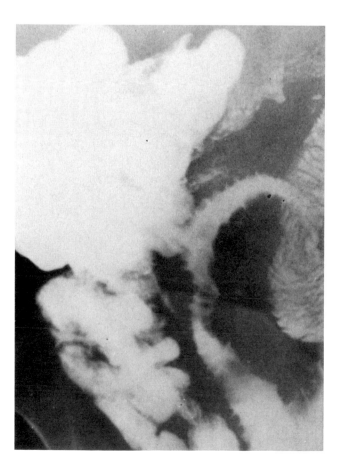

Figure 7 Bowel wall thickening around an ileal loop displacing normal adjacent bowel equally on either side.

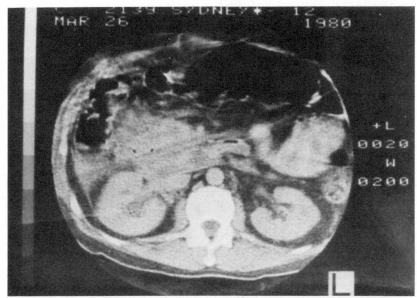

Figure 8a

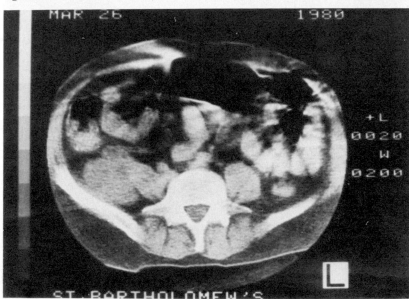

Figure 8b

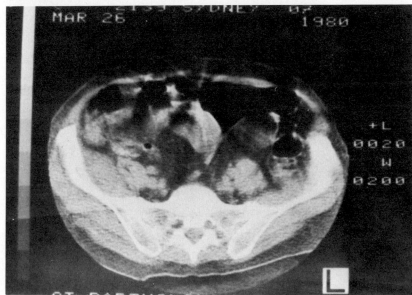

Figure 8 The patient presented with a fixed flexion of the right hip. (a) Computerized axial tomography shows a large abscess mass anterior to the right kidney. This was due to a perforation in small bowel Crohn's disease. (b) The abscess extended inferiorly and retroperitoneally to involve the right iliacus and psoas muscles. (c) Swollen right iliopsoas muscle.

Figure 8c

185

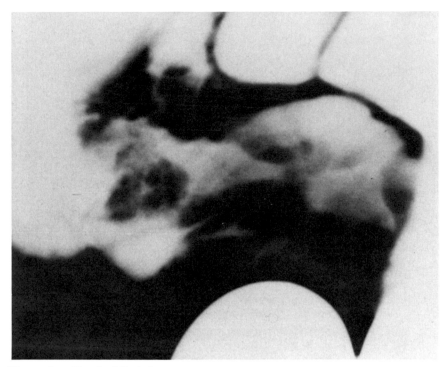

Figure 9a Terminal ileal disease.

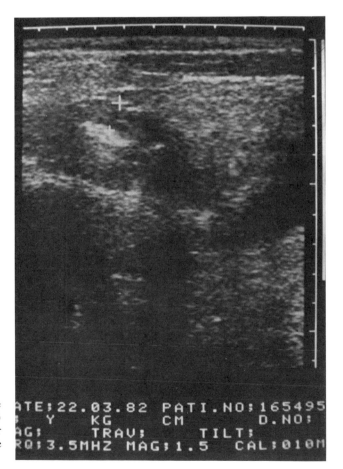

Figure 9b Ultrasonography in a transverse plane to the terminal ileum (using an Aloka SS 250 real-time scanner) clearly defines a sonolucent zone 10 mm thick (see the caliper markers) which represents the thickened bowel wall. The luminal contents are echogenic.

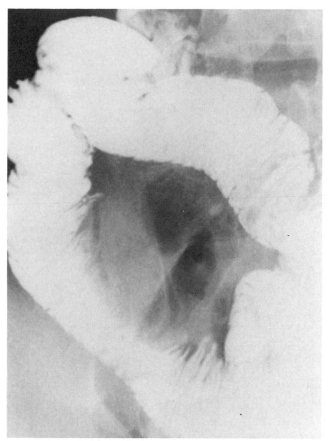

Figure 10a Extrinsic compression of distal small bowel from a mass in the right iliac fossa.

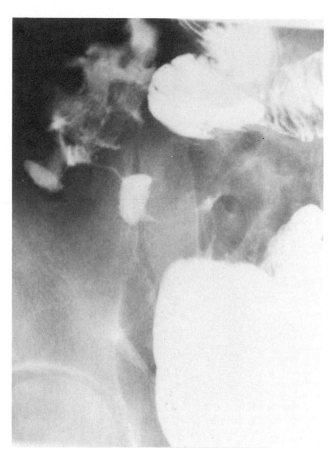

Figure 10b Diseased terminal ileum with stricturing.

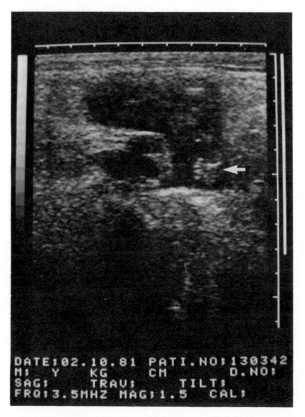

Figure 10c Ultrasonography in a oblique plane over the pelvic brim. A large poorly defined echogenic area inferiorly (arrow) represents the lumen of the ileum in (a). The remainder of the mass was a mixture of acute inflammatory change, mesenteric thickening, and a small abscess.

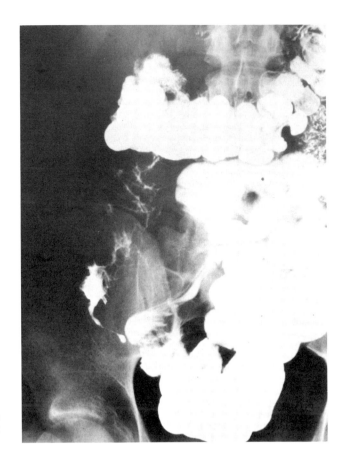

Figure 11a There is a large mass in the right iliac fossa displacing the small bowel and compressing the ascending colon. The appendix is normal.

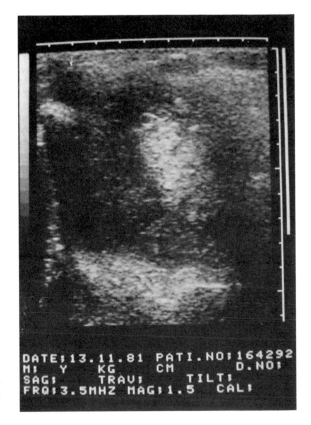

Figure 11b Ultrasonography in the sagittal plane showing an echogenic area of gas in the bowel lumen surrounded by a large poorly demarcated sonolucent area. A very large abscess was drained at operation.

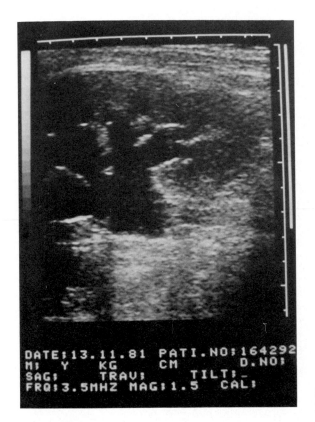

DATE:13.11.81 PATI.NO:164292
M: Y KG CM D.NO:
SAG: TRAV: TILT:-
FRQ:3.5MHZ MAG:1.5 CAL:

Figure 11c Obstructed right kidney with marked hydrone-phrosis.

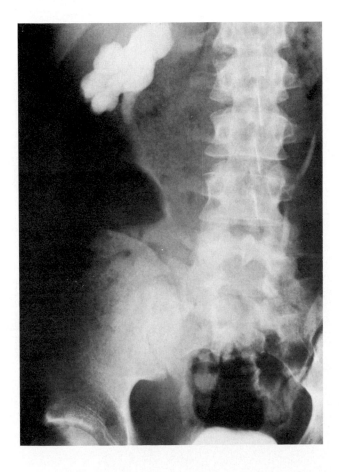

Figure 11d This was confirmed on an intravenous urogram. Note the compression and displacement of the abdominal ureter by the abscess.

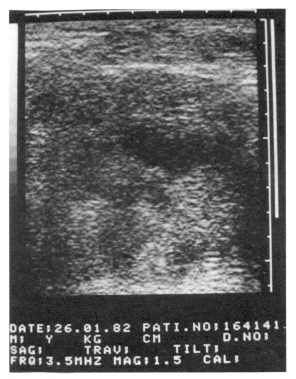

Figure 12a Sonolucent band extending across the pelvic brim into the right side of the pelvis.

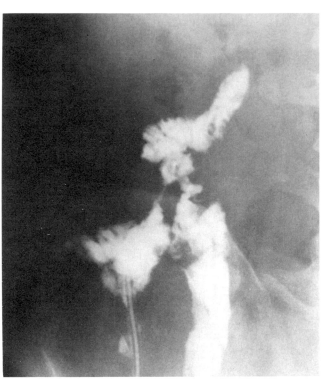

Figure 12b Sinogram confirms a abscess cavity in the right iliac fossa that communicates with small bowel.

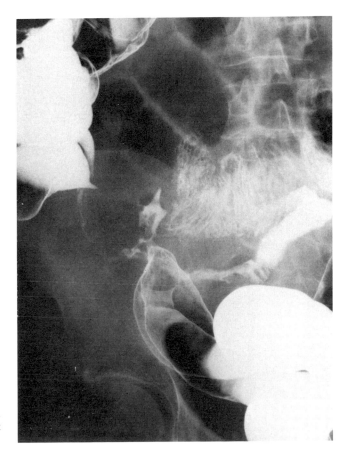

Figure 13 Ileosigmoid fistula, with extensive ileal disease and virtually no involvement of the colon except for the fistula site.

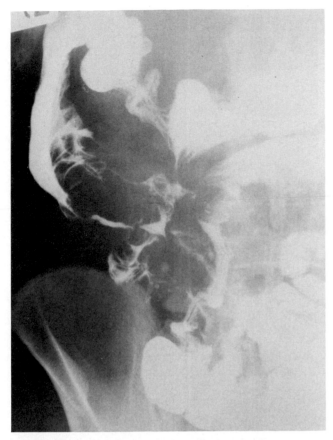

Figure 14 Multiple fistula between ileum and colon.

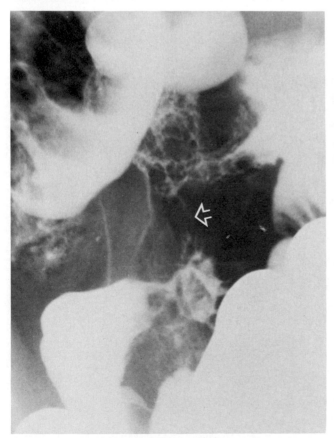

Figure 15a Fistula between distal small bowel and transverse colon (arrow) shown on small bowel meal.

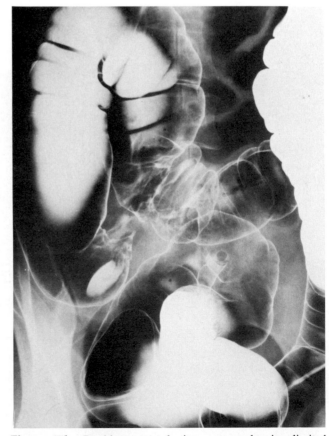

Figure 15b Double-contrast barium enema showing limited disease around the site of the fistula. The small bowel has not filled.

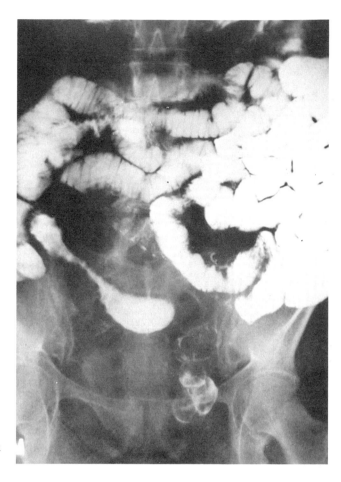

Figure 16a Premature filling of the sigmoid colon during a small bowel examination.

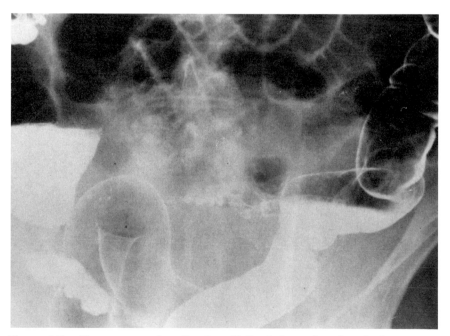

Figure 16b The presence of an ileosigmoid fistula is confirmed on barium enema. (From Ref. 69.)

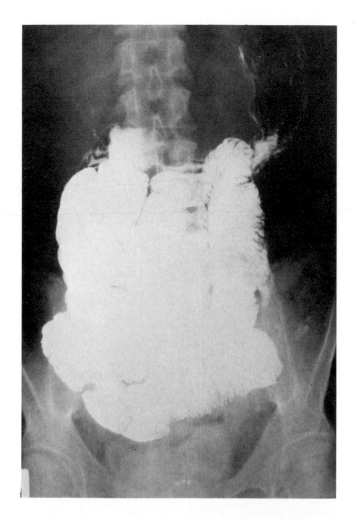

Figure 17a Following a limited small bowel resection this patient had intermittent discharge of bowel contents from a small sinus opening. The small bowel examination did not show any fistula.

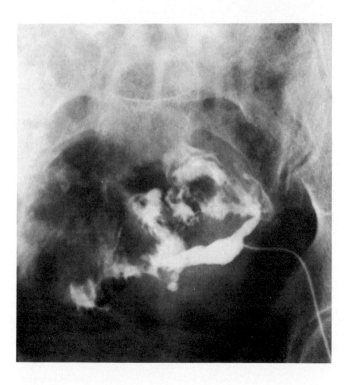

Figure 17b Sinogram using a fine polythene catheter to enter the small cutaneous opening demonstrated two short tracks leading into small bowel.

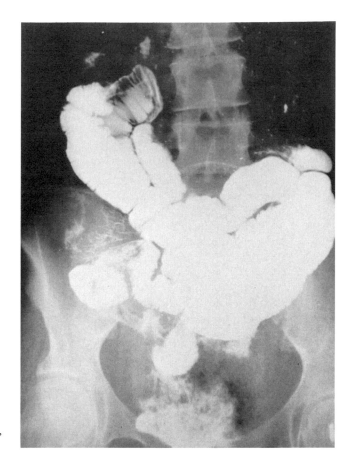

Figure 18a Premature filling of the distal small bowel, suggesting an ileosigmoid fistula.

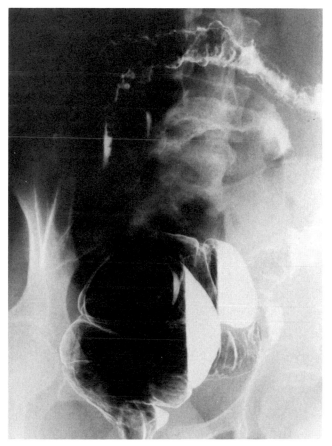

Figure 18b The fistula did not fill on double-contrast barium enema, but its presence was confirmed at operation.

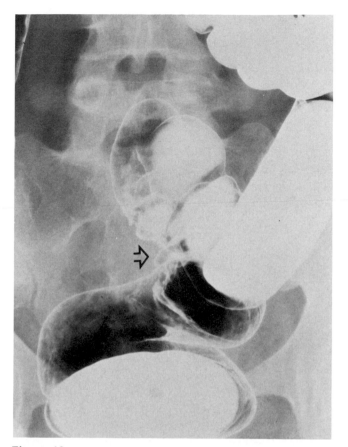

Figure 19

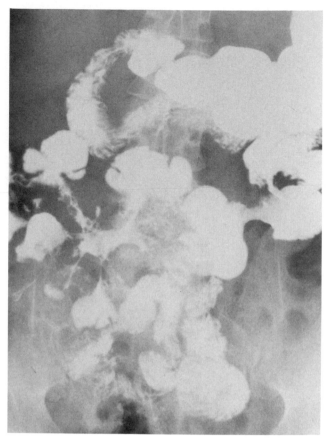

Figure 20

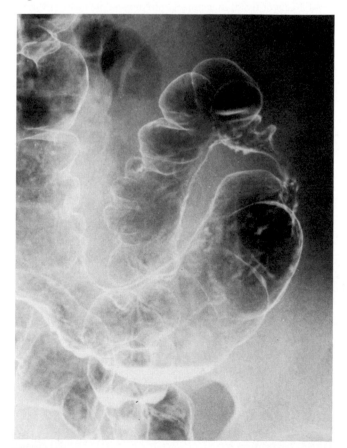

Figure 21

Figure 19 Deformity of the lateral wall of the sigmoid (arrow) due to adherent diseased small bowel with contiguous spread of the Crohn's disease.

Figure 20 Multiple ileal fistulas arranged in a radial fashion. This patient presented with an episode of severe gastrointestinal hemorrhage.

Figure 21 Colonic stricture. Note the angulation of the stricture, the presence of pseudodiverticula, and ulceration on the antimesenteric border.

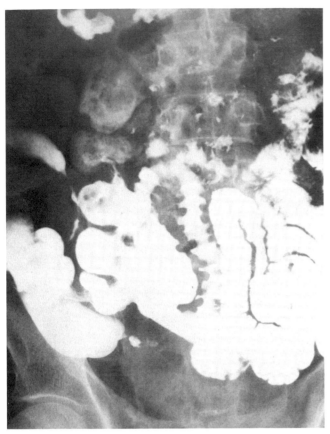

Figure 22a Distal ileal involvement with stricturing treated by resection.

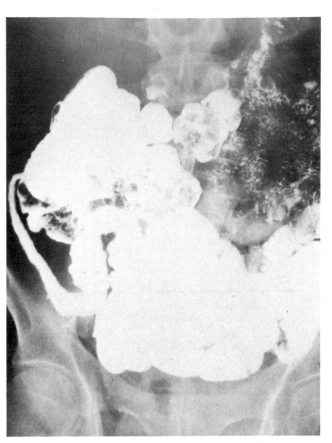

Figure 22b Seven years later there is recurrent disease in the distal 20 cm of ileum immediately proximal to the anastomeosis.

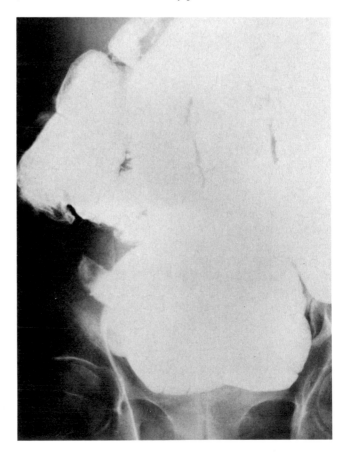

Figure 22c One year later the patient presented with small bowel obstruction. A very narrow stricture is seen at the anastomosis and required resection.

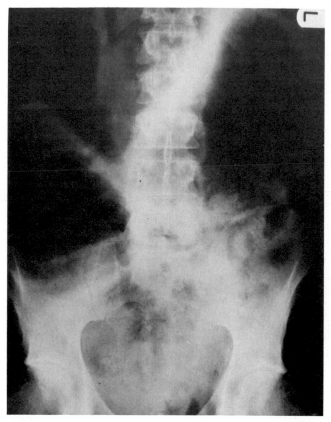

Figure 23

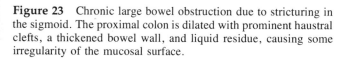

Figure 23 Chronic large bowel obstruction due to stricturing in the sigmoid. The proximal colon is dilated with prominent haustral clefts, a thickened bowel wall, and liquid residue, causing some irregularity of the mucosal surface.

Figure 24 (a) This patient presented with obstruction. There was no history to suggest Crohn's disease and a small bowel meal was performed. (b) This showed a number of strictures throughout the small bowel (arrows).

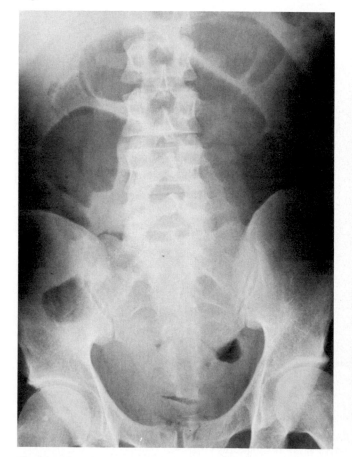

Figure 24a

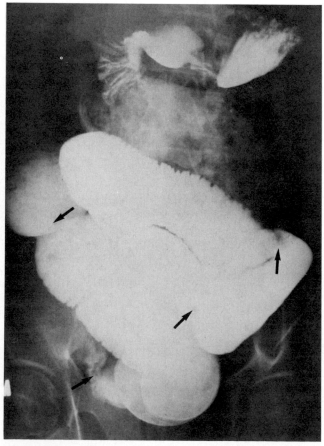

Figure 24b

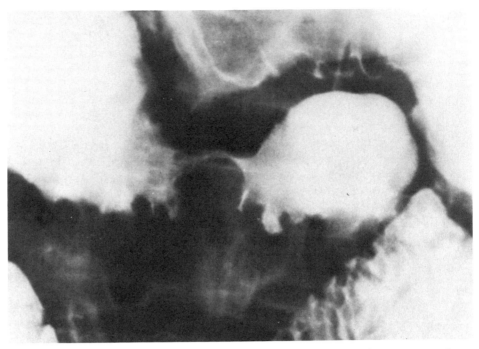

Figure 25 A short narrow stricture in the ileum in a patient with obstructive symptoms, shown on compression spot film during a small bowel enema.(From Ref. 70.)

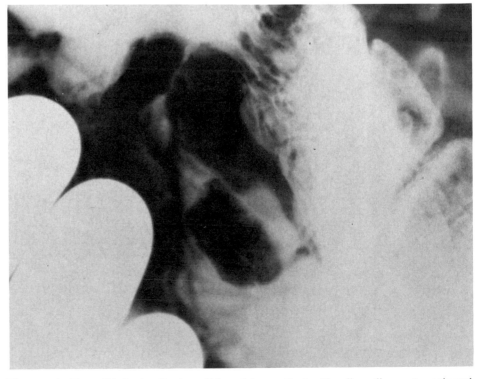

Figure 26 Enterolith in the distal small bowel in a patient with a ileocolic anastomosis and recurrent disease with stricturing at the anastomosis.

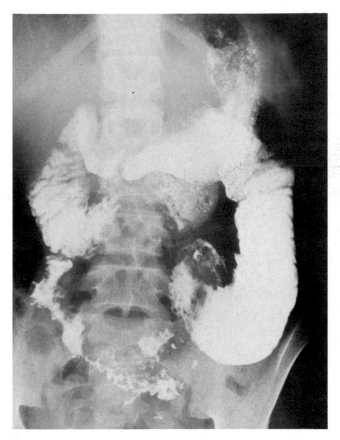

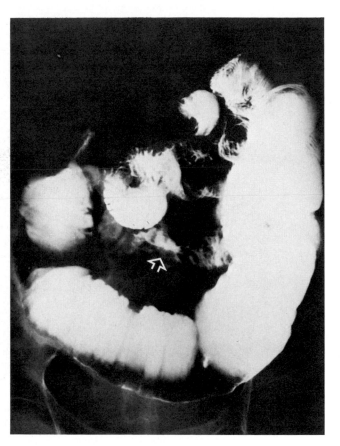

Figure 27 Jejunal dilatation proximal to a strictured sigment.

Figure 28 Recurrent disease (arrow) in a patient with an ileostomy. There is marked dilatation of the jejunum proximally.

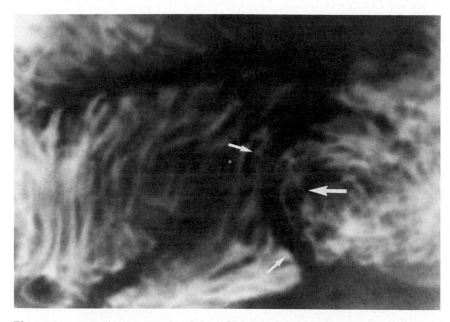

Figure 29 Adhesion between two loops of jejunum (arrows). Compression showed that the loops were fixed together. Note the normal gap separating the loops and retention of the fold pattern, although the folds are distorted running toward the fixed angulations.

199

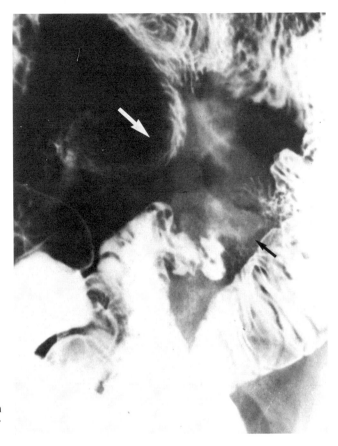

Figure 30 Large band adhesion (arrows) in a patient with an ileostomy and multiple operation for Crohn's disease. (From Ref. 69.)

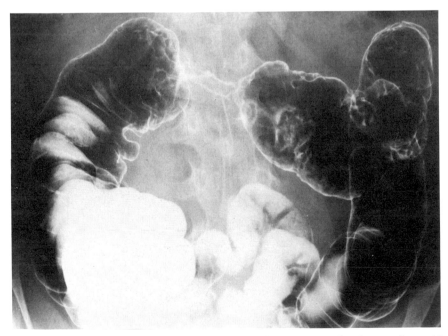

Figure 31 Suspicious annular stricture in the midtransverse colon in a patient with Crohn's disease and inflammatory polyps. Endoscopically, this proved to be benign.

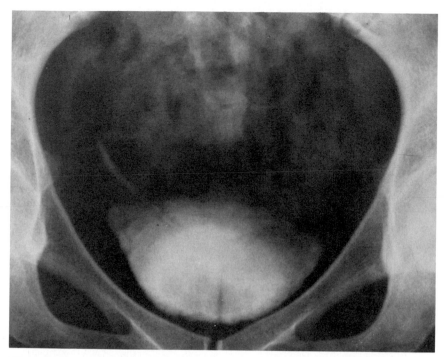

Figure 32a Air bubbles in the bladder in a patient with Crohn's disease complaining of pneumaturia.

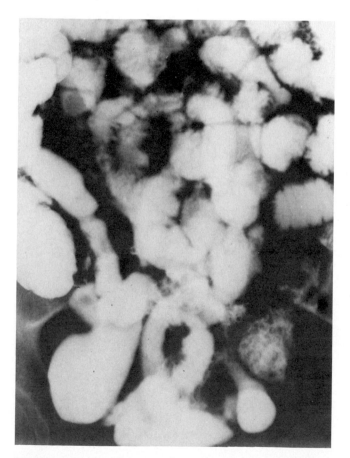

Figure 32b Ileal disease shown on small bowel meal. The presence of a fistula was confirmed at cystoscopy.

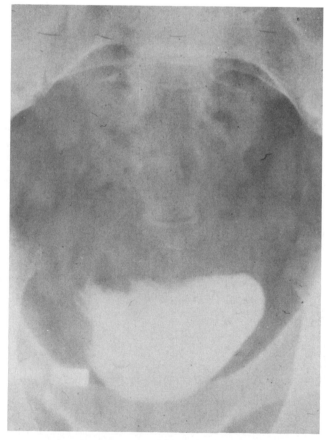

Figure 33 Illeal disease adherent to the bladder, causing deformity and a spiculated edge to the right side of the bladder.

6

Diagnostic Problems in Inflammatory Bowel Disease

MINIMAL CHANGE COLITIS

"Minimal change" describes a colitis that can be seen endoscopically, confirmed on biopsy, but is not visible on a good-quality double-contrast barium enema. The reasons for this vary with the type of colitis.

The earliest endoscopic abnormality in ulcerative colitis is loss of vessel pattern. This can occur before there is any gross alteration of the surface structure, so that the layer of barium coating the mucosa appears normal. Secondary changes in the configuration of the bowel wall also tend to be absent in such early stages (Figs. 1–3). Further evidence for minimal change in ulcerative colitis comes from comparisons with sigmoidoscopy and the assessment of the extent of colitis by colonoscopy.

About 3–12% of patients proven to have a proctitis at sigmoidoscopy may have a normal rectal mucosa at barium enema (1–3) (Fig. 4). Comparative studies with endoscopy as to the extent of the colitis are a little more difficult to interpret. Some allowance must be made for the problem of colonoscopic localization, as it may be difficult for the endoscopist to appreciate exactly which part of the colon is being observed. Experience with polyps suggests that there is often a considerable difference between the position assumed at colonoscopy and that shown radiologically. Nevertheless, there is definite evidence that radiology underestimates both the visual and histological extent of ulcerative colitis. Deliwari et al. (4) found that in 80 patients, colonoscopy showed more extensive disease than radiology in 6, and that in 8 histological changes were more extensive than the endoscopic abnormality. The type of barium enema was not stated. Warwick et al. (5) reported that in a group of 11 patients, biopsy in 8 showed more extensive disease than did radiology. In one patient total colitis was present when radiologically it seemed to extend only into the transverse colon. Endoscopy was abnormal in only 4 of these patients, and as pointed out by Laufer (6), the double-contrast examinations were perhaps not ideal. A comparative study in

22 patients using the instant enema showed that this underestimated the extent of colitis in 32% (7). The instant enema does not show the proximal colon well. The term "extensive colitis" is used to denote total histological involvement when the colitis appears to extend radiologically only to the hepatic flexure (Fig. 5). The validity of this concept has been proven by studying resected specimens (8). The instant enema is a limited examination, and this is one of its disadvantages.

In a recent study (9), comparisons of the extent of ulcerative colitis assessed by double-contrast barium enema, colonoscopy, and endoscopic biopsies revealed total colitis in 38 patients on histological or endoscopic evidence. In only 5 patients was the colitis total on double-contrast barium enema, in 29 partial colitis was thought to be present, and in 4 the barium enema was normal. In 17 patients the evidence for total colitis was purely histological.

These findings all suggest that there is a gradual transition in ulcerative colitis, from structural mucosal changes that can be seen radiologically, to vascular alterations that can be seen only on endoscopy, to a histological abnormality that is not visible on either. If this is accepted, it is then conceivable that a patient may have a colitis that is visible only endoscopically, because at no point is it severe enough to alter the mucosal surface. In a search for such patients only 10 could be found at St. Mark's and St. Bartholomew's hospitals in whom a double-contrast barium enema of adequate technical quality had been reported as normal, but colonoscopy performed within a month had been abnormal and shown a colitis of substantial extent. Sigmoidoscopy was normal in 8 of these patients, but rectal biopsy abnormal in 8 or 9. Seven had ulcerative colitis and 3 had Crohn's disease. Three observers compared the barium enemas of this group to 10 barium enemas of noncolitics and 10 with early but definite changes of colitis. In 4 patients with minimal change all three observers considered the barium enema to be normal (10), confirming that minimal change colitis exists.

The problem in Crohn's disease is slightly different. In its earliest manifestations small erythematous areas may be seen endoscopically, but as there is no ulceration typical "aphthoid ulcers" will not be visible radiologically. Hypertrophy of lymphoid follicles has been suggested as a preulcerative stage that can be recognized radiologically, but this may be seen in patients without colitis, and there is no good evidence linking this to Crohn's disease. Biopsies around the edge of these small lesions may be abnormal, but those of the mucosa in between quite normal. The diagnosis of this very early stage of Crohn's colitis therefore rests with the endoscopist.

Minimal change has several implications for the radiologist, the principal one being that even an excellent double-contrast barium enema does not exclude colitis. This does not mean that every patient requires colonoscopy. If sigmoidoscopy and rectal biopsy are normal, a normal double-contrast barium enema virtually excludes colitis and leaves only a very small group of patients with minimal change colitis and rectal sparing. Colonoscopy and biopsy are indicated only when there is some specific feature in either the patient's history or laboratory tests to suggest the presence of a colitis.

The true extent of a colitis can really only be demonstrated histologically. The clinical significance of "histological colitis" is somewhat uncertain. This has been the sole abnormality in only a few patients at St. Mark's and St. Bartholomew's hospitals (Fig. 2). On follow-up two have developed overt changes of colitis. Minimal change colitis would not appear to alter the risk factors for carcinoma in ulcerative colitis. Radiology has been used for many years to assess the extent of colitis, and its value in demonstrating "extensive colitis" as a risk factor has been clearly documented.

One of the indications for the instant enema is to show the extent of a colitis. Minimal change means that this will be underestimated to varying degrees. This does not invalidate the instant enema but qualifies the information that it gives. When a radiologist reports that a colitis extends to a certain point, this refers to the overt mucosal changes, not the most proximal extent of the histological abnormality.

DIFFER-ENTIATION OF ULCERATIVE FROM CROHN'S COLITIS

It is usually possible to make a diagnosis of Crohn's disease or ulcerative colitis from a visual inspection of the resected colon (11). The double-contrast barium enema provides a comparable although indirect view of the mucosa, and should also be able to distinguish these forms of colitis. However, in several series a definitive diagnosis could not be made in 10–15% of cases in colons resected for nonspecific inflammatory bowel disease confined to the large bowel (12–15). This difficulty reflects the overlapping pathological features of Crohn's disease and ulcerative colitis and indicates the lack of clear definitions of the diseases.

It is difficult to define a disease when the etiology is unknown. To identify a single disease within a group of similar disorders depends on being able to recognize a defining factor. This usually implies a knowledge of the etiology, as, for example, in the infective forms of colitis. Where the etiology is not known it is necessary to find a factor that is present in every patient with one form of the colitis, but in none with the other, or vice versa, before this could be recognized as a defining factor (16). Such a factor or group of factors has been searched for using numerical taxonomy and discriminant analysis (17). This showed that 5 of the 107 features investigated, a combination of 5 of these—mucous depletion histologically, abnormal anal canal, normal sigmoidoscopy, granular mucosa on barium enema, and tenesmus—could separate 109 patients into two clusters with only about a 4% misclassification. No defining feature was established. The absence of this means that any classification is somewhat arbitrary, as it will be affected by the number and nature of the criteria employed.

It seems likely that Crohn's disease and ulcerative colitis are different disorders with overlapping features. The degree of overlap may not be constant throughout the course of the disease. Price (15) has shown that most patients with indeterminate colitis had resections for fulminating disease. Once toxic megacolon has developed the diseases overlap macroscopically and histologically, so that the original nature of the colitis cannot be determined. When the colitis first presents there is often more overlap than after a while, when as repeat examinations will show, the colitis becomes more clearly defined (18). It is therefore important when reviewing the literature to look not only at the basis of the classification for distinguishing ulcerative colitis and Crohn's disease, but also at the stage of the colitis. Studies that are based on comparisons with resected colons will bias the radiological findings to those found in the more typical chronic stages of the disease, but if resections for acute disease are included, patients with toxic megacolon will increase the overlapping features.

One of the uses of the barium enema is to provide the clinician with some sort of idea as to the likely nature of the colitis. An opinion may have to be given before there are any other pathological data, in which case the only details given to the radiologist will be the clinician's impression as to the type of colitis. This will have been formed from the patient's history, clinical examination, and the appearance of the rectal mucosa at sigmoidoscopy. Specific forms of colitis should, of course, be excluded bacteriologically before radiological investigation. The main symptoms of colitis are diarrhea, rectal bleeding, and abdominal pain. Diarrhea is a prominent symptom of any form of colitis. Rectal bleeding is usually associated with ulcerative colitis (19), but is more common in Crohn's disease (20). Abdominal pain is more typical of Crohn's disease.

Clinical examination of the abdomen may reveal tenderness over the inflamed colon. The presence of a mass suggests Crohn's disease. Inspection of the anus is important. Some redness and small fissures may be found in any acute colitis, but the appearance of the chronic destructive changes of Crohn's disease is a frequent and valuable sign of Crohn's disease.

Sigmoidoscopy is undoubtedly the most important part of the examination. Early changes of proctitis are a granular, friable, or edematous mucosa, which progresses in acute disease to ulceration with mucopus. Studies in observer variation indicate that it is unwise to overinterpret the changes (21). The mucosa should first be classified as either normal or abnormal, and if abnormal, whether the disease is continuous or discontinuous. The severity is judged best from the presence of contact or spontaneous bleeding (21). Discontinuous disease indicates Crohn's disease, but the frequency of rectal sparing limits the value of sigmoidoscopy, so that it may be diagnostic in only 16–29% of cases of Crohn's disease (20,22).

The consensus view of the double-contrast features of ulcerative colitis is of a diffuse symmetrical disease with a granular mucosa that is continuous from its proximal extent to the distal colon (23) (Fig. 6). In contrast, Crohn's disease is considered an asymmetric disease, with discontinuous involvement and discrete mucosal ulceration (24,25) (Fig. 7). This neat division has recently been challenged (26,27) by reports of a diffuse superficial colitis in Crohn's disease that mimics ulcerative colitis. The absolute discriminatory value of some of the standard radiographic signs must be questioned. The individual signs are discussed in detail next.

Discriminatory Radiographic Signs 1. *Granularity.* Since its original description by Welin and Brahme (23), granularity has been considered the characteristic change in ulcerative colitis and specific to it, as it was not seen in Crohn's disease (24,25,28). One of the problems of this sign is that it describes a wide range of changes. Granularity can describe an amorphous coating with a fine (Fig. 8) to coarse texture, or a stippled effect. Only a broad definition, such as a diffuse superficial mucosal irregularity without overt ulceration, would encompass all the radiological appearances that are collectively termed "granularity." Its texture may relate to the endoscopic findings (29), but it is difficult to establish any histological connection (8) among its variations. Should Crohn's disease present with a diffuse superficial colitis without deep ulceration it would not be unreasonable to expect the mucosa to appear "granular" radiologically. This has been noted in the occasional patient (26), and recently four cases of Crohn's disease with a granular mucosa on double-contrast barium enema have been reported (27). In a review (22), of 54 patients presenting for the first time with colitis and without any small bowel disease, 10 of 29 of the patients finally considered to have Crohn's disease showed a granular type of mucosal pattern on double-contrast barium enema, and in 7 (24%) this was the sole abnormality. Sometimes there is a transverse component to the stippling (Fig. 9), which is suggestive of Crohn's disease, but in many there is no distinguishing feature to the granularity (Figs. 10–12). A granular mucosa may be typical of ulcerative colitis, but does not exclude Crohn's disease.

2. *Discrete ulceration.* This may be applied to an ulcer of any configuration that is surrounded by a flat normal mucosa. Rarely, isolated ulcers can be seen in ulcerative colitis, but then the surrounding mucosa is abnormal. Discrete ulcers, either aphthoid or punched out, set in normal mucosa are typical of Crohn's disease and may be the only manifestation (Figs. 13 and 14) or seen in part usually at the ends of an involved segment where the disease is merging into normal.

3. *Confluent ulceration.* This described ulceration where no flat mucosa can be seen between the ulcers as these are so numerous and closely packed. Any remaining mucosa becomes pseudopolypoid. Confluent ulceration may be seen in both ulcerative colitis and Crohn's disease, but in ulcerative colitis only during a severe attack (Figs. 15 and 16).

4. *Depth of ulceration.* The depth of an ulcer is measured in profile from the base of the ulcer to the summit of the adjacent mucosa. An ulcer less than 3 mm may be considered

shallow; and one more than 3 mm, deep. Deep ulceration in ulcerative colitis occurs only in fulminating disease; otherwise, it is found only in Crohn's disease, where fissuring-type ulcers extend down into thickened bowel wall (Fig. 17).

5. *Bowel wall thickness*. The thickness of the bowel wall may be measured from the mucosal surface to the properitoneal fat line (Fig. 18). The normal thickness is 2 mm, but may be increased up to 5 mm in Crohn's disease or ulcerative colitis (30) (Fig. 19). A thickness of more than 5 mm indicates Crohn's disease (Fig. 20). Confluent shallow ulceration may be seen in both, but in about 50% of Crohn's disease the wall thickness will exceed 5 mm, so this may be a useful discriminatory sign in this particular situation.

6. *Fistula*. Spontaneous enteroenteric fistulas never occur in ulcerative colitis (19), so they are diagnostic of Crohn's disease. Small anal fistulas may be seen in acute ulcerative colitis, but multiple anal fistulas are typical of chronic Crohn's disease (Fig. 21).

7. *Configuration of the bowel*. This may be altered by changes in smooth muscle tone or fibrosis. Any active colitis will alter the smooth muscle tone so that haustration is lost. Marked shortening of the colon is typical of ulcerative colitis, but is not a usual feature of Crohn's disease (31) (Fig. 22). Strictures may be found in both, but tend to be asymmetric in Crohn's disease, whereas in ulcerative colitis they are symmetric. Deformed haustration and pseudodiverticula are typical features of Crohn's disease.

8. *Distribution of the lesions*. Rectal sparing is more common in Crohn's disease than in ulcerative colitis, where it is seen in only about 5% of cases (19). Even if the rectum appears normal sigmoidoscopically and radiologically, rectal biopsy should be abnormal in ulcerative colitis, although it may be normal in Crohn's disease. Rectal sparing in ulcerative colitis may develop following healing of the disease by treatment with steroid enemas (Fig. 23). When an acute attack supervenes, the rectum often remains relatively unaffected in spite of severe disease in the sigmoid. The apparent sparing should not be taken as an indication of Crohn's disease.

A right sided-colitis implies Crohn's disease, as in ulcerative colitis the colitis would be in continuity with the distal colon. However, ulcerative colitis is not uniformly active (32). Segments of involved bowel may be more active than others. If the disease is active proximally but quiescent distally, the radiological changes will be more dramatic proximally and might at first glance, suggest right-sided colitis (Fig. 24).

Variations in activity may also account for the reports of skip lesions in ulcerative colitis (33). As with the reports of right-sided ulcerative colitis, these have been exaggerated by the use of single-contrast barium enemas, which failed to show the early changes of colitis in less active segments of the bowel. A skip lesion in ulcerative colitis on a double-contrast barium enema is very rare (Fig. 25) (26), and should always make one question the diagnosis.

By contrast, variations in activity and asymmetrical involvement are characteristic features of Crohn's disease. Lesions at different stages are often close together, so that apthoid ulcers may be adjacent to deep ulceration with pseudodiverticular change. The lesions vary, both transversely across the lumen of the bowel and longitudinally. One side of the lumen may be ulcerated when the other is normal, transverse asymmetry; or along the length of the bowel two abnormal segments may be separated by normal bowel, a skip lesion (Fig. 26).

In conclusion, several statements can be made regarding the value of radiology in the distinction between ulcerative colitis and Crohn's disease.

1. The presence of one or more of the following features excludes a diagnosis of ulcerative colitis:

    a. Aphthoid/discrete ulceration
    b. Deep ulceration
    c. Pseudodiverticula

d. Asymmetric involvement—transversely or longitudinally

e. Spontaneous enteroenteric fistula

f. Multiple anal fistulas

These are typical findings in about three-quarters of patients with Crohn's colitis without small bowel involvement.

2. A granular mucosa on double-contrast barium enema is typical of ulcerative colitis but does not exclude Crohn's disease, as up to one-quarter of patients with Crohn's disease may present with a superficial diffuse colitis.

3. As a consequence of the above a definitive radiological diagnosis of ulcerative colitis is not possible.

4. With acute disease the two forms of colitis merge, so that when toxic megacolon has developed it may be impossible to differentiate them pathologically.

5. In time the features of the colitis become more typical, so that there is less difficulty radiologically in distinguishing long-standing colitis.

REFERENCES

1. Simpkins, K.C., Stevenson, G.W. (1972). The modified Malmo double contrast enema in colitis: as assessment of its accuracy in reflecting sigmoidoscopic findings. Br. J. Radiol. 45; 486.

2. Young, A.C. (1969). The instant enema in procto-colitis. Proc. R. Soc. Med. 56; 491.

3. Kinsey, I., Hornes, N., Antonisen, P., Riss, P. (1964). The radiological diagnosis of non specific haemorrhagic procto-colitis. Acta Med. Scan. 176; 181.

4. Deliwari, J.B., Parkinson, C, Riddel, R.H., et al. (1973). Colonoscopy in the investigation of ulcerative colitis. Gut 14; 426.

5. Warwick, R.R.G., Sumerling, M.D., Gilmour, M.B., et al. (1973). Colonoscopy and double contrast barium enema in chronic ulcerative colitis. Am. J. Roentgenol. 117; 292.

6. Laufer, I. (1977). Air contrast studies of the colon in inflammatory bowel disease. CRC Crit. Rev. Diagn. Imaging 9; 421.

7. Loose, H.W.C., Williams, C.B. (1974). Barium enema versus colonoscopy. Proc. R. Soc. Med. 67; 1033.

8. Bartram, C.I., Walmesley, K. (1978). A radiological and pathological correlation of the mucosal changes in ulcerative colitis. Clin. Radiol. 29; 323.

9. Gabrielsson, N., Granqvist, S., Sundelin, P., Thorgeirsson, T. (1979). Extent of inflammatory lesions in ulcerative colitis assessed by radiology, colonoscopy and endoscopic biopsies. Gastrointest. Radiol. 4; 395.

10. Elliot, P.R., Williams, C.B., Lennard-Jones, J.E., et al. (1982). Colonoscopic diagnosis of minimal change colitis in patients with a normal sigmoidoscopy and normal air-contrast barium enema. Lancet, 1; 650.

11. Morson, B.C., Dawson, I.M.P. (1979). *Gastrointestinal Pathology*. Blackwell Scientific Publications, Oxford, p. 542.

12. Schachter, H., Rappaport, H., Goldstein, H.J., et al. (1970). Ulcerative and granulomatous colitis—validity of differential diagnostic criteria: a study of 100 patients treated by total colectomy. Ann. Intern. Med. 72; 841.

13. Kent, T.H., Ammon, R.K., Denbesten, L. (1970). Differentiation of ulcerative colitis and regional enteritis of colon. Arch. Pathol. 89; 20.

14. Glotzer, D.J., Gardner, R.C., Goldman, H., et al. (1970). Comparative features and course of ulcerative and granulomatous colitis. N. Engl. J. Med. 282; 582.

15. Price, A.B. (1978). Overlap in the spectrum of non-specific inflammatory bowel disease—"colitis indeterminate." J. Clin. Pathol. 31; 567.

16. Lennard-Jones, J.E. (1971). Definition and diagnosis. Regional enteritis (Crohn's disease). *Skand. Int. Symp.* p. 105.

17. Hywel-Jones, J., Lennard-Jones, J.E., Morson, B.C., et al. (1973). Numerical taxonomy and discriminant analysis. Q. J. Med. 42; 715.

18. Kirsner, J.B. (1975). Problems in the differentiation of ulcerative colitis and Crohn's disease of the colon: the need for repeated diagnostic evaluation. Gastroenterology 68; 187.

19. Lennard-Jones, J.E., Lockhart-Mummery, H.E., Morson, B.C. (1968). Clinical and pathological differentiation of Crohn's disease and procto-colitis. Gastroenterology 54; 1162.

20. Mekhjian, H.S., Switz, D.M., Melynk, C.S., et al. (1979). Clinical features and natural history of Crohn's disease. Gastroenterology 77; 989.

21. Baron, J.H., Connell, A.M., Lennard-Jones, J.E. (1964). Variation between observers in describing mucosal appearances in procto-colitis. Br. Med. J. 1; 89.

22. Donoghue, D., Bartram, C.I., Dawson, A.M., et al. (1982). Differential features of ulcerative and Crohn's colitis. (To be published.)

23. Welin, S., Brahme, F. (1961). The double contrast method in ulcerative colitis. Acta Radiol. 55; 257.

24. Laufer, I., Hamilton, J. (1976). The radiological differentiation between ulcerative and granulomatous colitis by double contrast radiology. Am. J. Gastroenterol. 66; 259.

25. Kelvin, F.M., Oddson, T.A., Rice, R.P., et al. (1978). Double contrast barium enema in Crohn's disease and ulcerative colitis. Am. J. Roentgenol. 131; 207.

26. Bartram, C.I. (1977). Radiology in the current assessment of ulcerative colitis. Gastroenterol. Radiol. 1; 383.

27. Joffe N. (1981). Diffuse mucosal granularity in double contrast studies of Crohn's disease of the colon. Clin. Radiol. 32; 85.

28. Brahme, F. (1967). Granulomatous colitis: roentgenologic appearance and course of lesions. Am. J. Roentgenol. 99; 35.

29. Laufer, I., Mullens, J.E., Hamilton, J. (1976). Correlation of endoscopic and double contrast radiography in the early stages of ulcerative and granulomatous colitis. Radiology 118; 1.

30. Bartram, C.I., Herlinger, H. (1979). Bowel wall thickness as a differentiating feature between ulcerative colitis and Crohn's disease of the colon. Clin. Radiol. 30; 15.

31. Marshak, R.J. (1975). Granulomatous disease of the intestinal tract. Radiology. 114; 3.

32. Morson, B.C. (1980). Pathology of ulcerative colitis. In *Inflammatory Bowel Disease* Kirsner, J.B., Shorter, R.G. (Eds.). Lea & Febiger, Philadelphia, p. 282.

33. Margulis, A.R., Goldbergh, I., Lawson, T.L., et al. (1971). The overlapping spectrum of ulcerative colitis and granulomatous colitis. A roentgenographic-pathologic study. Am. J. Roentgenol. 113; 325.

FIGURES 1 THROUGH 26

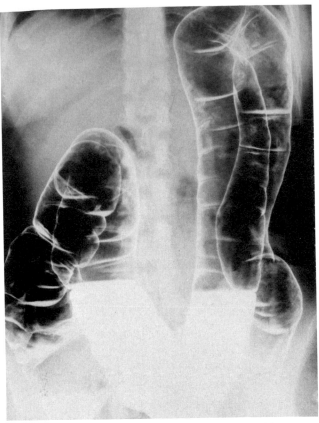

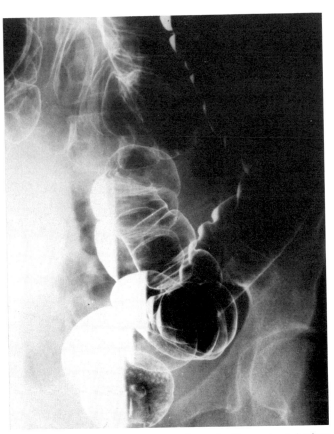

Figure 1 Minimal change colitis. Normal double-contrast barium enema. Colonoscopy showed total early ulcerative colitis.

Figure 2 The colon was normal on double-contrast barium enema and colonoscopy, but biopsies showed extensive minimal ulcerative colitis.

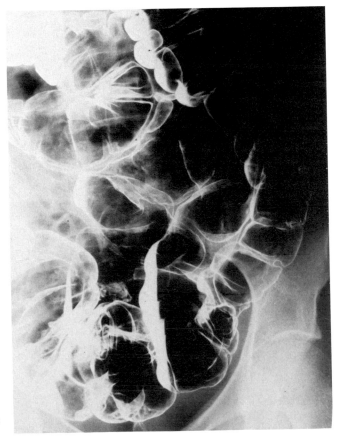

Figure 3 Minimal change colitis to the splenic flexure shown on endoscopy.

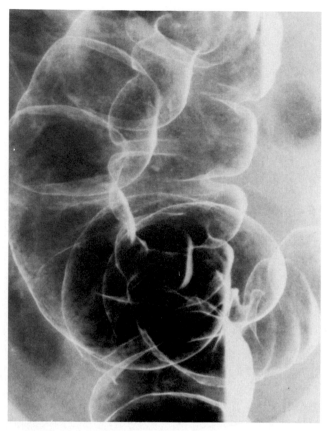

Figure 4 Proctitis on sigmoidoscopy. Radiologically, the rectal mucosa appears normal.

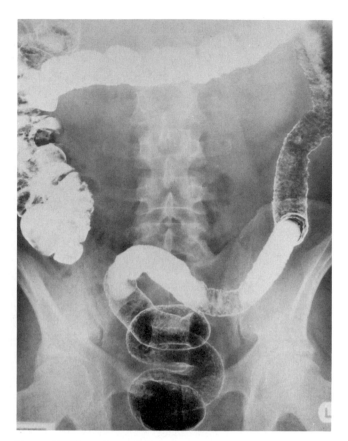

Figure 5 Extensive colitis on instant enema. Total histological involvement, although radiologically the colitis extends proximally only to the hepatic flexure.

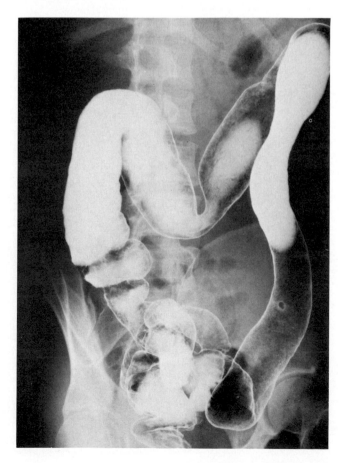

Figure 6 Typical ulcerative colitis with a granular mucosa and diffuse involvement in continuity.

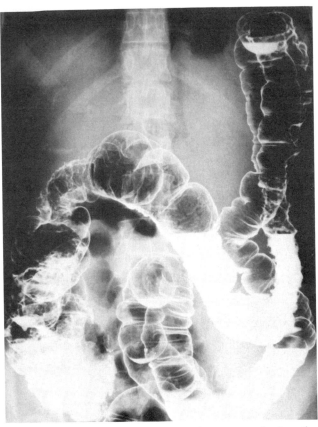

Figure 7 Typical Crohn's disease. Patchy asymmetric ulceration with rectal sparing.

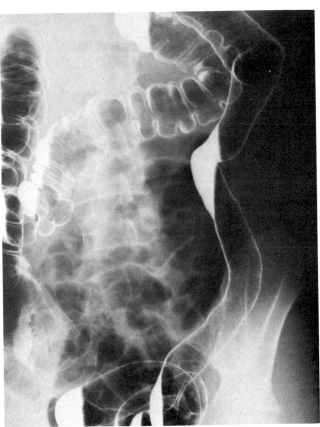

Figure 8 Ulcerative colitis with a fine granular mucosa extending in continuity from the rectum to its proximal extent in the splenic flexure.

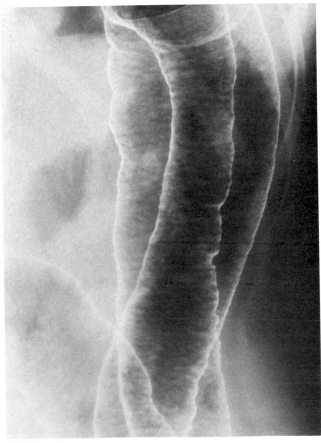

Figure 9 "Transverse" stippling in Crohn's disease.

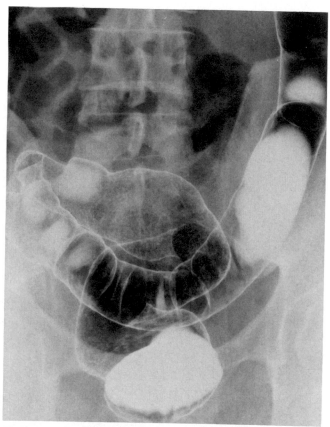

Figure 10 Distal colitis with a granular mucosa in Crohn's disease.

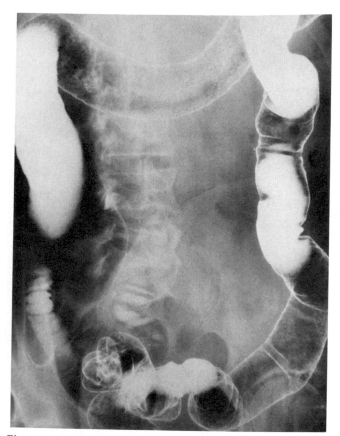

Figure 11 Total colitis with a granular mucosa in Crohn's disease.

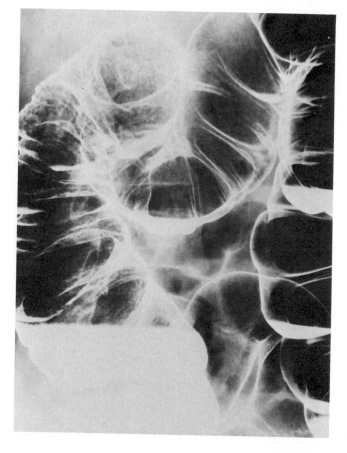

Figure 12 "Right-sided" colitis with a granular mucosa in Crohn's disease.

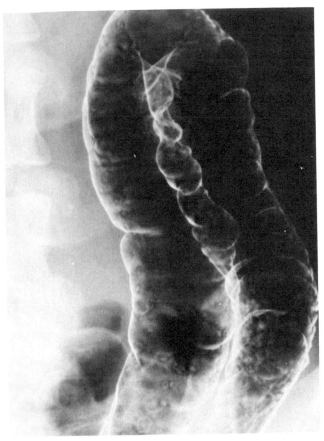

Figure 13 Aphthoid ulceration in Crohn's disease throughout the colon.

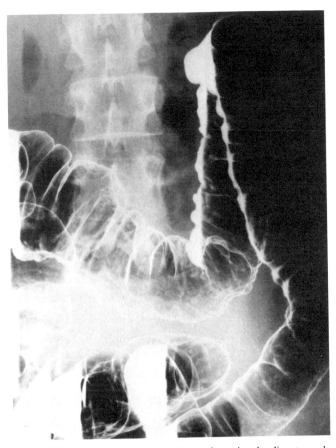

Figure 14 Aphthoid and some linear ulceration leading to early pseudodiverticula formation in Crohn's colitis.

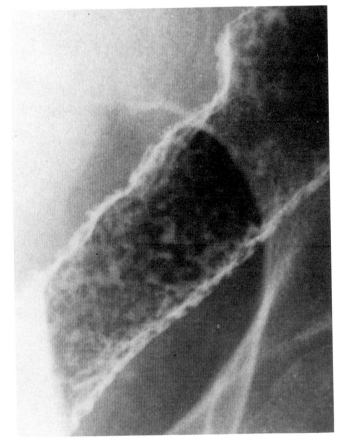

Figure 15 Superficial confluent ulceration in ulcerative colitis.

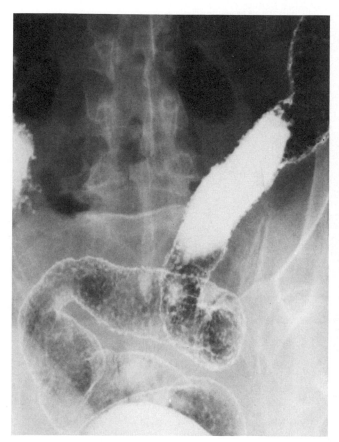

Figure 16 Superficial confluent ulceration in Crohn's disease.

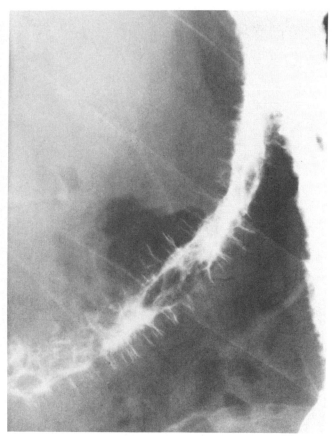

Figure 17 Deep fissuring ulcers in Crohn's disease.

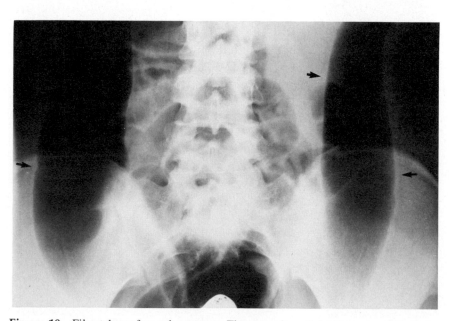

Figure 18 Film taken after colonoscopy. The properitoneal fat line around the colon shows very clearly (arrows).

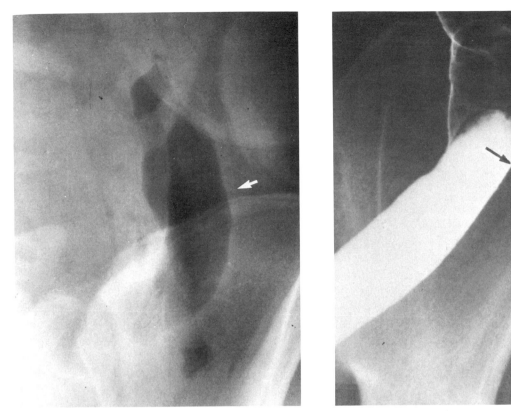

Figure 19 Bowel wall thickness of 4 mm in ulcerative colitis. Arrows show the serosal surface of the bowel wall outlined by properitoneal fat.

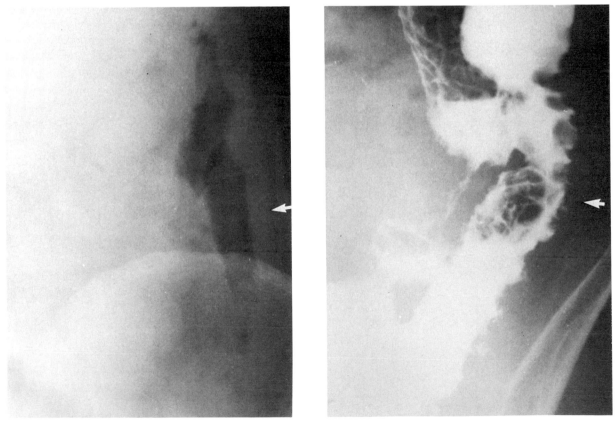

Figure 20 Bowel wall thickness of 8 mm in Crohn's disease. Arrows show the serosal surface of the bowel wall outlined by properitoneal fat.

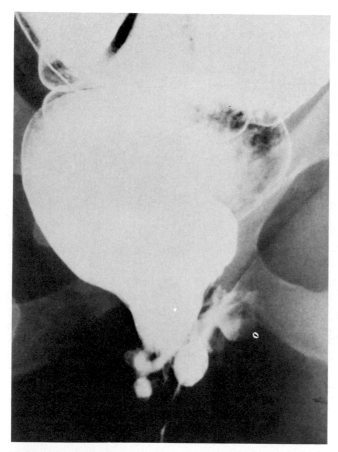

Figure 21 Multiple anal fistula in Crohn's disease.

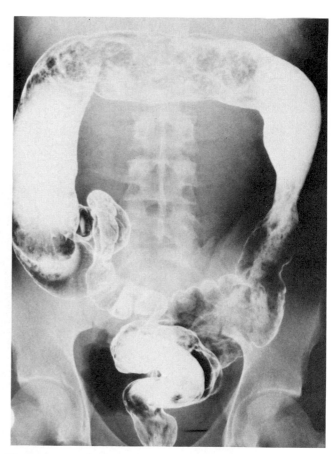

Figure 22 Crohn's disease in a inactive stage with a tubular colon and some shortening, although the bowel is not as narrow as would by typical for ulcerative colitis. Note that the sigmoid is of normal width but the haustra asymmetric and there is rectal sparing—features favoring Crohn's disease.

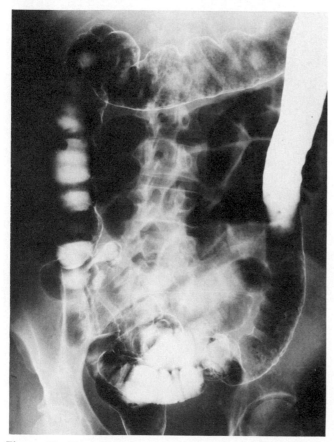

Figure 23 Total ulcerative colitis with rectal sparing.

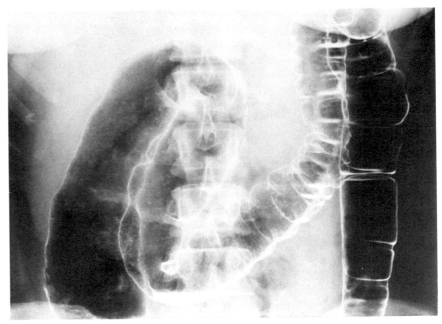

Figure 24 ''Right-sided'' colitis in ulcerative colitis. The descending color appears normal radiologically. Endoscopic and histological changes in the proximal colon were typical of ulcerative colitis.

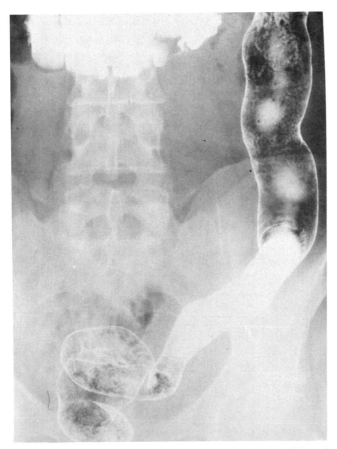

Figure 25 There is a short segment of apparently normal bowel just below the left iliac crest in a patient with ulcerative colitis. Histologically, the colitis was in continuity and this is a rare radiological ''skip'' lesion in ulcerative colitis, due to a localized variation in activity of the colitis.

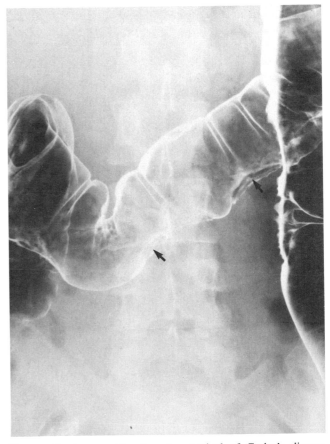

Figure 26 Asymmetric ulceration typical of Crohn's disease (arrows).

7

Differential Diagnosis of Inflammatory Bowel Disease

Having distinguished ulcerative colitis from Crohn's disease, there remains the problem of differentiating other disease processes that may simulate colitis radiologically, and separating the nonspecific forms from ulcerative colitis or Crohn's disease. For example, radiology plays an important part in the diagnosis and investigation of ischemic colitis. The infective forms of colitis are diagnosed bacteriologically, but an exact diagnosis is not always easy and other factors must be considered. The geographical location of the patient affects the probable nature of a colitis, so that, where Crohn's disease might be diagnosed in the West, tuberculosis would be diagnosed in Asia. Amoebiasis is rare outside endemic areas, but a simplistic approach is impossible with widespread emigration and population movements. The infective forms of colitis are important to diagnose, as they are often readily treatable and must be excluded before a final diagnosis of ulcerative colitis or Crohn's disease is made. The radiological findings may not be diagnostic but can be suggestive, and this is very helpful to alert the clinician to the possibility of an infective colitis, so that more intensive investigation can be undertaken.

ISCHEMIC COLITIS

There are a number of causes of ischemic colitis (see Table 1), which although diverse all have a common effect on the bowel—namely, to lower the blood flow below a critical level necessary to maintain its structure and function. Any interruption of the flow of oxygenated blood leads to a complex reaction that is dependent on the severity and length of the ischemia, the adequacy of collaterals, and the ability of affected cells to survive ischemia and to regenerate. Pathologically, ischemia may be divided into an acute phase, with hemorrhage and necrosis, and a reparative phase, with epithelial regeneration, granulation tissue formation, and chronic inflammation with mural fibrosis, which may then leave residual pathology with paramural fibrosis and stricture formation (1).

Table 1 Factors Reducing Mucosal Blood Flow

Large artery occlusion	Non-occlusive	Veno-occlusive	Raised intra-luminal pressure
Atherosclerosis	Cardiac failure	Oral contraceptives	Obstruction
Thrombosis	Shock		
Embolus	Diabetes mellitus	Thrombotic states	
Aortic aneurysm	Rheumatoid arthritis		
Buerger's disease	Collagen disorders		
Mesocolon hematoma	Intravascular coagulation		

The colon has a relatively poor blood supply, particularly at the splenic flexure, which is the junction of the superior and inferior mesenteric systems. Ischemic changes are commonest at this site, but as can be seen from Table 2, any part of the colon, and also the rectum, may be involved.

The layers of the bowel wall are not uniformly affected by ischemia. The mucosa and submucosa are most susceptible. The muscularis is more resistant and the serosa least affected. In the acute stages of ischemia submucosal hemorrhage and edema produce swelling of the mucosa, so that "thumbprinting" may be visible on plain films and barium enema (2,3) (Figs. 1 and 2). The ischemia of the muscle layer may be insufficient to cause necrosis, but does result in marked spasm, which does not respond to intravenous relaxants. The radiological changes of acute mucosal ischemia are therefore thumbprinting and narrowing of the affected part of the bowel. The spasm is more marked than is seen in ulcerative colitis, with rapid contractions that make filling of the bowel difficult. Some distension of the affected segment may be possible with air insufflation. This may obliterate the thumbprinting (Figs. 2b,c and 3), which is a useful finding if there is any problem distinguishing thumbprinting from ulceration or deformed haustration in acute ulcerative colitis (4).

The instant enema is a useful investigation for the diagnosis of acute ischemic colitis. Mucosa ulceration, which can be discrete or deep (Fig. 4a), indicates more advanced mucosal damage and the patient's condition should be monitored by repeat plain films, as the gangrenous stage of ischemia can be complicated with toxic megacolon (Fig. 4b) or perforation (5,6). Gas within the bowel wall indicates necrotizing colitis, and is probably due to *Clostridium perfringens,* which are normal commensals in the large bowel, invading the necrotic bowel wall (7) (Fig. 5).

Most patients resolve without complication and a follow-up barium enema at 4–6 weeks will be normal. This then confirms a transient attack of ischemic colitis (2,5) in which the

Table 2 Segment of Large Bowel Involved in 358 Cases of Ischemic Colitis

Segment	Number of cases	
Right colon	24	(6.7%)
Transverse colon	54	(15%)
Splenic flexure	84	(23.5%)
Descending colon	99	(27.5%)
Sigmoid colon	75	(21%)
Rectum	22	(6.3%)

Source: Ref. 1.

initial damage was minimal and complete cellular reparation was possible. If the damage was greater, the reparative phase will be delayed and may be complicated by stricture formation (3,5) (Figs. 6 and 7). The strictures are fibrotic, short, and typically at the splenic flexure. They are often fusiform in shape with prominent sacculation. The mucosa looks smooth radiologically, although the resected specimen often shows patchy ulceration. The remaining colon is normal. This, taken in conjunction with the configuration and site of the stricture, are distinguishing features from Crohn's disease. If the patient gives a typical history of acute ischemic colitis several weeks before, there is little doubt as to the diagnosis. The strictures tend to improve in time, so to establish the permanent configuration of the stricture another barium enema should be performed within 4–6 months.

The division of ischemic colitis into acute transient, gangrenous, and stricture formation phases is a valuable concept (5) which can be used to classify most cases. However, the condition may not present in a typical fashion in the elderly, and low-grade chronic ischemia may be more common that is realized. Any segmental lesion with narrowing and some mucosal irregularity could be due to ischemia and requires endoscopy with biopsy for confirmation (Figs. 8 and 9).

Ischemic colitis may complicate large bowel obstruction. The mechanism for this is probably a rise in intraluminal pressure which reduces the blood flow through the bowel wall (8). Obstruction due to carcinoma is the commonest cause of this, but it has been reported in obstruction from Hirschsprung's disease, adhesions, or an incarcerated hernia. An instant enema will show the level of obstruction and the most likely cause.

INFECTIOUS COLITIS

Salmonella or shigella infection is a common cause of severe diarrhea in endemic areas, or may occur anywhere in small outbreaks. The diagnosis is established from stool culture. Only if this is omitted or there is some technical failure should the infectious nature of the colitis be overlooked and the patient referred for a barium enema.

Shigella infection affects predominately the rectosigmoid; salmonella infection, the terminal ileum (Fig. 11). In one-third of salmonella cases the whole colon is involved (9). Severe infections may affect both the small and large bowel. Plain films will then show an extensive ileus of the small and large bowel (10) (Fig. 10).

The intensity of the colitis varies. Pathologically, there is acute inflammation with hyperemia and edema of the mucosa, which may slough creating ulcers. These vary in configuration and "collar-stud" ulcers have been reported radiologically (11,12). In shigella infection the ulceration is usually in the rectosigmoid (Fig. 12), whereas it is more likely to be diffuse in salmonella infection (9,11) (Fig. 13). Both may have a radiologically diffuse or segmental colitis (10,11). Spasm and mucosal edema complicate the radiological picture so that ischemic colitis can be simulated as well as inflammatory bowel disease (IBD). Toxic dilatation of the colon has been reported in salmonella colitis (13). Shigella infections may become chronic, with intermittent episodes of exacerbation followed by remission. The colon may become shortened and tubular, as in chronic ulcerative colitis, with strictures and spasm causing segmental contractions.

Infectious colitis remains a hazard, both diagnostically and directly, to those involved in performing the barium enema. There is no specific feature on which to base the diagnosis, so one must rely on routine bacterial screening of all patients with diarrhea to exclude cases with infectious colitis. Patients with inflammatory bowel disease may pick up an incidental infectious colitis, and again, only routine bacterial screening will detect this (14).

Yersinia   Yersinia is an infection caused by a small gram-positive coccobacillus which is common in birds, hares, pigs, and dogs. The disease presents with an acute ileitis, fever, and diarrhea. The diagnosis may be confirmed by isolating the bacterium from the stool or serologically from a rising titer of antibodies (15).

Radiological abnormalities are usually present in the terminal ileum. Typical changes (15) include a disordered coarse fold pattern in the terminal ileum (Fig. 14), or short longitudinal ulcers (Fig. 15). The ulcers may be oval or aphthoid and the terminal ileum dilated and hypercontractile. Thickening of the bowel wall and indentations from enlarged lymph nodes may be seen. The changes have been divided into three stages (16):

1. A nodular phase lasting up to 3 weeks with ulceration and enlarged lymph nodes.

2. An edematous stage with thickened folds lasting for 4–5 weeks.

3. A period of resolution, which may last for several months, where follicular lymphoid hyperplasia is seen in the terminal ileum.

Discrete ulceration has been reported in the colon (16), and although this may not be exactly the same as aphthoid ulceration in Crohn's disease (17), it must be considered in the differential diagnosis.

Antibiotic-Associated Colitis The administration of a broad-spectrum antibiotic, particularly clindamycin, lincomycin, or ampicillin, may be associated with diarrhea in 6.6–20% of cases (18,19). The development of a pseudomembranous colitis is rare. An incidence of 2% has been reported (19). Recently, it has been shown that the causative organism is *Clostridium difficile* (20). The actual damage to the colon is due to the production of a cytopathic endotoxin.

The pseudomembrane affects the entire large bowel, and only rarely involves the small intestine (21). As the rectum is usually involved, the diagnosis and appearance of the membrane can be studied by sigmoidoscopy. The typical appearance is of multiple slightly raised yellowish plaques up to 6 mm in diameter which are firmly attached to a congested mucosa. In severe cases the membrane may be confluent. Underlying mucosal necrosis may then lead to ulceration.

In severe cases plain film changes highly suggestive of pseudomembranous colitis (22) are present. The whole colon may be slightly distended with an irregular mucosal edge and thickened haustral clefts (Fig. 16). The changes on sigmoidoscopy should avoid any confusion with severe ulcerative colitis; also, the plain film changes are not exactly similar. An irregular mucosal edge may be due to a pseudomembrane or ulceration, but when the mucosa is ulcerated in ulcerative colitis, haustra are always absent, so that the presence of broad haustral clefts would be quite atypical for ulcerative colitis in this situation.

In most patients a barium enema is unnecessary for diagnosis or management. If performed it will demonstrate the state of the pseudomembrane (23). Small plaques may be present (Fig. 17), or the mucosa may appear edematous with some ulceration (Fig. 18), or shaggy or irregular where the membrane is confluent.

Herpetic Colitis Visceral reactions with cutaneous herpres zoster may be more common than is realized, as gastrointestinal examinations are seldom performed when the patient has a cutaneous eruption. However, several cases have been reported (24) in which the mucosal changes coincided with the cutaneous stage. During the vesicular phase, small polygonal raised lesions may be seen in the segment of bowel related to that dermatome. These are similar to urticaria in configuration (Fig. 20). In the ulcerative stage small ulcers may be seen in the mucosa. These heal but may leave some residual narrowing.

Histoplasmosis There are a few reports of ileocolitis due to primary infection with *Histoplasma capsulatum* (25). Strictures are common, but ulceration and polypoid change may be seen. The diagnosis is confirmed by demonstrating *Histoplasma* on methenamine silver stains.

Amebiasis The protozoon *Entamoeba histolytica* is worldwide in distribution. Although infestation reaches endemic proportions only in the tropics, sporadic cases have been reported in patients who have never left Northern countries (26). *Entamoeba* has two life cycles, a noninvasive one where it exists as a cyst in the bowel and can transmit the disease, and an invasive one where the parasite excretes a cytolytic enzyme which enables it to invade intestinal epithelium. In endemic areas about 20% of the population harbor the cyst, but only a small number develop invasive amebiasis (27).

Invasion of the epithelium produces small yellowish nodules, which rupture, leaving discrete oval ulcers. These tend to lie transversely and have overhanging edges and a hyperemic border. Ulceration may be diffuse, or more commonly scattered throughout the colon with concentrations at the flexures, cecum, and rectum.

Radiologically, several forms of invasive amebiasis are recognized (27):

1. *A colitis with an ulcerated mucosa, narrowing of the lumen, and loss of haustration.* Involvement of the colon is usually patchy, so that skip lesions may be present. A typical appearance in the cecum is deformity causing a funnel shape and a shaggy mucosal outline (Fig. 19).

2. *Ameboma.* These are chronic localized lesions due to secondary infection and fibrosis. Radiologically, these present as a stricture, and may be confused with malignancy or diverticulitis. Compared to a cancer the lesion tends to be longer, with tapering ends. The most reliable indication of an ameboma is its rapid response to antiamebic therapy. Multiple amebomas are present in about half of all cases. Their situation in descending order of frequency is: cecum, ascending colon, rectosigmoid, transverse colon, and descending colon. The incidence of ameboma is 1.5–8.4% (27) (Fig. 21–23).

3. *Fulminating colitis and toxic megacolon.* Plain films will show extensive mucosal ulceration. Thumbprinting and changes suggesting ischemic colitis have been reported (29), but once toxic megacolon has developed the changes in the colon will be similar whatever the cause. The value of the plain film is to show the severity of the colitis. Barium enema is contraindicated (Fig. 24).

4. *Appendicitis.* If this is secondary to amebiasis, there will probably be signs of amebiasis elsewhere in the colon.

Complications of amebiasis include perforation (Fig. 25) and fistula formation (30). The most serious is embolic spread to the liver, which occurs in about 15% of untreated cases (31). In amebic hepatitis there is a nonspecific inflammatory reaction involving the portal tracts. Ameba are found only in abscesses which form from the coalescence of small areas of necrosis in the liver parenchyma. The abscess is surrounded by a zone of hyperemia. Bleeding into it results in the "anchovy sauce" content. The abscess may rupture into the peritoneal or pleural cavity, or progress to a chronic state with a fibrous capsule. Focal liver involvement may be detected by isotope scanning, ultrasonography, or computerized axial tomography.

The sigmoidoscopic appearances of amebiasis are really nonspecific. Radiology may be suggestive, but the only certain method to prevent confusion with IBD is to examine the fresh stool for trophozoites and to perform indirect hemagglutination tests (32).

Tuberculosis Gastrointestinal disease may be due to ingested bovine bacilli, which pass through the small intestinal mucosa to form a primary focus in the draining lymph nodes. Ulceration is then a secondary phenomenon from retrograde spread. Secondary infection may occur from the ingestion of infected sputum, hematogenous spread, or reinfection in a previously sensitized individual.

In the first half of the century most intestinal tuberculosis was secondary to pulmonary disease. Nowadays the majority of patients have a normal chest x-ray (33) and the disease is a primary bovine infection. This is rare in the West but remains common in patients from endemic areas in Asia.

Any part of the gastrointestinal tract may be involved, but the commonest site is the ileocecal region, as this contains the largest collection of lymphoid tissue in the form of the Peyer's patches. Intestinal tuberculosis may present with weight loss, fever, abdominal pain, diarrhea in 30%, a mass in 40%, and ascites in 60% (34). The diagnosis must be established bacteriologically from culture, guinea pig inoculation, or histology. Histologically, tubercle bacilli and caseating granulomas are present in all layers of the bowel wall and regional lymph nodes, except in very chronic lesions with extensive fibrosis. The granulomas may then have become hyalinized or have disappeared. The pathological distinction from other forms of strictures is then very difficult (35). Tuberculosis may be diagnosed from endoscopic biopsy, but numerous biopsies should be taken, as these are frequently negative (36). The definitive diagnosis is from the examination of resected bowel and lymph nodes following laparotomy.

Radiologically, Crohn's disease has many similarities to tuberculosis, but there are some signs that may enable the radiologist to alert the clinician to the possibility of tuberculosis. In the ulcerative stage, the ulcers are typically oval and lie in a circumferential plane (Figs. 26 and 27). The ulcers may be large and deep with a shaggy base (Fig. 28). Stellate lesions may occur (37), but it is unusual to find a longitudinal ulcer except when a Peyer's patch is involved (38). Spasm associated with a transverse ulcer produces a short hourglass type of stricture that is unusual in Crohn's disease (Figs. 27a,29, and 31). In the hypertrophic form there is very extensive fibrosis with loss of normal tissue planes in the bowel wall, which has become grossly thickened (Fig. 30). This may be seen in association with ulceration, but often the mucosa is relatively smooth. Pipe stem narrowing may be seen. In the ileocecal region a typical appearance is dilated, rigid, incompetent ileocecal valve, a dilated terminal ileum with no fold pattern, except for possibly a thickened longitudinal fold, and contracted cecum with some radiating folds to the site of an old ulcer (Fig. 32) (39). Smooth-walled strictures may be seen in Crohn's disease, but typically ulceration is present in some part of the diseased segment.

Diffuse involvement of the colon, or segmental disease other than in the proximal part (Fig. 28), is rare and may be confused with other conditions such as carcinoma or amebiasis (40,41) (Figs. 33 and 34). Ascites is a common finding, and in one series was present in 52% of patients (34). It may be due to serious involvement in "wet" peritonitis or possibly extensive lymph node disease with lymphatic obstruction. The presence of ascites, small bowel distention, and an absent cecal shadow (suggesting a right iliac fossa mass) have been considered a triad of plain film changes highly suggestive of tuberculosis (34). In the dry type of peritonitis there are extensive caseous nodules and adhesions affecting the omentum and small bowel, which results in separation of loops of small bowel, with rigid walls and thickening of the folds (Figs. 35 and 36) (42).

Complications of tuberculosis include obstruction, perforation or fistula formation, hemorrhage (34,37), and malabsorption from extensive small bowel disease (43). In patients from tropical areas parasitic infestation of the small bowel is common (34), and accounts for some radiological abnormalities.

There is considerable overlap between Crohn's disease and tuberculosis, both in presentation and radiological appearances. The absence of cobblestoning (35), and the presence of deep shaggy ulcers, transverse ulcers, hourglass strictures, or deformity of the ileocecal region with a smooth mucosa are features that suggest tuberculosis. All patients from endemic areas should not be accepted as having Crohn's disease purely on radiological grounds. In these patients the diagnosis should be accepted only after bacteriological and histological exclusion of tuberculosis, as the therapeutic implication of misdiagnosis is so important.

Schistosomiasis Infestation of the large bowel is commonest with *Schistosoma mansoni*, but may occur in *S. japonicum* or *S. haematobium* (44). After the cercaria have penetrated the skin, they are carried to the liver, where the adult worms develop. These then migrate in the mesenteric veins to lay their eggs in the intestinal wall. The pathological changes result from an inflammatory reaction due to the presence of eggs in the intestinal wall. In *S. mansoni* this is usually in the distal colon and rectum.

The initial colitis is followed by ulceration and possible stricture formation. Typically, the patient is left with multiple inflammatory polyps. In *S. mansoni* these tend to be small (Fig. 37), but may be large in *S. japonica* or *S. haematobium* (45). Involvement of the terminal ileum has been described (46). The diagnosis is confirmed by finding bilharzial granulomas on rectal biopsy.

Lymphogranuloma Venereum   Lymphogranuloma inguinale or venereum (LGV) is due to a psittacosis-related virus and is confirmed by a positive skin test (Frei test) and a complement fixation test. It is commonest among poor black populations in the tropics. A papule forms at the site of infection and is followed in 4–8 weeks by an acute purulent lymphadenitis. A proctocolitis may then develop in females, but is uncommon in males except in homosexuals where the rectum has been infected directly. This is followed by a chronic phase with stricturing complicated by perianal abscesses and fistula.

Barium examination is usually performed only in the chronic stage. The rectum is narrowed with multiple fistulous tracts (47) (Fig. 38). Rectovaginal fistula are common. Strictures tend to be long and tubular with tapering ends. The anorectal region is usually involved, but strictures may extend up into the sigmoid (Fig. 39) and can occur proximally in the colon with intervening skip areas of normal bowel (48). The lumen of the strictures may be smooth or ulcerated. Lateral pelvic views should be taken to exclude a fistula to the vagina. The rectosigmoid is often straightened on the anterioposterior view and seen to be displaced anteriorly on the lateral view, due to inflammatory changes in the presacral space.

Miscellaneous Parasitic Infestations

1. *Trichuriasis*. Double-contrast studies may show the coiled worm lying on the mucosal surface. The male parasite is tightly coiled into a "target" pattern, whereas the female is more unfurled (49).

2. *Strongyloides stercoralis colits* (50). Edema, loss of haustration, ulceration, and stricture formation have been described due to filariform invasion of the wall of the large bowel.

3. *Chagas' disease*. This is a systemic infection due to the protozoan *Trypanosoma cruzi*. It is prevalent in South America. *T. cruzi* produces a neurotoxin that gradually destroys ganglion cells in the myenteric plexi. Gross dilatation of the colon and esophagus are common in Brazil (51).

RADIATION ENTERITIS   Radiation damage to the bowel may simulate other conditions, such as Crohn's disease, ischemia, or neoplasia, and manifest several years after therapy. This delay complicates its diagnosis. Although the details of the original radiotherapy may be known, it is not always a simple matter to exclude recurrent disease or the development of some other pathology when symptoms develop many years later.

The incidence of radiation enteritis depends on the total amount of radiation to the bowel and the period over which it was administered. The minimum tolerance dose is defined as the radiation dosage that would cause complications in 5% of patients within 5 years of therapy (TD/5/5). For the colon and small bowel this is 4500 rad, and for the rectum 5500 rad (52). Although less sensitive, the rectum and sigmoid are affected most because of their proximity and fixation within the most common field of radiation, which is for carcinoma of the cervix.

Radiation causes an acute inflammatory reaction with hyperemia and edema of the mucosa. This usually resolves after the cessation of therapy. Later and more severe reactions include mucosal ulceration and sclerosis of the bowel wall (53).

Ulceration as a result of radiation damage is very variable. The ulcers may be single or multiple, superficial or deep. Penetration of an ulcer through the bowel wall leads to perforation, peritonitis, or fistula formation. The bowel wall, often also the mesentery, becomes thickened, pale, and indurated with a telangectatic serosa and mucosa, which has a typical appearance endoscopically. Histologically, there is a marked hyaline degeneration of connective tissue with an increase in fibrous tissue, which are responsible for the increase in bowel wall thickness. These changes in the vessel walls lead to an endarteritis which can cause infarction of part of the bowel.

Radiation Changes in the Small Intestine During radiotherapy the small bowel will often show an ileus on plain films. It is rare for barium studies to be required, but an atonic, dilated bowel with thickened folds due to edema has been reported (54).

Later changes involve the mesentery and the bowel. The fold pattern is spiky; the transverse folds are thickened and seem to be compressed together, leaving narrow intervening furrows of barium. This appearance has been described as a picket fence (54). The bowel wall is rigid and there is wide separation of the bowel loops (Figs. 40 and 41). Nodular defects are common and may cause confusion with recurrent tumor. These nodules are due to submucosal fibrosis and edema, and may disappear spontaneously (54). Ulceration is usually superficial and not visible radiologically. This is unlike Crohn's disease, where superficial ulceration is usually visible in association with mucosal edema. Deep ulceration is rare, but may result in free perforation or abscess formation. Adherence at the site of perforation produces a fistula, which may be to either the small or large bowel or to the bladder. Massive adhesions and multiple strictures lead to obstruction, which is the commonest clinical problem. Surgery is very difficult in these patients, as long segments of bowel have to be resected. The changes are always more extensive than is suggested radiologically. Anastomoses are liable to breakdown, as endarteritis in even minimally affected bowel leads to a poor blood supply and delayed healing.

Radiation Changes in the Large Bowel Acute radiation colitis causes spasm and mucosal edema (Fig. 42) which may mimic ischemic colitis, or if localized, even a carcinoma (55,56). Endoscopically, there is no evidence of submucosal hemorrhage, and unlike ischemic colitis, the changes do not resolve in a few days. If the mucosa ulcerates, the appearance is difficult to distinguish from ulcerative colitis, but radiation ulcers tend to be wider, deeper, and more irregular.

As in the small bowel, the development of chronic changes may be delayed for several years. Implant therapy often results in tubular narrowing of the rectosigmoid (Fig. 43). This can lead to colonic obstruction, but ulceration on the anterior wall of the rectum with abscess or fistula formation to the vagina, bladder, or small bowel (55,56) is a much more common problem.

Two cases of severe total colitis have been reported (56). Whether this was due solely to radiation damage, or that radiation changes were superimposed on ulcerative colitis, is uncertain (Fig. 44). The commonest clinical problem is rectal bleeding. This is due to telangiectasia, which is a typical finding in chronic radiation enteritis. Double-contrast barium enema will exclude strictures and similar factors but will not show telangiectasia,, which requires endoscopic confirmation.

NEOPLASIA-SIMULATING COLITIS Malignancy does not always present with a polypoid mass or an annular shouldered stricture. More diffuse changes can simulate IBD, particularly Crohn's disease (54). A diffusely infiltrating scirrhous type of primary carcinoma is very rare in the large bowel (58). This can produce a long strictured segment. There may be some shouldering and mucosal irregularity to suggest a malignant origin, but these tumors can look benign (Fig. 45). Secondary malignancy is more common. This causes extrinisic deformity of the bowel from tumor growth and its associated desmoplastic response. The mucosa becomes thrown into spiculated folds and the bowel wall straightened and fixed (Fig. 46). Pseudodiverticular formation may occur with eccentric fibrosis (Fig. 47). Mucosal ulceration and nodular masses indicates tumor growth into the lumen. The distribution of these changes depends on the site of the primary (59). For example, gastric cancer spreads along the gastrocolic ligament to involve the superior border of the transverse colon (Fig. 47). The involved bowel is usually clearly demarcated from normal. Its distribution, often along one border, and the essential difference between spiculation and ulceration should enable the radiologist to suggest secondary malignancy rather than IBD.

Primary lymphoma of the colon is rare. It may present with diffuse nodularity. This can simulate ulceration radiologically (Fig. 48), or if umbilicated, an aphthoid type of ulceration (Figs. 50 and 51). Biopsy is obviously essential to establish the diagnosis.

IDIOPATHIC ULCERATION

This encompasses solitary ulcer of the rectum syndrome (60), and a number of cases of non specific ulceration in the colon have been reported (61). The presence of an ulcer with or without deformity, surrounded by otherwise normal bowel, would be suggestive of Crohn's disease, but there has been no histological evidence to support this in any of these cases.

The solitary ulcer syndrome may be found in young adults of either sex, and presents with rectal bleeding, the passage of mucus, or perineal pain (60). The ulcer is usually on the anterior wall, is flat, and is covered with a white slough. No ulcer may be present and the mucosa shows only a localized roughened inflamed area. Radiologically, the flat ulcer is not always seen; a nodular mucosa, deformity, or polypoid changes may be seen instead (62) (Figs. 49 and 52). There is evidence that the condition is due to rectal prolapse, secondary to the puborectalis remaining contracted during defecation.

The cecum is the commonest site for nonspecific ulceration in the colon. The presentation may mimic appendicitis. Perforation or hemorrhage are significant complications. Barium enema may show a pool of barium at the site of the ulcer with surrounding deformity (63), but the terminal ileum is normal. These "cecal ulcers" may be the result of inflammation within a diverticulum (64). Discrete ulcers have been reported in other parts of the colon. These may be related to certain drugs, and oral contraceptives, phenylbutazone, and oxyphenylbutazone have been implicated (65). An ischemic mechanism is likely (66).

Rarely, the deformity surrounding a nonspecific ulcer may cause an appearance resembling an annular carcinoma (67). Whatever the underlying mechanism or configuration of the ulcer, endoscopic biopsy will be required to provide histological evidence that it is not due to Crohn's disease or tuberculosis.

CATHARTIC COLON

Purgative abuse may present clinically with diarrhea, potassium loss, and steatorrhea. Melanosis coli is a common finding with prolonged cascara usage, and is readily detected endoscopically. Macroscopically, the mucosa may become abnormal and take on the texture of a snake skin (68) (Fig. 53). The anthraquinones (cascara, senna, and bisacodyl) are neurotoxic and will eventually damage the myenteric plexus, resulting in smooth muscle atrophy (69). This is the most likely explanation for the changes in the configuration of the colon that are found in the "cathartic colon."

The radiological changes are more prominent in the proximal half of the colon, which is dilated, atonic, and featureless with absent haustration. Transient segmental contractions, termed "pseudostrictures," (70) may be seen (Fig. 54). The ileocecal valve may be patulous with reflux into the terminal ileum. If the mucosa is also abnormal, the distinction from chronic ulcerative colitis is difficult (71). The colon is not shortened and narrowed as in ulcerative colitis and the distal part of the large bowel tends to be normal in cathartic colon.

Cathartic colon may be first suspected by finding melanosis coli. The diagnosis is supported by a history of purgative abuse, typical radiological changes, and the exclusion of colitis by rectal biopsy.

BEHÇET'S DISEASE

The original triad of oral and genital ulceration with ocular inflammation that was described by Behçet is now recognized as part of a multisystem disease in which colitis may be a manifestation. Barium enema may show diffuse collar-stud-type ulceration with loss of haustration (72), or deep discrete undermining ulcers, which are surrounded by normal mucosa and haustration (73). The depth of the ulcer distinguishes Behçet's ulceration from apthoid ulceration in Crohn's disease, and leads to the main problem of intestinal involvement, which is perforation (73,74). Hemorrhage and fistula formation are other complications (74).

The ileocecal region is the commonest site of involvement. The disease is subject to remissions and exacerbations, and complete resolution of colonic ulceration has been reported (73).

GONORRHEAL PROCTITIS

This may be indistinguishable sigmoidoscopically from idiopathic proctitis (75). Radiology plays no part in the diagnosis, which must be by Gram's stain and culture.

COLLAG-ENOUS COLITIS

This is a rare entity with collagenous thickening of the subepithelial basement membrane. Only two cases have been reported (76,77). Presenting symptoms are abdominal pain and diarrhea. Mucosal irregularity may be noted on barium enema and endoscopy (77). The diagnosis depends on demonstrating the typical collagenous changes, and the absence of any feature of ulcerative colitis or Crohn's disease.

COLITIS IN GLUTEN-SENSITIVE ENTEROPATHY

The jejunal mucosa can be abnormal in ulcerative colitis, but whether or not this relates to the colitis is disputed (78,79). The prevailing opinion seems to be that it does not, and any patient with coeliac disease who develops diarrhea when on a proper diet should be considered to have developed additional pathology (80) and ulcerative colitis or Crohn's disease have merely supervened on the coeliac disease (Fig. 55).

FABRY'S DISEASE

Fabry's disease is a rare glycosphingoloid lipodosis. The diagnosis is usually apparent from the family history, typical facies and rash, but gastrointestinal manifestations may predominate, with diarrhea as the main symptom.

Radiologically, the small bowel shows thickened folds, dilatation, and a granular texture in the ileum. Confusion could arise with coeliac disease. In the colon, loss of haustration is the predominate feature and could be confused with chronic ulcerative colitis or the cathartic colon (81). The diagnosis is confirmed by the absence of α-galactosidase enzymatic activity.

SUMMARY

The colon exhibits a limited number of responses to the various causes of colitis. Changes in the mucosal surface, alteration in the configuration of the bowel, and the disribution of the lesions may be used to describe the colitis radiologically. Its classification tends to fall into

Table 3 Differential Diagnosis of IBD

Similar to Ulcerative colitis (granular mucosa, superficial ulceration in continuity)	Similar to Crohn's disease (discrete, deep ulceration; asymmetric ulceration, fibrosis)	Inflammatory polyposis (sessile, filiform polyps)	Toxic megacolon (dilatation, ulceration)
Infective colitis	Tuberculosis	Ulcerative colitis	Ulcerative colitis
Amebiasis	Ischemic colitis	Crohn's disease	Crohn's disease
Gonorrheal proctitis	Behçet's disease	Schistosomiasis	Ischemia
Cathartic colon	Yersinia		Amebiasis
Collagenous colitis	Herpetic colitis		Salmonella
Colitis in coeliacs	Amebiasis		
Fabry's disease	Idiopathic ulceration		
	Neoplasia-simulating colitis		
	Lymphogranuloma venereum		

four main types: a colitis resembling ulcerative colitis, Crohn's disease, inflammatory polyposis, or toxic megacolon. The conditions that may be loosely grouped under these headings are shown in Table 3.

A particular feature or combination of changes may suggest one type of colitis and exclude another. For example, discrete ulceration is a typical but not specific feature of Crohn's disease (82) and is not found in ulcerative colitis. Its presence means that radiologically one can say that Crohn's disease is the most likely diagnosis and that ulcerative colitis can be excluded. In this way radiology focuses attention on the most likely cause of a colitis and provides a useful step along the diagnostic pathway. The final diagnosis depends on incorporating this knowledge with all the other clinical, endoscopic, histological, and bacteriological information.

REFERENCES

1. Alschibaja, T., Morson, B.C. (1977). Ischaemic bowel disease. J. Clin. Pathol. 30 Suppl. (R. Coll. Pathol.) 11; 68.
2. Boley, S.J., Schartz, S., Lash, J., Stenhill, V. (1963). Reversible vascular occlusion of the colon. Surg. Gynaecol. Obstet. 116; 53.
3. Lea Thomas, M. (1968). Further observations on ischaemic colitis. Proc. R. Soc. Med. 61; 341.
4. Bartram, C.I. (1979). Obliteration of thumbprinting with double contrast enemas in acute ischaemic colitis. Gastrointest. Radiol. 4; 85.
5. Marston, A., Pheils, M.T., Lea Thomas, M., Morson, B.C. (1966). Ischaemic colitis. Gut 7; 1.
6. Miller, W.T., Scott, J., Rosato, E.F., et al. (1970). Ischaemic colitis with gangrene. Radiology 94; 291.
7. Killiingback, M.J., Williams, K.L. (1961). Necrotizing colitis. Proc. R. Soc. Med. 54; 731.
8. Whitehouse, G.H., Watt, J. (1977). Ischaemic colitis associated with carcinoma of the colon. Gastrointest. Radiology 2; 31.

9. Margulis, A.F., Burhenne, H.J. (1973). *Alimentary Tract Roentgenology*. Mosby, St. Louis, 2nd ed. p. 1597.

10. Marshak, R.H., Lindner, A.E., Maklansky, D. (1980). *Radiology of the Colon*. Saunders, Philadelphia, p. 223.

11. Farman, J., Rabinowitz, J.G., Meters, M.A. (1973). Roentgenology of infectious colitis. Am. J. Roentgenol. 119; 375.

12. McElfatink, F.A., Wurtzeback, L.R. (1973). Collar-button ulcers of the colon in a case of shigellosis. Gastroenterology 65; 303.

13. Schofield, P.F., Mandal, B.K., Ironside, A.G. (1979). Toxic dilatation of the colon in salmonella colitis and inflammatory bowel disease. Br. J. Surg. 66; 5.

14. Dronfield, M.W., Fletcher, J., Langman, M.J.S. (1974). Salmonella infections and ulcerative colitis: problems of recognition and management. Br. Med. J. 1; 99.

15. Vantrappen, G., Agg, H.O., Ponette, E., et al. (1977). Yersinial enteritis and enterocolitis: gastroenterological aspects. Gastroenterology 72; 220.

16. Ekberg, O., Sjostrom, B., Brahme, F.J. (1977). Radiological findings in yersinial ileitis. Radiology 123; 15.

17. Williams, C.B., Waye, J.D. (1978). Endoscopy in inflammatory bowel disease. Clin. Gastroenterol. 7; 701.

18. Swartzberg, J.E., Maresca, R.M., Remington, J.S. (1977). Clinical study of gastrointestinal complications associated with clindamycin therapy. J. Infect. Dis 135 (Suppl.); 99.

19. Lusk, R.H., Fekerty, F.R., Silva, J., et al. (1977). Gastrointestinal side effects of clindamycin and ampicillin therapy. J. Infect. Dis. 135 (Suppl.); 111.

20. Bartlett, J.G., Moon, N., Chang, T.W., et al. (1978). Role of *Clostridium difficile* in antibiotic associated pseudomembranous colitis. Gastroenterology 75; 778.

21. Price, A.B., Davies, D.R. (1977). Pseudomembranous colitis. J. Clin. Pathol. 30; 1.

22. Stanley, R.J., Melson, L., Tedesco, F., Saylor, J. (1976). Plain film findings in severe pseudomembranous colitis. Radiology 118; 7.

23. Stanley, R.J., Melson, G.L., Tedesco, F.J. (1974). The spectrum of radiographic findings in antibiotic related pseudomembranous colitis. Radiology 111; 519.

24. Menuck, L., Brahme, F., Amberg, J., Sherr, H. (1976). Colonic changes of herpes zoster. Am. J. Roentgenol. 127; 273.

25. Haws, C.C., Long, R.F., Caplan, G.E. (1977). Histoplasma capsulatum as a cause of ileocolitis. Am. J. Roentgenol. 128; 692.

26. Morton, T.C., Neal, R.A., Sage, M. (1951). Indigenous amoebiasis in Britain. Lancet 1; 766.

27. Cardoso, J.M., Kimura, K., Stoopen, M., et al. (1977). Radiology of invasive amoebiasis. Am. J. Roentgenol. 128; 935.

28. Cockshott, P., Middlemiss, H. (1979). *Clinical Radiology in the Tropics*. Churchill Livingstone, Edinburgh, p. 115.

29. Hardy, R., Scullen, D.R. (1971). Thumbprinting in a case of amoebiasis. Radiology 98; 147.

30. Pelaez, M. Villazon, A., Zaraboso, R.S. (1966). Amoebic perforation in the colon. Dis. Colon Rectum 9; 356.

31. Cockshott, P., Middlemiss, H. (1979). *Clinical Radiology in the Tropics*. Churchill Livingstone, Edinburgh, p. 130.

32. Tucker, P.C., Webster, P.D., Kilpatrick, L.M. (1975). Amoebic colitis mistaken for inflammatory bowel disease. Arch. Intern. Med. 135; 681.

33. Theoni, R.F., Margulis, A.R. (1979). Gastrointestinal tuberculosis. Semin. Roentgenol. 24; 283.

34. Kolawole, T.M., Lewis, E.A. (1975). A radiological study of tuberculosis of the abdomen. Am. J. Roentgenol. 123; 348.
35. Morson, B.C., Dawson, I.M.P. (1979). *Gastrointestinal Pathology.* Blackwell Scientific Publications, Oxford, 2nd ed. p. 278.
36. Franklin, G.O., Mohapatru, M., Perillo, R. (1979). Colonic tuberculosis diagnosed by colonoscopic biopsy. Gastroenterology 76; 362.
37. Carrera, G.F., Young, S., Lewicki, A.M. (1976). Intestinal tuberculosis. Gastrointest. Radiol. 1; 147.
38. Prout, W.G. (1968). Multiple tuberculosis perforations of the ileum. Gut 9; 381.
39. Brombart, M., Massion, J. (1961). Radiological differences between ileo-caecal tuberculosis and Crohn's disease. Am. J. Dig. Dis. 6; 589.
40. Tischler, J.M.A. (1979). Tuberculosis of the transverse colon. Am. J. Roentgenol. 133; 229.
41. Balthazar, E.J., Bryk, D. (1980). Segmental tuberculosis of the distal colon: radiographic features in 7 cases. Gastrointest. Radiol. 5; 75.
42. Stassa, G. (1967). Tuberculous peritonitis. Am. J. Roentgenol. 101; 409.
43. Eerbeloff, L., Novis, B.H., Bank, S., Marks, I.N. (1973). The radiology of tuberculosis of the gastrointestinal tract. Br. J. Radiol. 46; 329.
44. Azar, J.E., Schraibman, I.G., Pitchford, R.J. (1958). Some observations on *Schistosoma haematobium* in the human rectum and sigmoid. Trans. R. Soc. Trop. Med. Hyg. 60; 231.
45. Medina, J.T., Seaman, W.B., Guzman-Acosta, C., Diaz-Bonnet, R.B. (1965). The roentgen appearances of *Schistosoma mansoni* involving the colon. Radiology 85; 682.
46. Cockshott, P., Middlemiss, H. (1979). *Clinical Radiology in the Tropics.* Churchill Livingstone, Edinburgh, p. 111.
47. Annamunthodo, H., Marryatt, J. (1961). Barium studies in the intestinal lympho-granuloma venereum. Br. J. Radiol. 34; 53.
48. Marryatt, J. (1961). Lymphogranuloma venereum. In *Tropical Radiology,* Middlemiss, H., Heinemann, London, p. 229.
49. Fisher, R.M., Cremin, B.J. (1970). Rectal bleeding due to *Trichuris trichiura.* Br. J. Radiol. 43; 214.
50. Drasin, G.F., Moss, J.P., Cheng, S.H. (1978). Strongyloides stercoralis colitis: findings in four cases. Radiology 126; 619.
51. Cockshott, P., Middlemiss, H. (1979). *Clinical Radiology in the Tropics.* Churchill Livingstone, Edinburgh, p. 119.
52. Rubin, P., Casarett, G. (1972). A direction for clinical radiation pathology. In *Frontiers of Radiation Therapy and Oncology,* Vol. 6, Vaeth, J.N. (Ed.). University Park Press, Baltimore, p. 1.
53. Halls, J.M. (1956). Radiation damage of the small intestine. Clin. Radiol. 16; 173.
54. Mason, G.R., Dietrich, P., Friedland, G.W., Hanks, G.E. (1970). The radiological findings in radiation induced enteritis and colitis. Review of 30 cases. Clin. Radiol. 21; 232.
55. Roswit, B. (1974). Complications of radiation therapy: the alimentary tract. Semin. Roentgenol. 9; 51.
56. Novak, J.M., Collins, J.T., Donowitz, M., et al. (1979). Effects of radiation on the human gastrointestinal tract. J. Clin. Gastroenterol. 1; 9.
57. Meyers, M.A., Oliphant, M., Teixidor, H., Weiser, P. (1975). Metastatic carcinoma simulating inflammatory colitis. Am. J. Roentgenol. 123; 74.
58. Meyers, M.A. (1980). Patterns of spread of malignancy in the colon: In *Radiology of the Colon,* Marshak, R.H., Lindiner, A.E., Maklansky, D., Saunders, Philadelphia, p. 335.

59. Wolf, B.S., Marshak, R.H. (1963). Linitus plastica or diffusely infiltrating type of carcinoma of the colon. Radiology 81; 502.

60. Rutter, K.R.P., Riddell, R.H. (1975). The solitary ulcer syndrome of the rectum. Clin. Gastroenterol. 4; 505.

61. Brock, A.L., Reynolds, J.D.H., Wood, W.G. (1979). Nonspecific ulcers of the colon: a case presentation of ulceration of the transverse colon. J. Clin. Gastroenterol. 1; 241.

62. Feczko, P.J., O'Connell, D.J., Riddell, R.H., Frank, P.H. (1980). Solitary rectal ulcer syndrome: radiologic manifestations. Am. J. Roentgenol. 135; 49.

63. Brodey, P.A., Hill, R.P., Baron, S. (1977). Benign ulceration of the caecum. Radiology 122; 323.

64. Lloyd-Williams, K. (1960). Acute solitary ulcers and acute diverticulitis of the caecum and ascending colon. Br. J. Surg. 47; 351.

65. Bernardino, M., Lawson, T.L. (1975). Discrete colonic ulcers associated with oral contraceptives. Am. J. Dig. Dis. 21; 503.

66. Lawson, T.L. (1980). Ischaemic colitis and discrete colonic ulceration secondary to oral contraception. In *Radiographic Atlas of Colon Disease,* Greenbaum, E.I. (Ed.). Year Book Medical Publishers, Chicago, p. 253.

67. Gardiner, G.A., Bird, C.R. (1980). Nonspecific ulcers of the colon resembling annular carcinoma. Radiology 137; 331.

68. Morson, B.C., Dawson, I.M.P. (1979). *Gastro-intestinal Pathology.* Blackwell Scientific Publications, Oxford, p. 697.

69. Smith, B. (1972). Pathology of cathartic colon. Proc. R. Soc. Med. 65; 288.

70. Marshak, R.H., Gerson, A. (1960). Cathartic colon. Am. J. Dig. Dis. 5; 724.

71. Urso, F.O., Urso, M.J., Lee, C.H. (1975). The cathartic colon: pathological findings and radiological/pathological correlation. Radiology 116; 557.

72. Stanley, R.T., Tedesco, F.J., Melson, G.L. et al. (1975). The colitis of Behçet's disease: a clinical-radiographic correlation. Radiology 114; 603.

73. Baba, S., Maruta, M., Ando, K., et al. (1976). Intestinal Behçet's disease: report of five cases. Dis. Colon Rectum 19; 428.

74. Smith, G.E., Kime, L.R., Pitcher, J.L. (1973). The colitis of Behçet's disease: a separate entity. Am. J. Dig. Dis. 18; 987.

75. Kilpatrick, Z.M. (1972). Gonorrheal proctitis. N. Engl. J. Med. 287; 967.

76. Lindstrom, C.G. (1976). "Collagenous colitis" with watery diarrhoea — a new entity? Pathol. Eur. 11; 87.

77. Bogomoletz, W.V., Adnet, J.J., Birembaut, P., Feydy, P., Dupont, P. (1980). Collagenous colitis: an unrecognized entity. Gut 21; 164.

78. Salem, S.N., Truelove, S.L. (1965). Small intestinal and gastric abnormalities in ulcerative colitis. Br. Med. J. 1; 827.

79. Binder, V., Soltoff, J., Gudman-Hoyer, E. (1974). Histological and histolochemical changes in the jejunal mucosa in ulcerative colitis. Scand. J. Gastroenterol. 9; 293.

80. Kumar, P.J., Donoghue, D.P., Gibson, J. et al. (1979). The existence of inflammatory bowel lesions in gluten-sensitive enteropathy. Postgrad. Med. J. 55; 753.

81. Rowe, J.W., Gilliam, J.I., Warthin, T.A. (1974). Intestinal manifestations of Fabry's disease. Ann. Intern. Med. 81; 628.

82. Max, R.J., Kelvin, F.M. (1980). Nonspecificity of discrete colonic ulceration on double contrast barium enema study. Am. J. Roentgenol. 134; 1265.

FIGURES 1 THROUGH 55

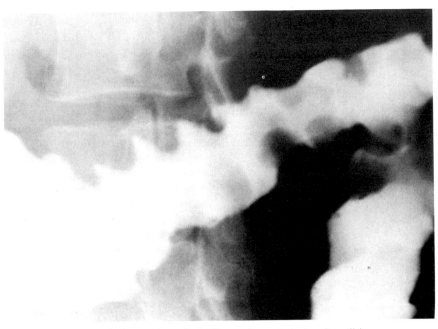

Figure 1 Thumbprinting at the splenic flexure in acute ischemic colitis.

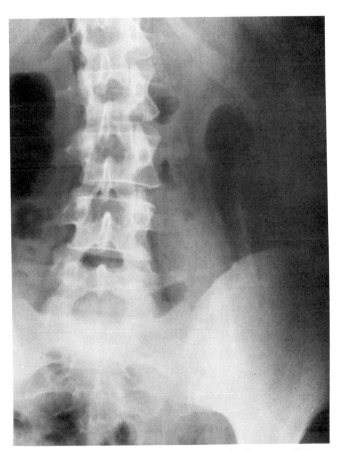

Figure 2a Plain film with gas in the splenic flexure outlining a narrowed bowel with thumbprinting.

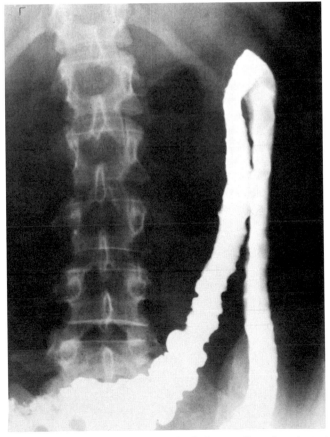

Figure 2b Narrowing and thumbprinting confirmed on instant enema.

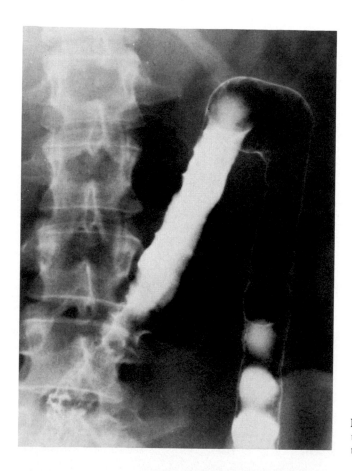

Figure 2c The descending colon was in considerable spasm, unrelieved by intravenous relaxants. Air insufflation could temporarily obliterate the thumbprinting.

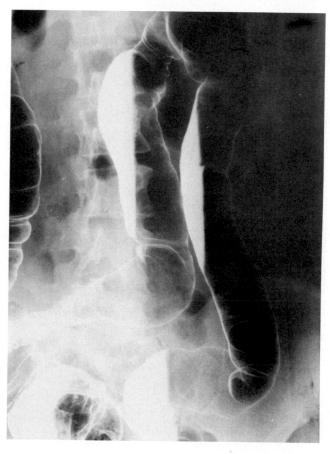

Figure 2d A repeat barium enema 1 month later shows a normal colon, confirming transient ischemic colitis. (From Ref. 4.)

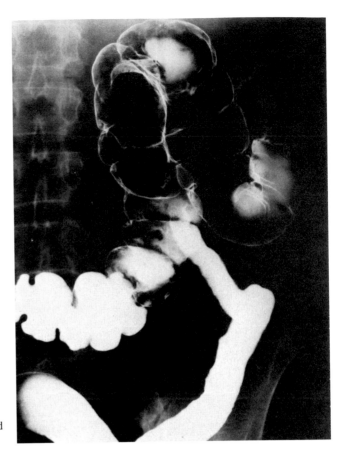

Figure 3a Typical acute ischemic colitis with narrowing and some thumbprinting of the mucosa in the descending colon.

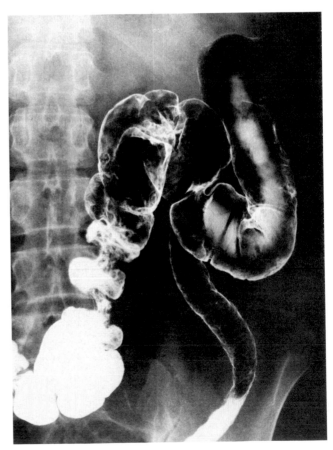

Figure 3b Some distention of the bowel was possible with air insufflation, which obliterated the thumbprinting and excluded gross ulceration.(From Ref. 4.)

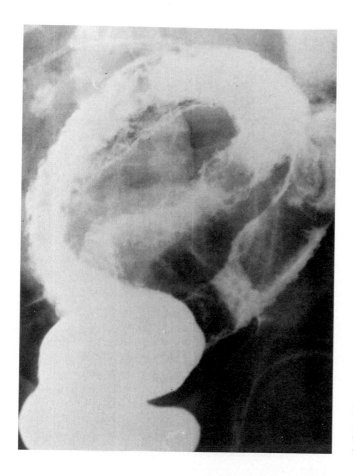

Figure 4a An elderly patient presenting with severe abdominal pain and rectal bleeding. An instant enema showed ulceration in the sigmoid. Distal rectum normal on sigmoidoscopy. Biopsy of the ulcerated bowel was typical of ischemic colitis.

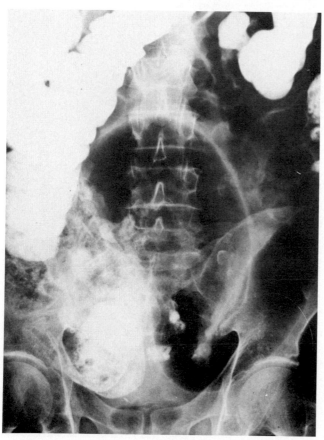

Figure 4b Several days later toxic megacolon developed in the sigmoid.

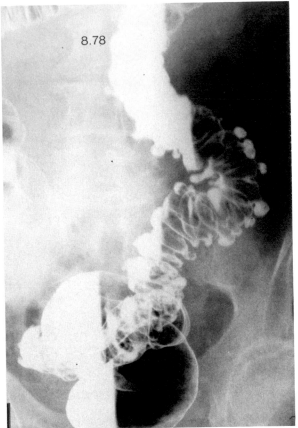

Figure 5a

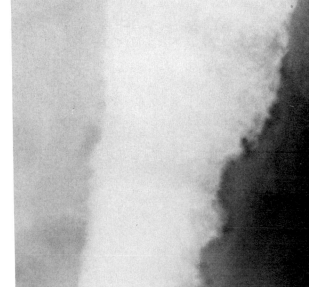

Figure 5b

Figure 5c

Figure 5a Barium enema showing diverticular disease only.

Figure 5b Six months later the patient presented with rectal bleeding. Sigmoidoscopy showed patchy ulceration and an instant enema revealed discrete aphthoid-type ulceration in the descending colon. The muscle changes were less prominent and hardly any of the diverticula filled.

Figure 5c The patient was admitted 2 weeks later in a toxic state. Plain abdominal radiographs showed free air and numerous small gas bubbles in the wall of the descending colon. Examination of the resected specimen confirmed ischemic colitis with necrotizing enterocolitis.

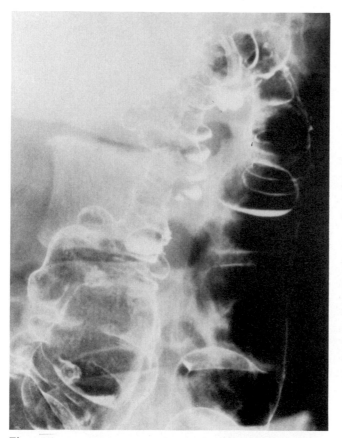

Figure 6

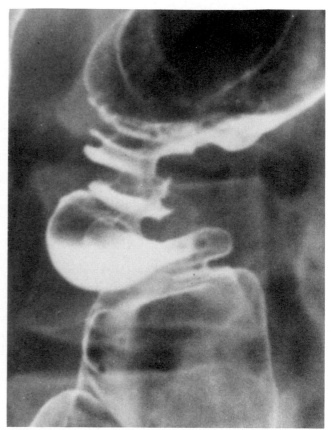

Figure 7

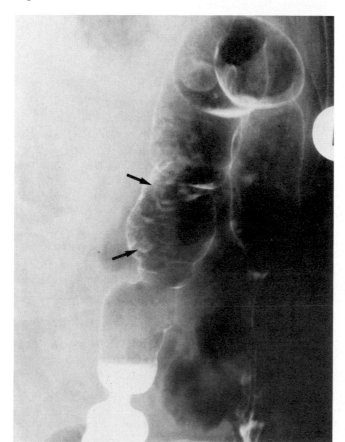

Figure 8

Figure 6 Long ischemic stricture at the splenic flexure with marked sacculation and pseudodiverticula formation. The adjacent colon is normal and there is no overt ulceration.

Figure 7 Short ischemic stricture in the descending colon. Note also the prominent sacculation and absence of ulceration.

Figure 8 Patient with rectal bleeding. A polyp was present in the lower descending colon, but colonoscopy showed that the patient was bleeding from an area of ischemic colitis in the distal transverse colon. Radiologically, this has caused some patchy mucosal irregularity, suggesting superficial ulceration (arrows) but no narrowing of the bowel.

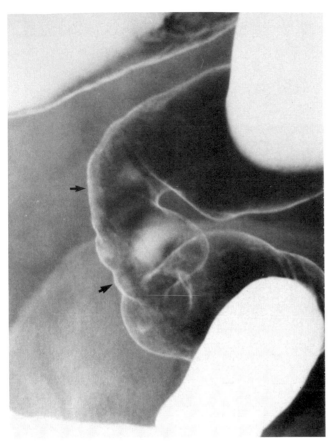

Figure 9 Localized segment of ischemic colitis found on colonoscopy.. Persistent narrowing with minimal mucosal irregularity (arrows) are the only radiological indications of this.

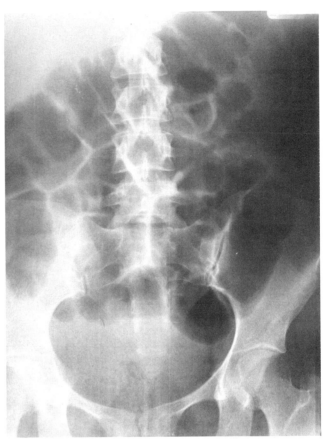

Figure 10 Small and large bowel ileus in a patient with acute paratyphoid B infection.

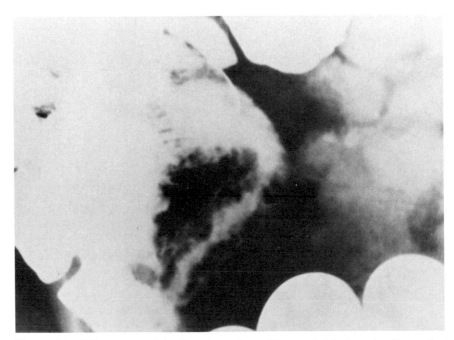

Figure 11 Enlargement of the Peyer's patches with superficial ulceration in a patient with salmonellosis.

242

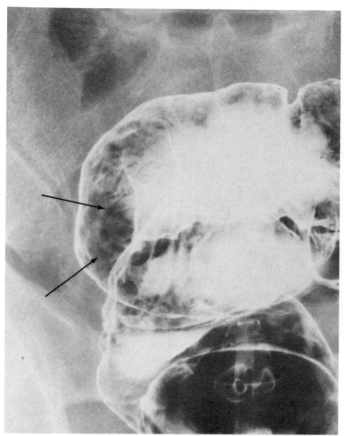

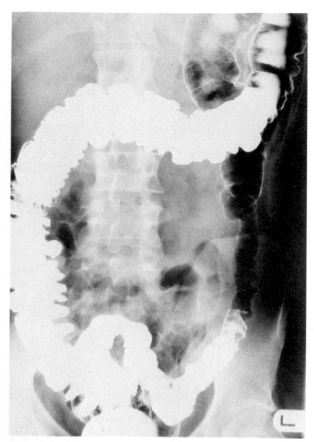

Figure 12 Superficial ulceration in the rectosigmoid (arrows) in early shigella. (Courtesy of Dr. R. Kottler, Groote Schuur Hospital, Capetown, South Africa.)

Figure 13 Instant enema in a patient with mild proctitis sigmoidoscopically, and a negative stool culture, who later proved to have salmonella. Confluent granular mucosa in the descending colon.

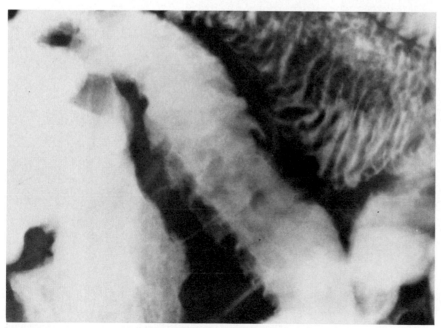

Figure 14 Yersinia of the terminal ileum with disorganized thickened folds (Courtesy of Dr. D. Nolan, Radcliffe Hospital, Oxford.)

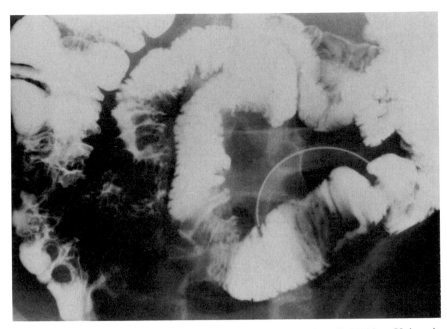

Figure 15 Short longitudinal ulcers in yersinia. (Courtesy of Dr. P. Mahieu, Universite Catholique de Louvain, Brussels, Belgium.)

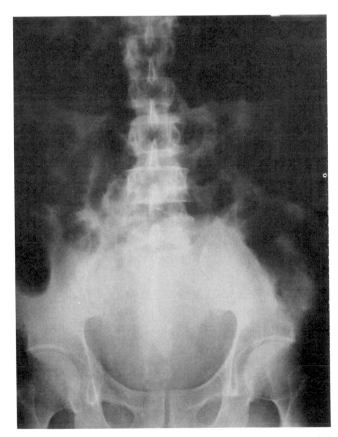

Figure 16 Plain film in pseudomembranous enterocolitis showing a small and large bowel ileus. The haustral clefts are thickened and the mucosa slightly irregular. (Courtesy of Dr. L. A. Berger, Royal Free Hospital, London.)

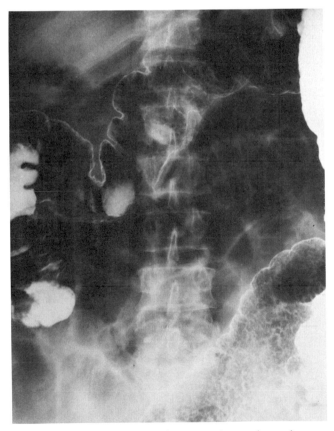

Figure 17 Double-contrast barium enema in pseudomembranous colitis showing a rather irregular nodular mucosa due to small plaques with a confluent membrane in parts. (Courtesy of Dr. L. A. Berger, Royal Free Hospital, London.)

244

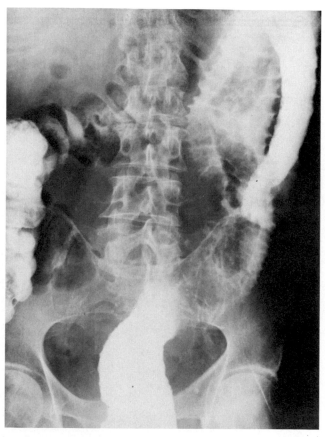

Figure 18 Pseudomembranous colitis with edematous mucosal folds in the distal large bowel and some superficial ulceration. The inflammatory changes are more prominent than the membrane in this case.

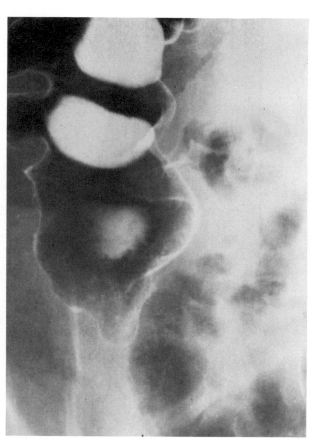

Figure 19 Cecal amebiasis. Typical funnel-shaped deformity with superficial ulceration.

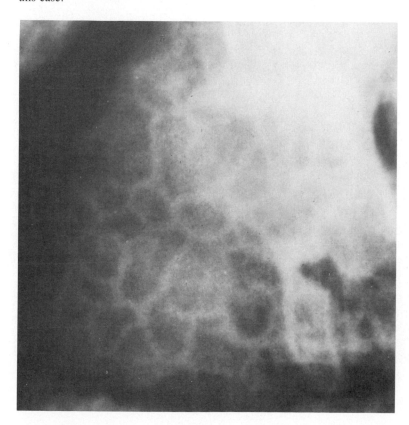

Figure 20 Mosaic pattern which could be due to urticaria or vesicule formation in herpetic colitis.

245

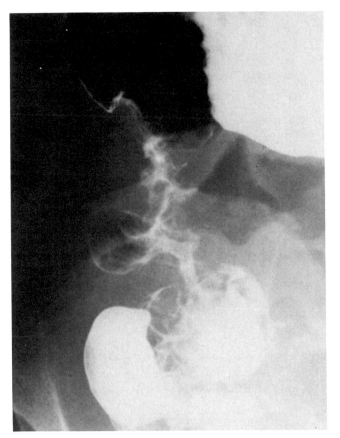

Figure 21 Ameboma in the ascending colon.

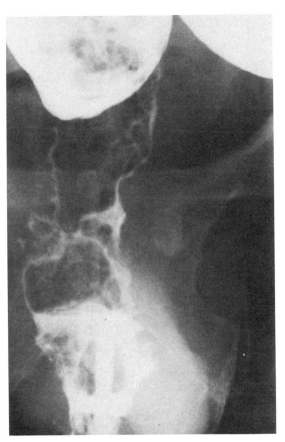

Figure 22 Narrowing and irregular ulceration in the rectum due to an ameboma.

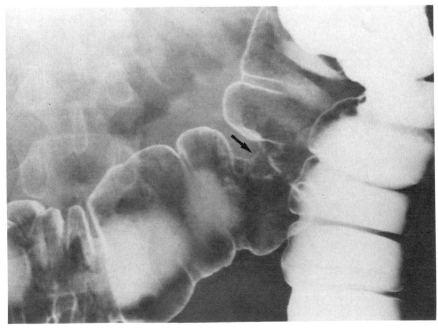

Figure 23 Small localized ameboma (arrow.)

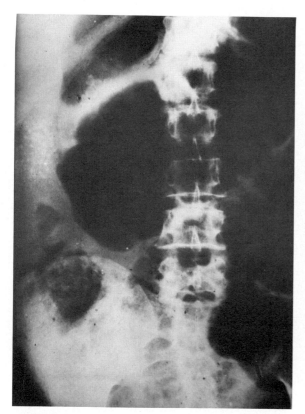

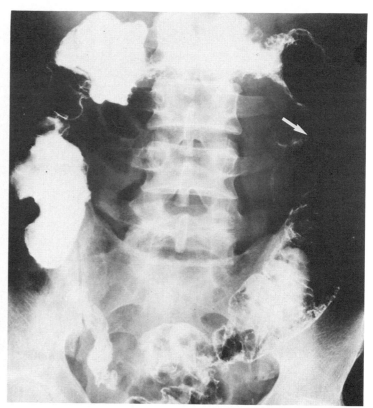

Figure 24 Toxic dilatation in amebiasis. (Presented by Dr. Aggarwal, New Delhi, India.)

Figure 25 Total colitis with ulceration and perforation in the descending colon (arrow) due to amebiasis.

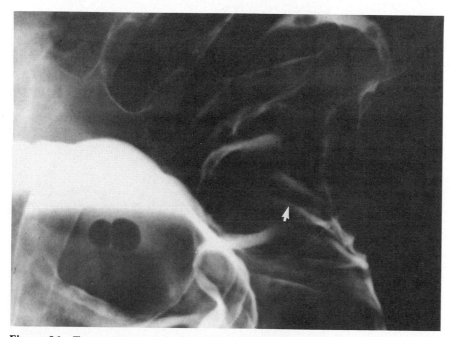

Figure 26 Transverse ulceration in tuberculosis (arrow).

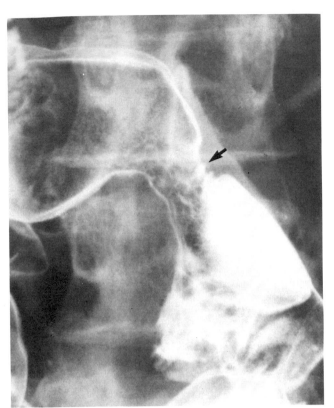

Figure 27a

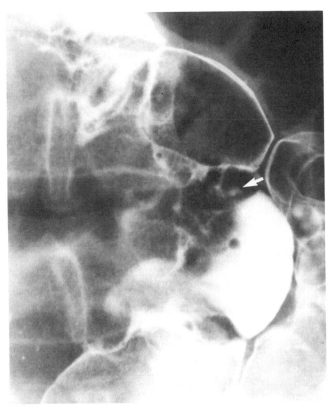

Figure 27b

Figure 27   Ileal tuberculosis with short strictures associated with transverse ulcers (arrow).

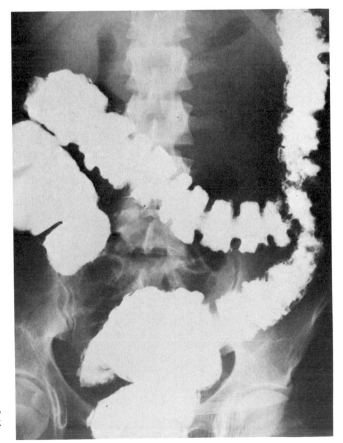

Figure 28   Extensive colitis due to tuberculosis, with large, deep, shaggy ulcers. (Courtesy of Dr. D. Silk, Central Middlesex Hospital, London.)

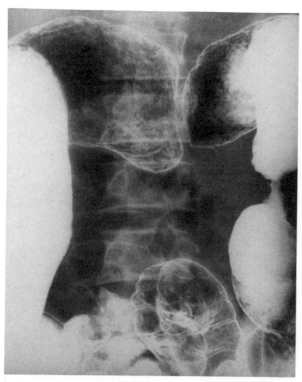

Figure 29 Two colonic strictures. The transverse colon stricture is very narrow and would be a most unusual configuration for Crohn's disease. (Courtesy of Dr. Aggarwal, New Delhi, India.)

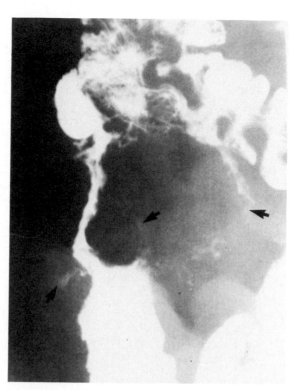

Figure 30 Hypertrophic ileocecal tuberculosis. A dilated terminal ileum leads into a very narrowed cecum and ascending colon. Several fistulous tracts outline the grossly thickened bowel wall (arrows).

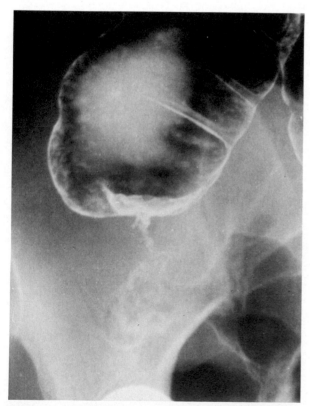

Figure 31 Clearly defined narrow stricture in the ascending colon without any adjacent mucosal disease, which would also be unusual in Crohn's disease. The deformed cecum and patulous ileocecal valve is typical of tuberculosis.

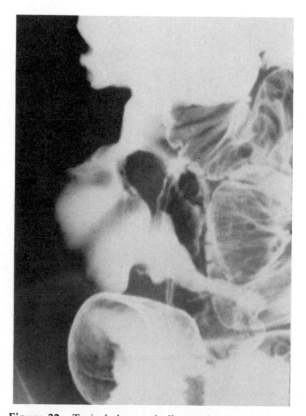

Figure 32 Typical changes in ileocecal tuberculosis.

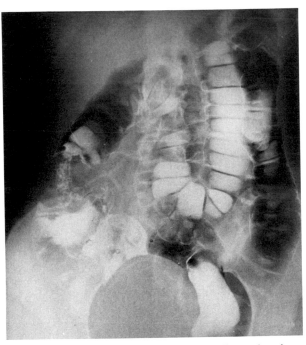

Figure 33 Annular stricture in the ascending colon due to tuberculosis, but radiologically more typical of amebiasis or carcinoma with the shouldered edges. (Courtesy of Dr. Aggarwal, New Delhi, India.)

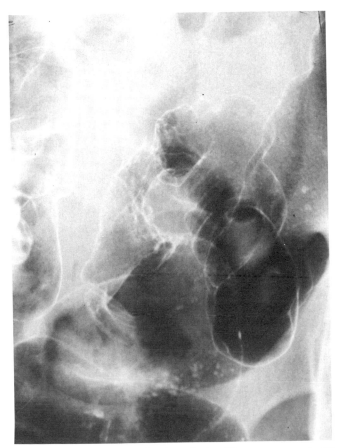

Figure 34 Rectosigmoid tuberculosis. The appearances are atypical and could be due to amebiasis or Crohn's disease.

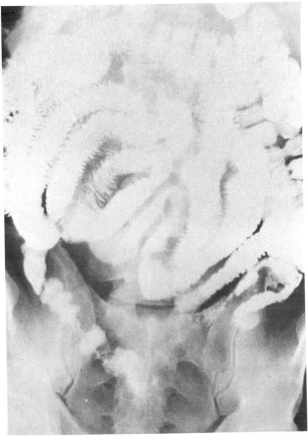

Figure 35 Tuberculous mesenteritis.

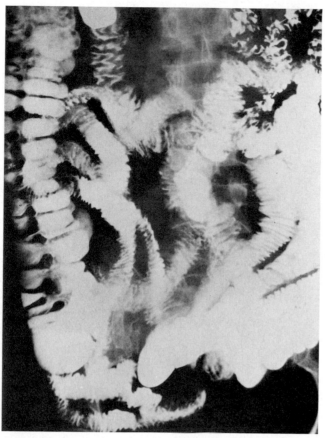

Figure 36 Tuberculous mesenteritis with a tuberculous abscess in the right iliac fossa causing localized displacement of loops.

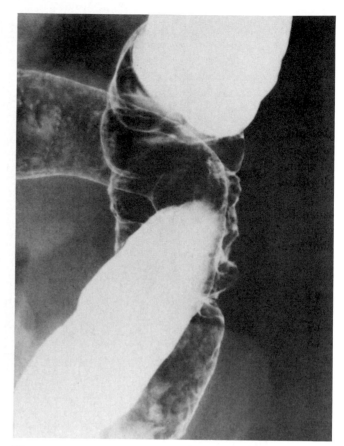

Figure 37 Inflammatory polyps due to schistosomiasis.

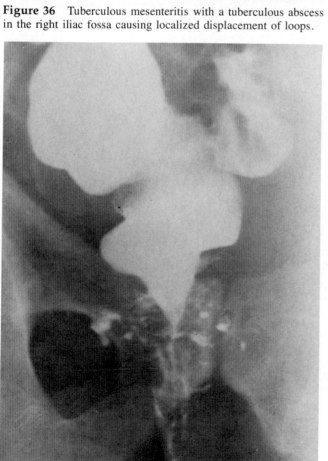

Figure 38 Lymphogranuloma venereum with rectal stricturing and multiple fistula.

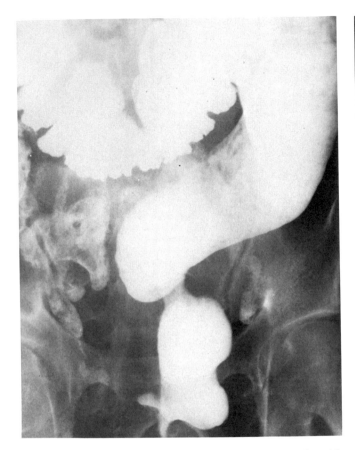

Figure 39 Lymphogranuloma venereum with rectosigmoid strictures.

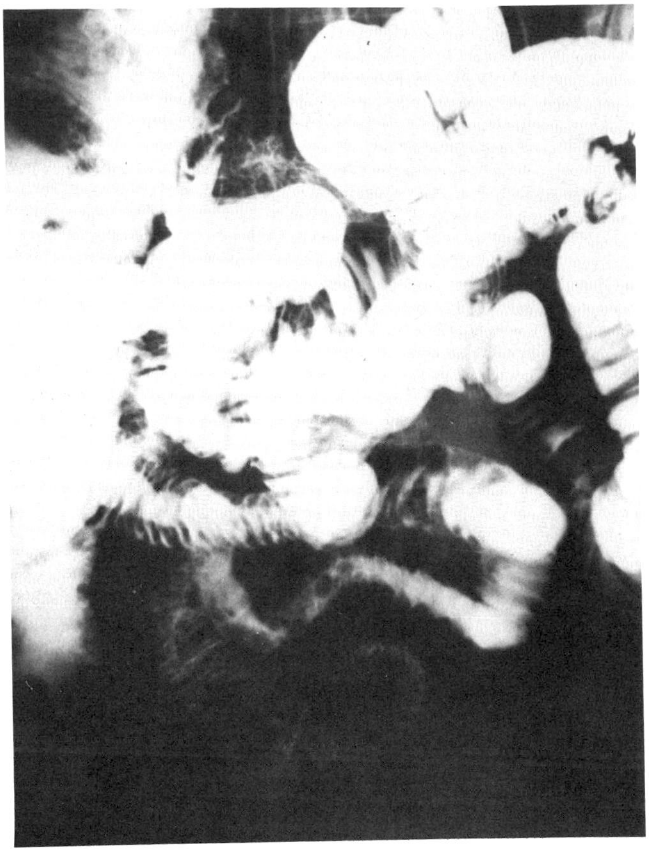

Figure 40 Typical radiation changes in distal ileum.

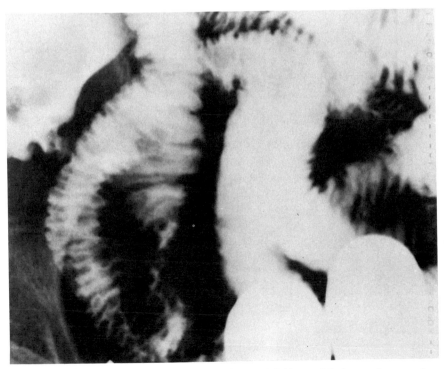

Figure 41 Early radiation changes with thickened folds, nodularity, and narrowing, with wide separation of distal ileal loops.

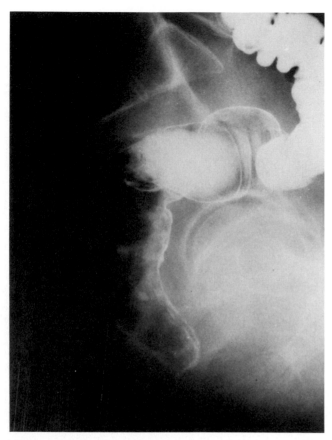

Figure 42 Radiation proctitis with widening of the postrectal space and a granular mucosa.

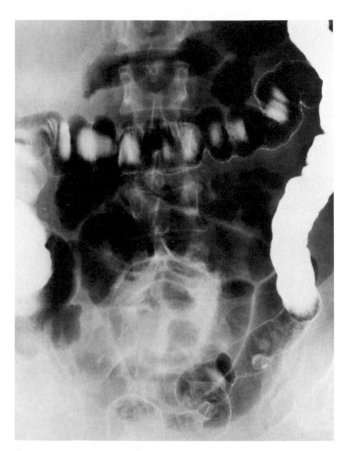

Figure 43 Colitis, probably ulcerative, which developed following radiation therapy for a carcinoma of the uterus.

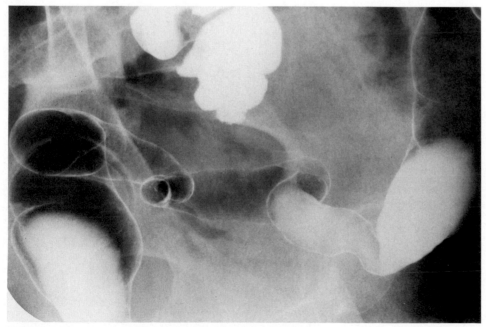

Figure 44 Sigmoid strictures following radiation therapy.

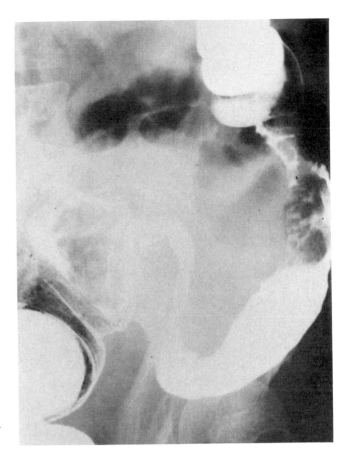

Figure 45 Scirrhous carcinoma producing a relatively smooth stricture, although the ends are shouldered and there is nodular mucosal irregularity proximally.

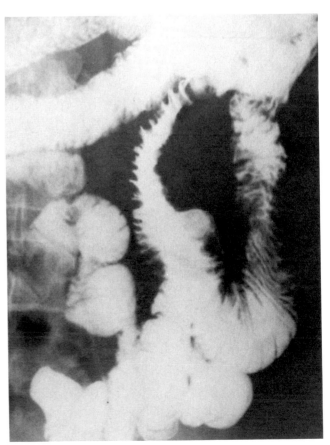

Figure 46 Secondary carcinoma in the small bowel mesentery. Spiculated folds with fixation and straightening of the bowel wall.

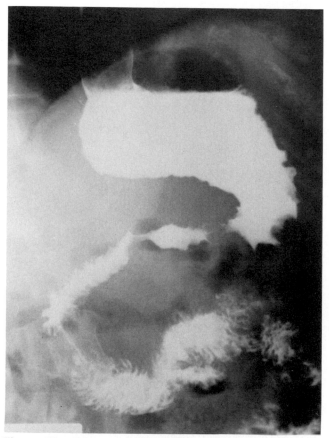

Figure 47a Primary gastric carcinoma.

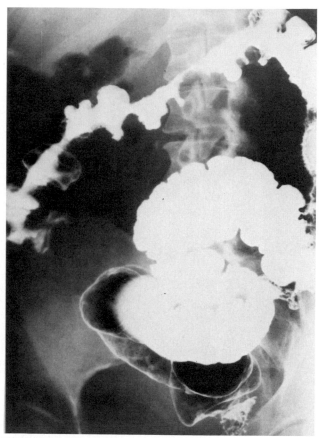

Figure 47b Secondary involvement mainly of the transverse colon with mucosal irregularity, straightening, and pseudodiverticula formation, and of the rectum with narrowing and ulceration.

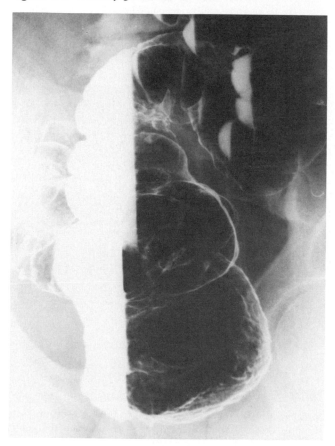

Figure 48 At sigmoidoscopy the changes were typical of a proctitis with diffuse ulceration. Radiologically, the changes are compatible with superficial ulceration. Lymphoma found on biopsy.

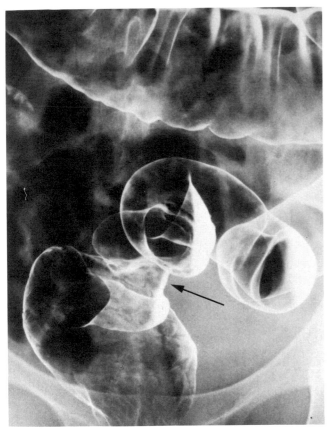

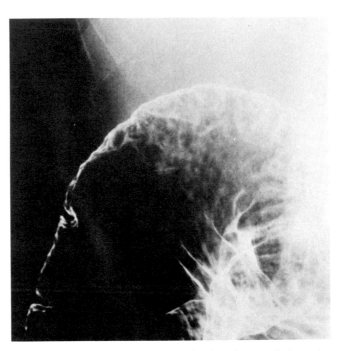

Figure 49 Solitary ulcer of the rectum. The wall is deformed at the site of the ulcer (arrow).

Figure 50 Another case of nodular lymphoma of the colon where the lesions are smaller and could be confused with aphthoid ulcers.

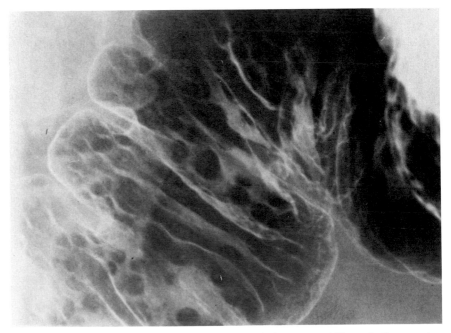

Figure 51 Nodular lymphoma of the colon. The lesions are umbilicated. Compared to aphthoid ulceration in Crohn's disease, the lesions are too elevated and the central umbilication too small and clearly defined.

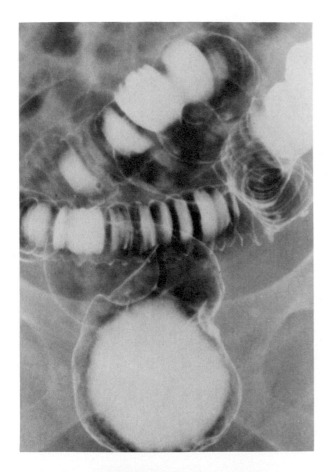

Figure 52 Polypoid lesions at the edges of a solitary ulcer due to cystic changes in the mucosa.

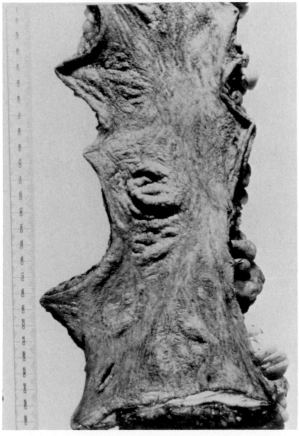

Figure 53 The ''snake skin'' appearance of a cathartic colon.

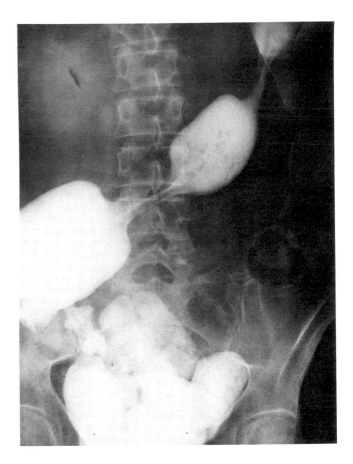

Figure 54 Transient "pseudostrictures" in cathartic colon.

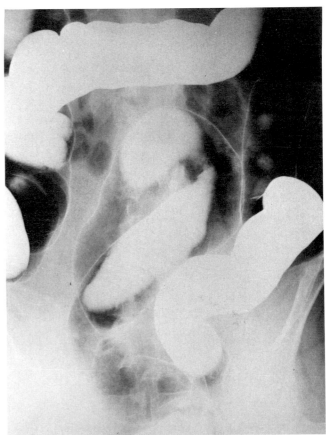

Figure 55 Colitis in a patient with adult coeliac disease. In this case the nature of the colitis was uncertain.

8

Pediatric and Neonatal Inflammatory Bowel Disease

PEDIATRIC INFLAM-MATORY BOWEL DISEASE

With improved diagnosis and awareness the onset of inflammatory bowel disease (IBD) in children is becoming more widely recognized. Both Crohn's disease and ulcerative colitis may develop early in life. Their onset in neonates is very rare, and in one series only 7.5% were below the age of 7 years when the disease developed. The usual age range at diagnosis is 9–14 years (1,2).

Presenting features include diarrhea, fever, weight loss, lethargy, anorexia, and abdominal pain. The important difference between IBD in adults and children is in the general effect that it has on a child. Marked delay in growth and puberty are common in children with severe IBD, and often present one of the most difficult aspects of management. A mean delay in diagnosis of almost 2 years has been reported (1), and because of the effects that this may have on the development of the child, failure to diagnose and treat IBD is more significant in children than in adults.

Other disorders, particularly infective colitis or cow's milk allergy (3), must be excluded before a child is investigated for IBD. Unfortunately, it is technically more difficult to confirm colitis histologically in a child than it is in an adult. Sigmoidoscopy and rectal biopsy can be performed in children, but this requires heavy sedation. Once the child has been sedated it is almost as simple to perform colonoscopy. This has the advantages of examining all the colon and being able to biopsy any site, which is often essential to diagnose Crohn's colitis. Although a barium enema might show the presence of colitis, the lack of histological confirmation of the type of colitis is a major disadvantage. If a child is suspected of having colitis, endoscopy with biopsy is the initial examination of choice. Once the diagnosis has been established, barium enema can be used to follow its progress, or to provide a pictorial view of the colitis should colonoscopy have been incomplete for any reason.

Barium studies remain the only method of examining the small bowel, so it is particularly important that these are performed and interpreted completely. Oral metoclopramide should always be given, with the dose adjusted according to the patient's age. Also, the volume of barium should be varied from 150 to 250ml at between 90 and 100 wt./vol. Overcouch films cannot be relied on for diagnosis, as so many of the loops of small bowel overlap. Careful examination of the small bowel, using manual compression with a lead glove, is the only reliable method of excluding or demonstrating a small segment of Crohn's disease (4,5) (Fig. 1).

A recent review of 29 children suspected of having IBD (5) suggested that most of the diagnostic inaccuracies were due to technically inadequate examinations.

Twenty-six small bowel examinations and 17 enemas had been performed. Comparison with the final diagnosis in these children showed that a correct diagnosis had been achieved in 22 of 26 of the small bowel examinations (85%), but in only 8 of 17 of the barium enemas (47%). Five of the small bowel examinations were grossly inadequate (Fig. 2), and compression studies had been performed only in a very few. In 2 children lymphoid nodular hyperplasia of the terminal ileum had been called Crohn's disease (Fig. 3), and in neither had compression films been taken. In the majority too little barium had been given with no accelerating agent, so that there was an insufficient volume of barium in the small bowel. Invariably this led to poor mucosal definition and sometimes to gross flocculation. Eleven children had double-contrast barium enemas, but 6 were technically inadequate (Fig. 4). Poor bowel preparation was common. The other major problem was the use of barium suspensions which were unsuited to double-contrast examination, resulting in cracking or poor coating of the mucosa. Comparison with colonoscopy showed that ulcerative colitis had been missed in 3 patients and Crohn's disease in 3 as a result of technically inadequate examinations. Good double-contrast barium enemas can show aphthoid ulceration (Figs. 5 and 7). The sensitivity of the examination in children should correspond to that in adults.

Bowel preparation depends on the age of the child. In the very young, clear fluids and a saline enema may suffice, whereas older children need phosphate enemas and some purgation (Table 1). In ulcerative colitis or extensive Crohn's an instant enema may be used.

The technique of the barium enema is important. A soft rubber catheter, such as a small Foley, is inserted per rectum and the barium suspension (100% wt/vol) is injected via a syringe. The volume obviously depends on the size of the child, but in those under 7 years, 50–100 ml will be sufficient to fill the bowel to the transverse colon. Air is then insufflated

Table 1 Bowel Preparation for Children

Age (yr.)	Day before barium enema	Day of barium enema
0–1	Feed until midnight	Water or fruit juice 4 a.m.; ½ sachet (5 ml) Fletcher's phosphate enema[a]
1–4	Clear fluids only; X-prep[b] 1 mg/kg body weight	Fletcher's phosphate enema: ¾ sachet 1–2 yr, 1 sachet 2–4 yr
Over 4	Clear fluids only; X-prep 1 mg/kg body weight	Saline enema: 150 ml, 5 yr 300 ml, 5 10 yr 500 ml, over 10 yr

[a] Pharmax Ltd., Bourne Rd., Bexley, Kent DA5 1NX, U.K.

[b] Napp Laboratories Ltd., Hill Farm Ave., Watford WD2 7RA, U.K.

gently and the child turned from side to side. Should there be any spasm, an intravenous relaxant should be given. Two or three spot films in different projections are then taken (Figs. 6 and 8).

The radiological changes of IBD are the same in children as in adults. The suggestion that an earlier onset of disease is associated with more severe disease may in part reflect the use of inadequate methods of diagnosis; for example, only gross colitis will be apparent on poorly prepared single-contrast enemas. Unfortunately, a large proportion of children with IBD seen in hospital practice do have advanced disease. This is associated with failure to thrive and delayed bone age.

The bone age is assessed by comparing film of the nondominant hand and wrist of the patient to a set of standard films in a reference book. Progress can be monitored by repeat assessments of bone age. Surgery at an early stage with resection of the involved bowel removes the "toxic effect" of the disease and allows growth (6). If this is delayed, the epiphyses may fuse before adequate growth is possible, so surgery should be considered earlier rather than later in the pediatric age group.

NEONATAL NECROTIZING ENTERO-COLITIS

Necrotizing enterocolitis (NEC) affects about 5% of premature infants, usually within the first week of oral feeding. It presents with abdominal distension, rectal bleeding, and bilious vomiting. The cause is uncertain. A number of factors may be involved, such as oral feeding with infection or endotoxins producing mucosal injury and ischemia when there is altered host defense. NEC can occur following exchange transfusions, in congenital obstructions, or in Hirschsprung's disease. The disease process seems to be similar to that in premature infants.

Early plain film changes may suggest a small bowel obstruction with gaseous distension of the small bowel and little or no gas in the colon (7,8). Dilated fluid-filled loops, loss of bowel wall definition, and a generalized ileus are other possible findings. These are relatively nonspecific and a definite diagnosis of NEC should be made when gas is seen in the bowel wall (Fig. 10) (9). This may be seen in almost any part of the intestine, but the ileocecal region is most commonly affected. Gas may tract into the portal vein (Fig. 9a, b), or bowel wall necrosis lead to perforation which can be free, with air in the intraperitoneal cavity, or sealed when a peritonitis develops with localized ileus and free fluid widening the gap between bowel loops. Intramural and portal vein gas does not always relate to the severity of the NEC or its disappearance to clinical improvement (8).

The benign form of pneumatosis intestinalis is very rare in neonates, and in most cases where air is seen in the bowel wall will be due to NEC. Confusion may occur with the meconium plug syndrome, Hirschsprung's disease, or the inspissated milk syndrome (10). Obstruction develops several days after artificial feeds, and mottled masses outlined by gas may be seen in the colon. If there is any doubt as to the diagnosis, barium enema can be considered. In NEC the affected segment is narrowed and ulcerated, and obstruction from itraluminal collections excluded. Naturally, a barium enema is contraindicated if gas is seen in the bowel wall.

NEC is a serious condition with a high mortality. Parenteral nutrition and antibiotic therapy have recently been found to be successful unless perforation has occurred, when surgery will be needed. Stricture formation is common and is due to fibrosis following extensive submucosal damage.

Routine barium enema is advised several weeks following recovery to exclude a stricture (11). These can resolve spontaneously, so that unless the stricture is causing marked obstruction, a futher examination should be performed a month or two later to assess the stricture's progress.

REFERENCES

1. Walker-Smith, J. *Diseases of the Small Intestine in Childhood.* Pitman, London, p. 285.
2. Berger, L.A., Wilkinson, D. (1974). The investigation of colitis in infancy.
3. Gryboski, J.D. (1967). Gastrointestinal milk allergy in infants. Paediatrics 40; 354.
4. Silverman, F.N. (1966). Regional enteritis in children. Aust. Paediatr. J. 2; 207.
5. Chong, S.K.F., Bartram, C.I., Campbell, C.A., et al. (1982). Chronic inflammatory bowel disease in childhood. Br. Med. J. 284; 101.
6. O'Donoghue, D.P., Dawson, A.M. (1977). Crohn's disease in childhood. Arch. Dis. Child. 52; 627.
7. Kogutt, M.S., (1979). Necrotizing enterocolitis of infancy. Early roentgen pattern as a guide to prompt diagnosis. Radiology 130; 367.
8. Danerum, A., Woodward, S., de Silva, M. (1978). The radiology of neonatal necrotizing enterocolitis: a review of 47 cases and the literature. Paediatr. Radiol. 7; 70.
9. Bell, R.S., Graham, C.B., Stevenson, J.K. (1971). Roentgenologic and clinical manifestations of necrotizing enterocolitis. Am. J. Roentgenol. 112; 123.
10. Friedland, G.W., Rush, W.A., Hill, A.J. (1972). Smythe's inspissated milk syndrome. Radiology 103; 159.
11. Tonkin, I.L.D., Buelland, J.C., Hunter, T.B., et al. (1978). Spontaneous resolution of colonic strictures caused by necrotizing enterocolitis: therapeutic implications. Am. J. Roentgenol. 130; 1077.

FIGURES 1 THROUGH 10

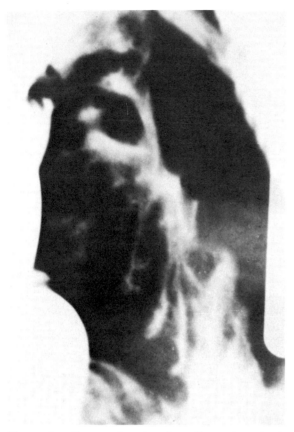

Figure 1a Compression view shows linear ulceration in the terminal ileum due to Crohn's disease.

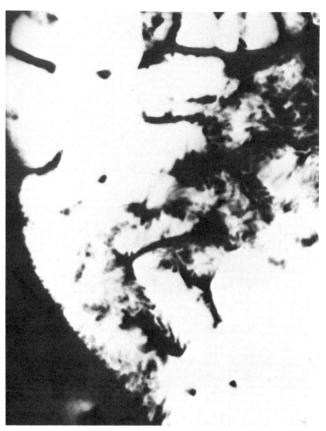

Figure 1b Small bowel meal. The cecum has filled and the small bowel appears normal, although the terminal ileum is not seen.

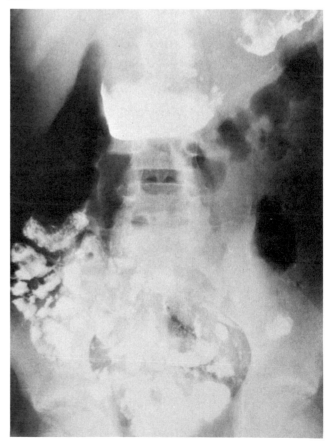

Figure 2 Technically inadequate small bowel examination due to flocculation of the suspension. Note the retention of barium in the stomach.

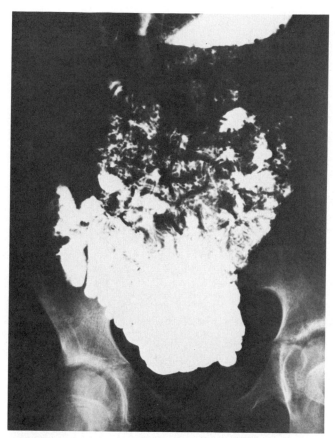

Figure 3a Small bowel examination. No abnormality seen.

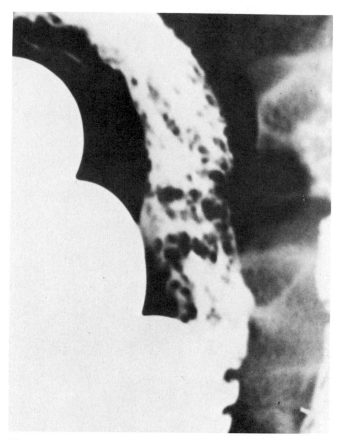

Figure 3b Compression view of the terminal ileum showing multiple 2-mm nodules; typical changes of follicular lymphoid hyperplasia.

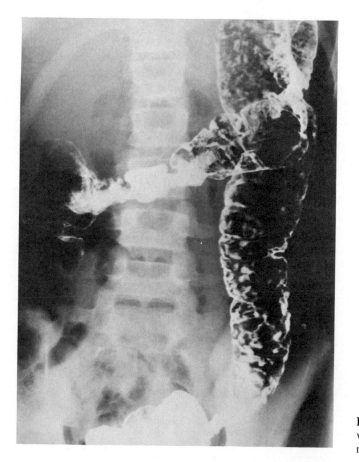

Figure 4 Technically inadequate double-contrast barium enema with extensive break up of the suspension, causing loss of all mucosal detail.

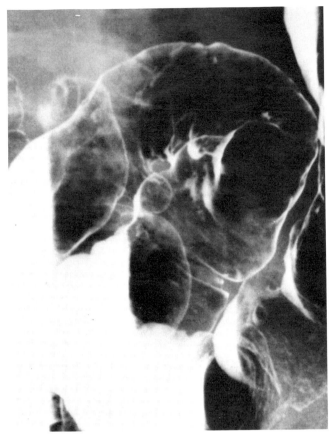

Figure 5 Aphthoid ulceration in the sigmoid colon.

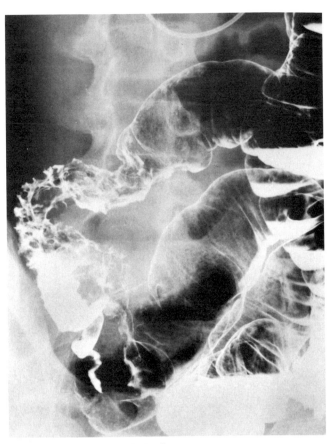

Figure 6 Ileocecal Crohn's disease.

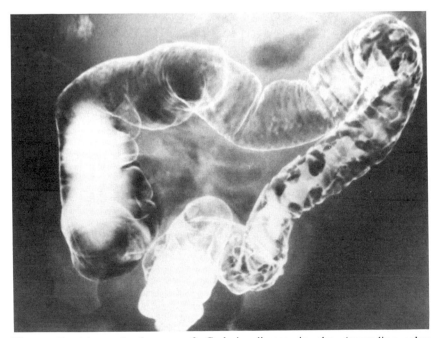

Figure 7 Advanced changes of Crohn's disease in the descending colon prevented full colonoscopy. Double-contrast barium enema showed aphthoid ulceration extending to the hepatic flexure.

266

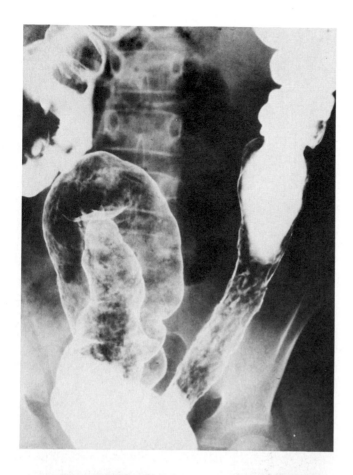

Figure 8a Instant enema showing linear ulceration in the lower descending colon.

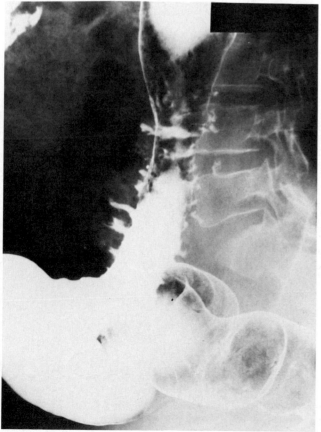

Figure 8b Several months later colonoscopy had been attempted and thought to show a stricture but the examination was incomplete. A repeat instant enema showed very deep ulceration penetrating the bowel wall, leading to perforation and abscess formation, which was confirmed at operation.

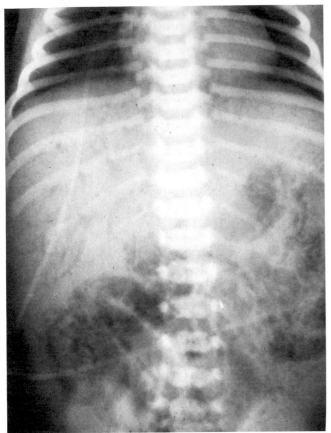

Figure 9 A severe case of NEC with extensive gas in the wall of the small bowel and portal veins.

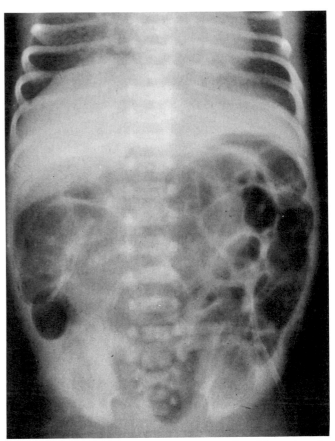

Figure 10a NEC with dilatation of the small and large bowel. Gas is just visible in the lateral wall of the caecum to confirm the diagnosis.

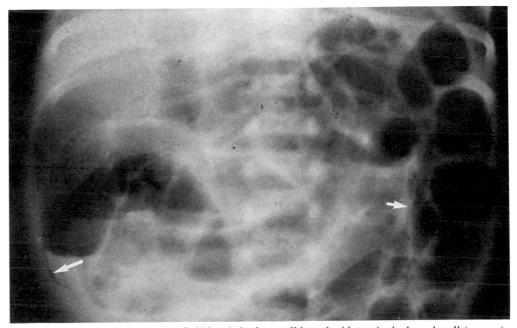

Figure 10b Erect view showing fluid levels in the small bowel with gas in the bowel wall (arrows).

9
Surgery of Inflammatory Bowel Disease

James P.S. Thomson / St. Mark's Hospital for Diseases of the Rectum and Colon, Hackney Hospital, and St. Bartholomew's Hospital Medical College, London, England

Operative treatment plays an important role in the management of many patients with inflammatory bowel disease. These patients are therefore best cared for by a surgeon and a physician working in close collaboration. Whereas in some patients the need for operation is abundantly clear, in others very careful consideration has to be given to this, often over a prolonged period, and then the radiologist, endoscopist, and pathologist, in addition, all contribute to the final opinion.

Ulcerative colitis (idiopathic proctocolitis) and Crohn's disease have many aspects in common, but they are fundamentally different. Ulcerative colitis, being confined to the large intestine, may be cured by total removal of the colon and rectum. In Crohn's disease operation may be curative, but because of the possible extensive nature of the disease and its liability to recurrence, this is not always the case. These two diseases will therefore be considered separately and this should serve to emphasize the importance of arriving at the correct diagnosis as soon as possible in a patient with inflammatory bowel disease.

ULCERATIVE COLITIS

Indications for Operation

Emergency.   Perforation, dilatation of the colon, and severe hemorrhage are indications for urgent operative treatment. In addition, patients with severe colitis who do not respond to potent drug therapy may also require emergency operation. This is the case when more than one of the following are present (1): persistent fever in excess of 38°C, more than eight bowel actions in 24 hrs, severe abdominal tenderness, serum albumin below 30 g/liter, prostration and malaise, and/or age over 60 years.

Elective.   Patients with recurrent acute attacks and persistent symptoms or ill health despite medical treatment will need operative treatment. Stool frequency and urgency due to a contracted rectum may be so severe that although the patient feels well, an ileostomy would be preferable. Other indications include malnutrition (low serum albumin), anemia, retardation of growth and development, and systemic complications (Table 1).

The other major indication for operation is the prevention or treatment of cancer. The cancer risk is not great, but those patients who have had extensive colitis for more than 10 years should be screened by means of endoscopy and biopsy for dysplasia and/or carcinoma.

Types of Operation   The operations available for the treatment of ulcerative colitis depend on whether or not the rectum is excised and whether or not a permanent stoma (ileostomy) is constructed. Preservation of the rectum means retention of bowel affected by ulcerative colitis and the small, but definite risk of cancer. On the other hand, removal of the rectum carries with it the risk of damage to the pelvic nerves that supply the bladder and sexual organs, and also means there will be a perineal wound, which in a small proportion of patients remains unhealed. The disadvantages of a stoma are obvious.

The operations are classified in Figure 1.

Proctocolectomy with Ileostomy.   The term "proctocolectomy" implies removal of the whole large intestine together with the anal canal. As previously stated, ulcerative colitis affects only the large bowel, so this procedure cures the patient. Proctocolectomy is therefore the standard elective operation.

The dissection of the rectum can be done very close to the bowel, (2), and this significantly reduces the risk of bladder and sexual dysfunction and if the perineal dissection is undertaken through the intersphincteric space (Fig. 2), a very small perineal wound is created. The details and complications of ileostomy are dealt with at the end of the chapter.

Subtotal Colectomy with Mucous Fistula and Ileostomy.   Excision of the rectum, even when carried out as described above, increases the morbidity and mortality of emergency operations for ulcerative colitis. For this reason in the acute situation a subtotal colectomy only is performed; the rectum, together with the distal sigmoid colon, are preserved—the latter to give length to the retained bowel, so that it may be exteriorized as a mucous fistula.

Very often this is a lifesaving procedure and when the patient has fully recovered, a decision has to be made about the retained bowel. The majority of patients will require rectal excision, but a few might be able to have the continuity of their bowel restored by an ileorectal anastomosis or with an ileal reservoir and anal anastomosis.

An instant enema of the rectum and distal sigmoid colon always shows a narrowed bowel, as it is defunctioned, but irregularity of the surface indicates active disease (Fig. 3).

Total Colectomy with Ileorectal Anastomosis.   Total coletomy with an ileorectal anastomosis sounds like an attractive procedure, but it must be remembered that the rectum is

Table 1   Systemic Complications of Ulcerative Colitis

Site	Complications
Joints	An arthropathy tending to affect large joints
	Sacroiliitis
	Ankylosing spondylitis
Skin	Erythema nodosum
	Pyoderma gangrenosum
Eyes	Iritis

practically always involved with disease. The patient will often require medication for the proctitis and as the average bowel frequency is three to six actions per 24 hr, medication with agents such as codeine phosphate or loperamide to reduce bowel frequency is often also required. Furthermore, the retained rectum carries an increased risk of cancer. These patients will therefore require long-term medical supervision and probably more than 25% will require a rectal excision at some stage. However, the majority of patients requiring operation for ulcerative colitis are not suitable for this procedure as the rectum is too severely inflamed.

In the assessment of patients for this operation the overall configuration of the rectum can be judged from the instant enema provided that a lateral pelvic and posterioanterior view are taken. If this appears narrow, the maximum rectal volume that can be tolerated may be measured by balloon inflation studies, 150 ml being the desired volume tolerated if this operation is to be functionally successful. Patients with reduced tolerance have a small, narrow rectum with increased postrectal space (Fig. 4). The exact interrelationship between radiology and balloon studies has not been established, but obviously there is a broad area of agreement.

An ileorectal anastomosis may be examined by an instant enema. Using intravenous relaxants and air insufflation, the anastomosis and distal small bowel can be visualized optimally (Fig. 5). Active disease may be seen within the rectum (Fig. 6). In patients who have had an anastomosis for many years, gross dilatation of the distal ileum may develop. This seems to be physiological, as no obstructive element may be present (Fig. 7).

Proctocolectomy with Ileal Reservoir and Anal Anastomosis. Parks and his colleagues (3) have described an operation which could, in time, radically change the surgical management of ulcerative colitis. All the diseased colon, together with the mucosa of the rectum, is removed, and the ileum joined to the anal canal at the level of the dentate line. In order that there be some capacity in the terminal ileum, a pouch is constructed from the ileum. A simple ileoanal anastomosis would result in severe and unacceptable fecal frequency and urgency. This *neorectum* requires catheterization to empty it in about half the patients, but in the other half spontaneous evacuation is possible. However, in nearly all patients, continence is entirely satisfactory. The initial results are most encouraging, but further experience is needed before its place in surgical management is completely defined.

In summary, proctocolectomy is the usual operation in the treatment of ulcerative colitis, but it should be avoided in the acute situation where subtotal colectomy is the treatment of choice. A few patients are suitable for total colectomy and ileorectal anastomosis if the rectal inflammation is not too great, but continued supervision is essential, and proctocolectomy with ileal pouch and anal anastomosis may in time become the elective operation of choice.

CROHN'S DISEASE

Indications for Operation The pattern of Crohn's disease varies considerably from patient to patient. This means that the indications for operation are less well defined than in ulcerative colitis. The main indications are:

1. Narrowing of lumen: severe colicky pain after food, subacute and acute intestinal obstruction
2. Perforation: generalized peritonitis, abscess formation, internal and external fistulas
3. Dilatation: toxic megacolon
4. Hemorrhage
5. Chronic ill health
6. Systemic complications
7. Anal disease

In the preoperative preparation of patients with Crohn's disease it is essential that the surgeon have as much information as possible about the extent of the disease. This means that radiological and endoscopic investigation (including biopsy) has to be thorough.

Types of Operation   Once a decision has been taken to operate on a patient with Crohn's disease the surgeon may find he or she has a relatively simple problem to deal with, such as resection of the terminal ileum, or may have an exceedingly complicated situation with internal fistulas and sepsis involving the resection of several lengths of small and large intestine and possibly the construction of a stoma. The various procedures include: resection with anastomosis, excision with exteriorization of the bowel ends, excision of the rectum (and colon) with a stoma, bypass procedures, and anal operations.

Resection with Anastomosis.   The diseased bowel is resected with a small margin (say 10 cm) of normal bowel. An end-to-end anastomosis is usually constructed. It is helpful to mark the site of the anastomosis with clips so that its site may be readily identified during any subsequent radiological investigation for possible recurrence. It is also helpful to measure the length of the remaining small intestine so that any tendency to malabsorption may be anticipated and again to assist in the interpretation of subsequent radiographs. Examples of this type of operative procedure would include resection of the terminal ileum and right colon with an end-to-end ileocolic anastomosis (right hemicolectomy), or a total colectomy with an ileorectal anastomosis.

Excision with Exteriorization of Bowel Ends.   On occasions, particularly in the presence of severe sepsis a staged procedure is safer. Thus the diseased bowel may be excised and a proximal ileostomy fashioned. The distal bowel may be brought to the surface as a mucous fistula, or the end oversewn and returned to the peritoneal cavity. Subsequently, after, say 4–6 months, at a further operation an end-to-end anastomosis may be carried out.

Excision of the Rectum with a Stoma.   The rectum and anal canal are usually removed for severe anal disease (see below). How much of the large intestine is involved will determine whether a terminal sigmoid colostomy, or a proctocolectomy with an ileostomy, is required. As with ulcerative colitis, a close rectal dissection is usually both possible and desirable.

Bypass Operations.   The bypassing of an area of Crohn's disease by constructing a side-to-side anastomosis was once popular. It is now the aim of most surgeons to resect the disease. However, when duodenal Crohn's disease is present this is not possible, so a side-to-side gastrojejunal anastomosis to bypass the lesion would be carried out.

Anal Operations.   The anal canal and perianal tissues are frequently the site of Crohn's disease. The overall incidence varies from 25 to 75%, the incidence increasing with the more distal involvement of the bowel. In a few patients anal disease may be the only manifestation. The characteristic features of anal Crohn's disease are as follows: Bluish coloration, Edematous tags, Ulceration, Abscess formation, Fistula, Stenosis.

The main principle in operations for anal Crohn's disease is to do the minimum to ease the patient's symptoms. It is not possible to cure anal disease by operation except by excision of the rectum, but with appropriate minor surgery, symptomatic improvement may be dramatic. Abscesses require drainage, but fistulas, provided that they are not painful, are best left alone. Ulceration is best managed with an anal dilator lubricated with local anesthetic or even steroid cream rather than by performing a sphincterotomy. Severe ulceration of the anal margin and extensive sepsis may demand fecal diversion and possible rectal excision.

The Severely Ill Patient with Abdominal Sepsis.   The patient with severe intra-abdominal sepsis with or without internal and external fistulas requires special mention. It is not usually possible to operate and resect the disease immediately without doing damage to surrounding, perhaps normal, bowel.

The first step is the control of the sepsis. Although antibiotics may help in this, their role should be considered as an adjuvant to the therapy. Usually, there is loculated pus; after this has been located, often now with the aid of ultrasonography or computerized tomography, it should be drained. The second step is to improve the nutritional state of the patient. Although this may be possible by the oral route, it is usually necessary to institute bowel rest and to provide the patient with parenteral nutrition. Once the sepsis is controlled and the patient is in a satisfactory nutritional state, investigation of the site of the disease and operation can proceed. It is essential that the surgeon allow adequate time for such an operation and makes a long abdominal incision so that there are no problems of access.

Prognosis. Contrary to the generally held view, operation for Crohn's disease can be undertaken with a very low overall morbidity and mortality rate (less than 5%). Recurrent disease, however, has a significant incidence. This is heralded by a return of symptoms and the diagnosis confirmed by radiology and endoscopy (Figs. 8 and 9). Further operation may be required if medical treatment does not control the symptoms and the indications are as previously stated. It is worth stating that occasionally the presence of obstructive symptoms is due to adhesions and not recurrent disease.

It would appear that the most important factor determining whether or not recurrence occurs is the length of time after primary resection. There are good figures from many sources and in those patients who have had a resection with an anastomosis at 10 years there is a recurrence rate of approximately 50%, whereas in those who have an excision with a stoma, the rate is very much lower, about 10%.

STOMAS The most usual stoma constructed in patients operated on for inflammatory bowel disease is an ileostomy, but very occasionally in patients with Crohn's disease a colostomy is constructed.

Ileostomy There are three principal types of ileostomy: terminal (spout) ileostomy, loop ileostomy, and continent ileostomy.

Terminal Ileostomy. A terminal ileostomy is usually placed in the right iliac fossa, but in order to get it well sited (away from bony prominences and previous scars) so that appliances may be satisfactorily worn, it may be necessary to put it on the left. To ensure that the effluent passes into the appliance, the ileostomy is constructed with a spout about 2.0 cm in length.

The volume of effluent in a 24-hr period varies considerably, but an average of approximately 500–700 ml is passed. In practical terms for the patient this means emptying the appliance three to four times a day. It should be remembered that the ileostomy effluent contained proteolytic enzymes, which if allowed to remain in contact with the skin will cause soreness.

Various complications occur in relationship to an ileostomy. The ileostomy itself can become necrotic, detached from the skin, or narrowed. If the appliance is too tight, ulceration may occur. Fistula formation usually means recurrent Crohn's disease. Prolapse and peri-ileostomy herniation can be difficult problems to manage, but fortunately they are rare.

Soreness of the surrounding skin was a great problem, but the newer types of appliance and the development of the nursing speciality *"Stoma Care Nurses"* has almost eliminated this. The causes include contact of the effluent on the skin, hypersensitivity to the appliance, too vigorous cleansing, and peristomal fungus infection.

Disturbances of function usually take the form of excessive action. One group of conditions causing this are those which cause diarrhea in normal people (e..g., infective episodes, transit disorders, malabsorption syndromes, including lactose deficiency, and sensitivity to antibiotics). More specific causes include paraintestinal sepsis, recurrent disease (Crohn's disease), and intestinal obstruction (Figs. 10–12).

Reduced action in the presence of colic usually means obstruction to the small bowel. This is an indication for laparotomy in 6–8% of patients within the first 2–3 years after initial surgery, and is the second most common specific cause of related death as recorded by the Ileostomy Association of Great Britain. Adhesions are the most common cause of the obstruction (Fig. 13), but a volvulus (Fig. 14), lateral space obstruction, or kinking of bowel around the rectal stump are other possibilities. Subacute episodes of obstruction are common and may be related to bolus obstruction; peanuts seem to be particularly troublesome in this respect. Most of these patients will have significant adhesions that can be demonstrated radiologically. The ileostomy enema shows only the distal small bowel. These adhesions may be situated in any part of the remaining small intestine and are demonstrated best by either a small bowel enema or meal (Fig. 15). Whatever the method the secret of showing adhesions lies in meticulous compression of all the small bowel loops; this may reveal fixation and angulation at the point of the adhesion.

There are various metabolic upsets which may present as an increased incidence of biliary and renal calculi or various electrolyte disturbances. Finally, there are a number of psychosocial problems, which depend very much on the age, sex, and personality of the patient (4).

Loop Ileostomy. A loop ileostomy (Fig. 16) is sometimes constructed proximal to an ileorectal anastomosis. it is closed when the anastomosis has soundly healed; this may be judged by means of a water-soluble enema examination.

Continent Ileostomy. The continent ileostomy was first described by Kock in the early 1970s (5). A pouch of terminal small intestine is constructed to act as a reservoir and a nipple valve constructed on the efferent limb leading to a flush ileostomy on the anterior abdominal wall (Fig. 17). In theory the patient does not need to wear an appliance and the reservoir is emptied approximately four times a day by passing a catheter. Unfortunately, only about half the patients had satisfactory results, so this operation is now being performed less and may be superseded by Park's ileal reservoir and anal anastomosis operation. These pouch operations are not suitable in patients with Crohn's disease, as the pouch could subsequently become the site of the inflammatory process (Fig. 18).

On plain films the pouch may contain gas and show a fluid level on the erect view, or a mottled mixture of gas and fluid which should not be confused with a pelvic abscess. (Figs. 19 and 20).

The most serious immediate problem is leakage from the pouch. If there is marked dehiscence with peritonitis, immediate reoperation with drainage and the establishment of a defunctioning loop ileostomy is necessary. A small leak with the formation of a fistula may close spontaneously if the pouch is drained continuously. In such situations a water-soluble contrast medium diluted with water (about 1:3) should be used to fill the pouch via a catheter through the valve and observed under screening to see the site of leakage (Fig. 21).

Later mechanical problems should be investigated using barium. Ideally, the patient should be fasted for several hours prior to the examination, and should always drain the pouch immediately before. The draining catheter may be left in situ and used to fill the pouch with about 150 ml of barium followed by air insufflation. The capacity of the pouch increases to about 500 ml 3–6 months after operation. Spot films should be taken to show the configuration of the pouch, a profile view of the nipple valve, and the distal small bowel if this has filled (Fig. 22). The commonest complication is reduction of the nipple valve (Fig. 23). This is usually partial, with retraction along the mesenteric wall, but may be complete if the pouch has become detached from the anterior abdominal wall (Fig. 24). Both result in incontinence and difficult intubation. Should intubation prove difficult at the time of the examination, the catheter should be left in the valve and contrast injected with spot films to show the valve itself. Nonspecific ileitis is uncommon; it presents with diarrhea and bleeding. Thickened mucosal folds or, rarely, ulceration may be seen in the pouch (Fig. 25).

Colostomy Rarely in some patients with Crohn's disease, a terminal colostomy is constructed following excision of the rectum. This is usually in the left iliac fossa and is similar to that constructed when the indication is carcinoma. The effluent is firmer and usually there are few problems with this type of stoma.

In summary, some of the important concepts of the surgical management of inflammatory bowel disease, particularly where there is relevance to the radiologist, have been described. Further detail must be culled from the larger surgical textbooks devoted to these topics (6,7).

REFERENCES

1. Lennard-Jones, J.E. (1976). Ulcerative colitis. In *Current Surgical Practice,* Vol. I, Hadfield, J., Hobsley, M. (Eds). Arnold, London, p. 185.
2. Parks, A.G., Lyttle, J.A. (1977). Intersphincteric excision of the rectum. Br. J. Surg. 64; 413.
3. Parks, A.G. Nicholls, R.J., Belliveau, P. (1980). Proctocolectomy with ileal reservoir and anal anastomosis. Br. J. Surg. 67; 533.
4. Thomson, J.P.S., Lennard-Jones, J.E. (1977). Life with an ileostomy. Clin. Gastroenterol. 6; 699.
5. Kock, N.G. (1973). Continent ileostomy. In *Progress in Surgery,* Vol. 12, Allgower, M., Bergentz, S.E., Calne, R.Y. (Eds)., Karger, Basel, p. 180.
6. Goligher, J.C. (1980). *Surgery of the Anus, Rectum and Colon.* Ballière Tindall, London.
7. Thomson, J.P.S., Nicholls, R.J., Williams, C.B. (Eds.) (1981). *Colorectal Disease.* Heinemann, London.

FIGURES 1 THROUGH 25

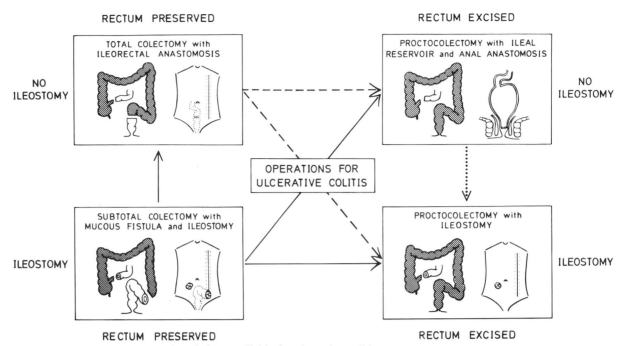

Figure 1 Scheme of the operative choices available for ulcerative colitis.

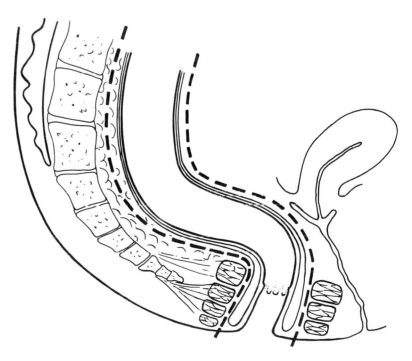

Figure 2 Plane for the perineal dissection of the rectum (dotted line) via the intersphincteric space.

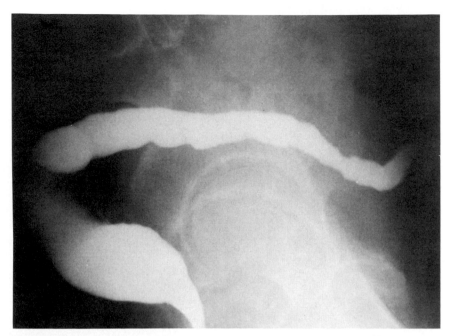

Figure 3 Retained rectum brought out onto the anterior abdominal wall as a mucous fistula. The rectum is narrowed as it is defunctioned. Mucosal irregularity would indicate active disease.

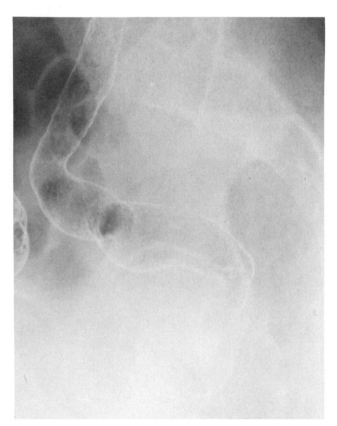

Figure 4 Instant enema with lateral view of the pelvis showing a narrowed rectum probably unsuitable for ileorectal anastomosis.

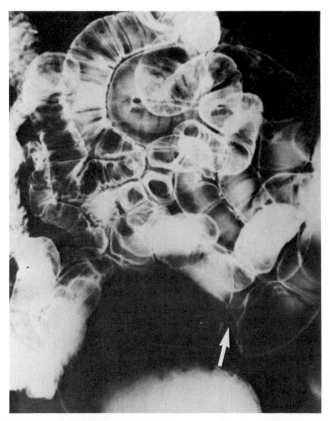

Figure 5 Instant enema with intravenous relaxant to show distal small bowel and anastomosis (arrow).

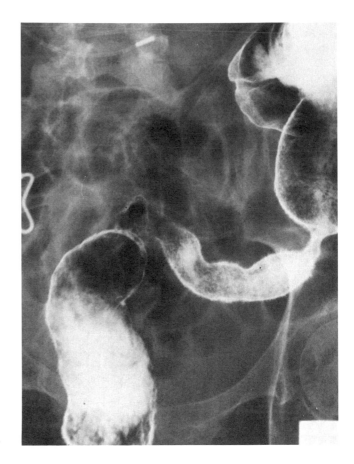

Figure 6 Active disease in the retained rectum.

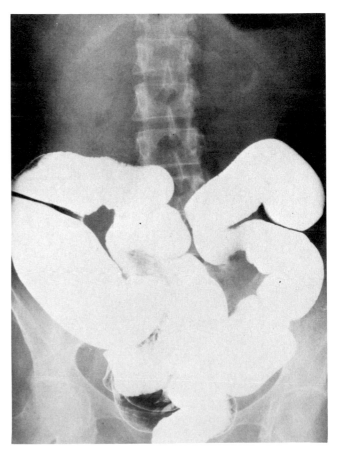

Figure 7 Ileal dilatation without obstruction in a long-standing ileorectal anastomosis.

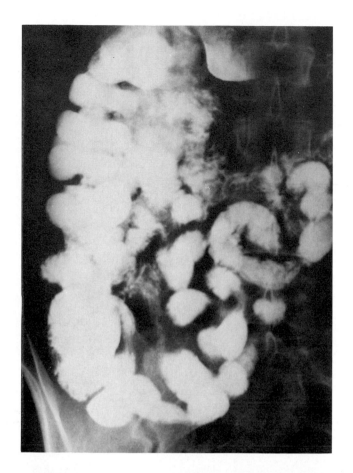

Figure 8a Right hemicolectomy — no recurrent disease.

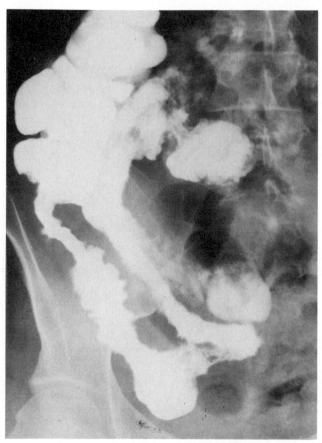

Figure 8b Two years later recurrent disease in the distal 20 cm of small bowel. Recurrent disease invariably affects the anastomosis and distal small bowel, and is best examined via the small bowel.

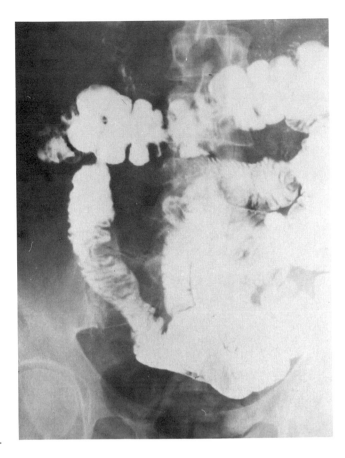

Figure 9a End-to-side anastomosis ileum to colon.

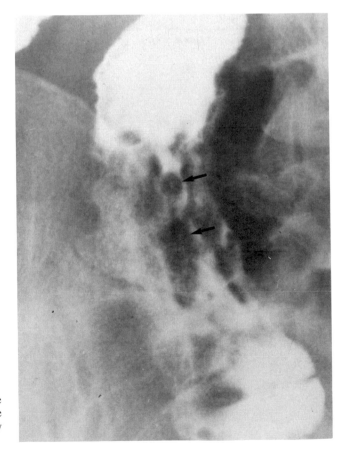

Figure 9b Compression views show aphthoid ulceration in the distal ileum (arrows).Compression or air reflux studies are important to show fine mucosal detail to demonstrate early recurrent disease.

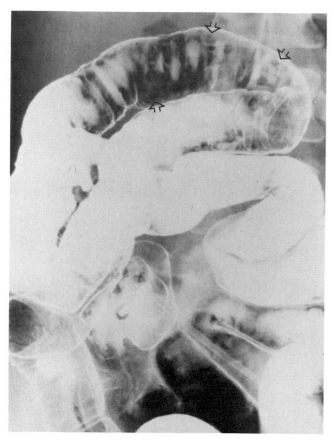

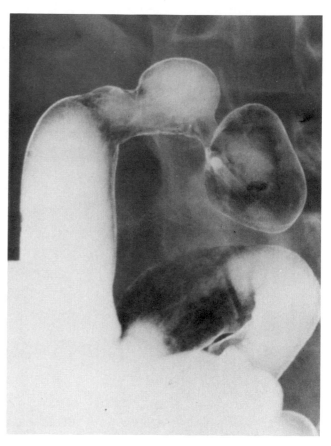

Figure 10 Ileostomy enema in a patient with Crohn's disease and high output. Endoscopic examination was normal, but the ileostomy enema showed aphthoid ulceration (arrows) in the ileum proximal to the reach of the endoscope.

Figure 11 Recurrent Crohn's disease with stricture formation.

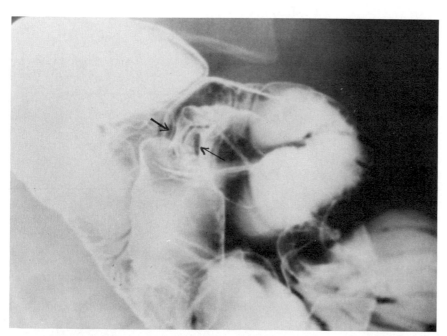

Figure 12 Ileostomy dysfunction with a short stricture immediately beneath the ileostomy (arrows).

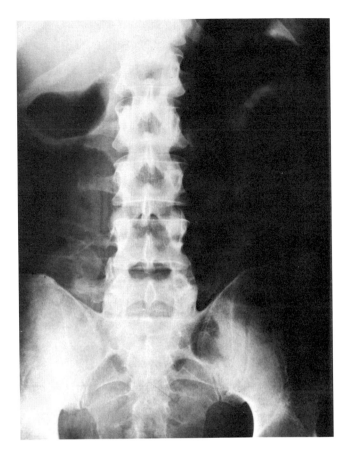

Figure 13a Small bowel obstruction in a patient with an ileostomy.

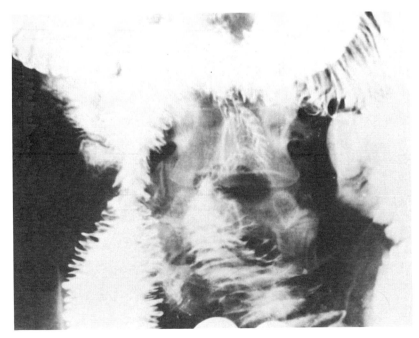

Figure 13b Extensive jejunal adhesions.

284

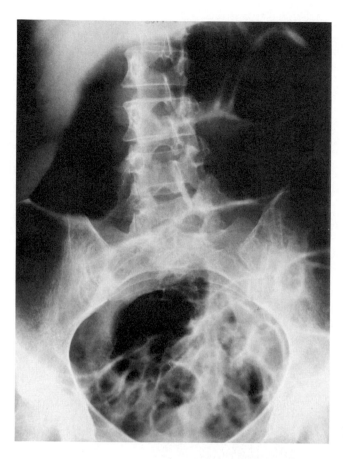

Figure 14a Small bowel obstruction in a patient with an ileorectal anastomosis.

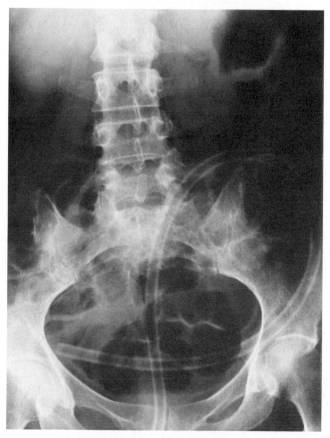

Figure 14b Passage of flatus tube outlining the volvulous. The bowel has been decompressed.

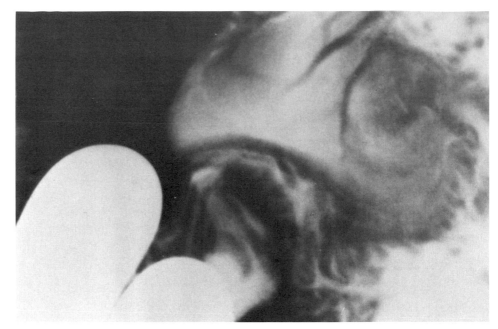

Figure 15a

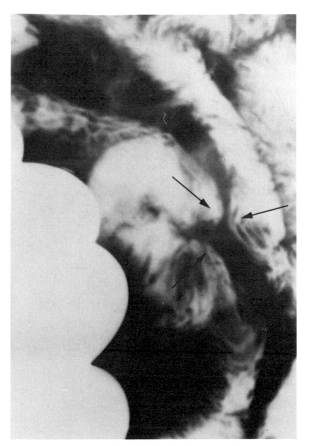

Figure 15b

Figure 15a and b   Small bowel adhesions in patients with ileostomies having obstructive symptoms. The adhesions (arrows) have been demonstrated on small bowel meals by the use of compression.

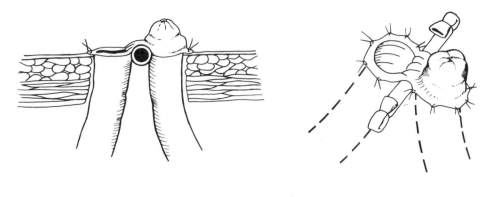

Figure 16 Construction of a loop ileostomy.

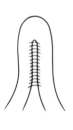 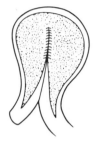 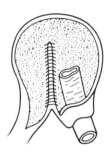 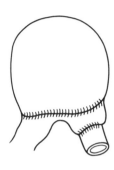

| 30 cm of ileum anastomosed along antimesenteric border | Bowel opened | Efferent limb intussuscepted to form valve 5 cm long | Valve and flap sutured to form reservoir |

Figure 17 Construction of Kock's ileostomy.

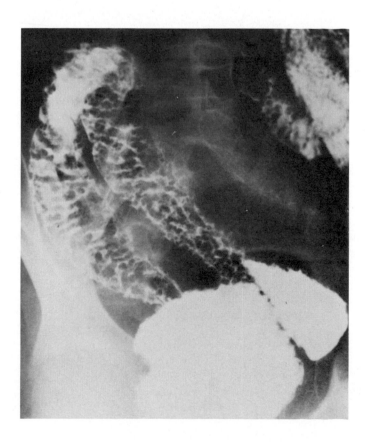

Figure 18 Recurrent Crohn's disease in a pelvic pouch.

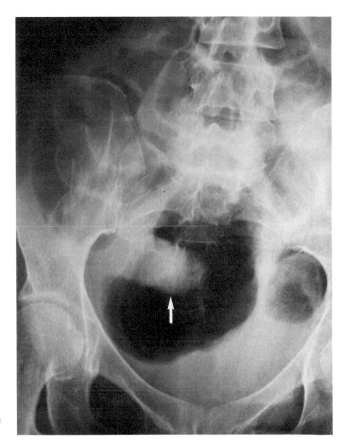

Figure 19 Koch's ileostomy on a plain film. The valve is visible (arrow) within the air-filled reservoir.

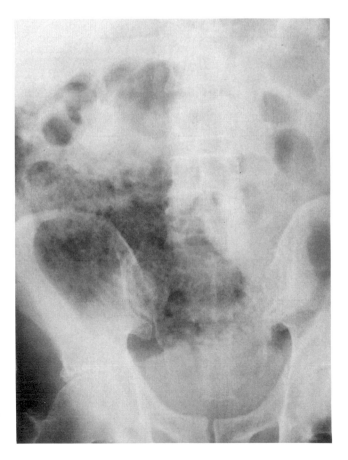

Figure 20 Large abscess cavity in the right iliac fossa. The cavity extends up to the edge of the abdominal cavity. It does not contain any valve and its borders are asymmetric.

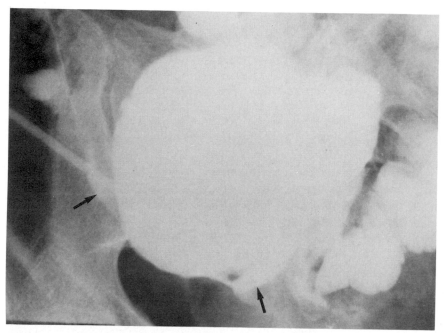

Figure 21a Water-soluble contrast enema of pouch showing a leak from the anastomosis at the junction of the afferent loop (arrows).

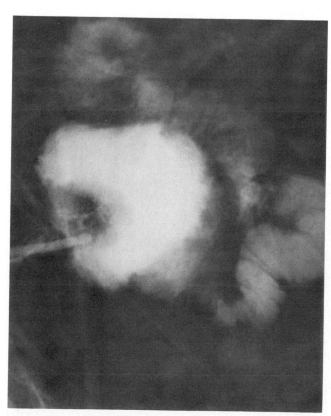

Figure 21b No leak 2 weeks later.

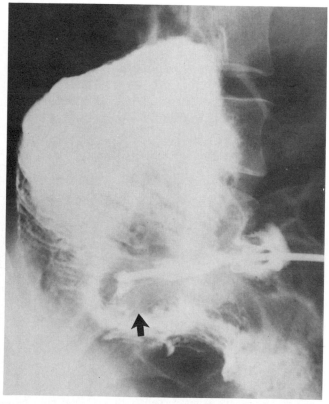

Figure 22 Normal Koch's ileostomy showing the valve (arrow) within the reservoir.

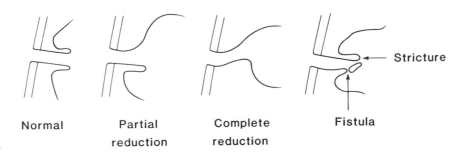

Normal   Partial reduction   Complete reduction   Stricture   Fistula

Figure 23   Complications of valve.

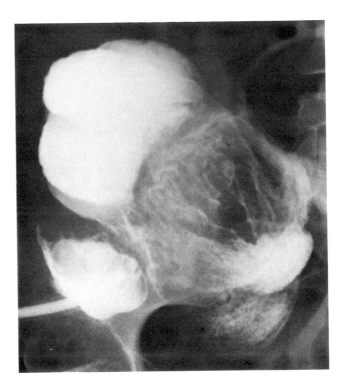

Figure 24   Complete reduction of the valve due to detachment of the reservoir from the abdominal wall.

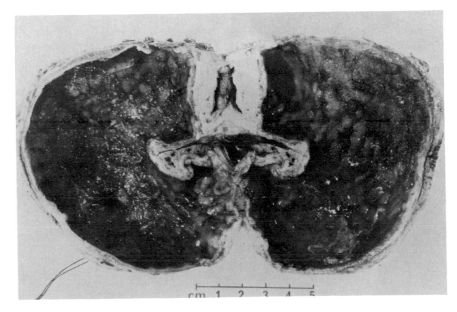

Figure 25   Resected pouch with gross inflammation and ulceration secondary to obstruction.

10

Rectal Biopsy in Ulcerative Colitis and Crohn's Disease

Ashley B. Price / Northwick Park Hospital, London, England

There are approximately 1.5 m of large bowel and 6.5 m of small intestine; an average rectal biopsy is less than 1 cm long. It is perhaps surprising, therefore, that the rectal biopsy has an important role in the diagnosis and management of inflammatory bowel disease. It is of most value in ulcerative colitis, for this is a mucosal disease originating in the rectum which may then spread proximally in a continuous manner. The sampling error, inherent in all biopsy procedures, is therefore small. By contrast, in Crohn's disease the sampling error is great not only because of the uneven pattern of intestinal involvement, but the inflammatory changes are transmural, and so partly deep to the grasp of the biopsy forceps. Even so, rectal biopsy can be diagnostic with only ileal disease and an apparently normal looking proctoscopic examination (1).

A biopsy in Crohn's disease or ulcerative colitis represent but a single moment in the time span of two chronic diseases. Only limited conclusions can be made about a film from looking at a single frame, so by analogy a single biopsy may not provide a complete answer. In some patients sequential biopsies are necessary to build up a dynamic view of the pathological changes. This improves the overall diagnostic yield from biopsy material as well as effectively monitoring the cause of the disease, the effect of treatment, and the onset of complications.

Colonoscopy and colonoscopic biopsy provide another dimension to the diagnostic role of biopsy work. The interpretation of histological signs is identical to that used for rectal biopsy. In particular, colonoscopy overcomes the sampling error which is such a limiting factor in the diagnosis of Crohn's disease. Moreover, the colonoscopist obtains a direct view of the mucosa in color which was previously only available after surgical resection.

*The drawings in this chapter are to complement the micrographs and are not exact replications.

Ultimately, the accuracy of diagnosis depends on the absolute discriminating value of the pathological criteria used (2). As the large bowel mucosa has only a limited range of responses to "injury," it is hardly surprising that the pathological features of Crohn's disease and ulcerative colitis, together with other "inflammatory" bowel disorders, show considerable overlap. The aim of this chapter is to emphasize the key features that make up a pathologist's diagnostic report.

TECHNICAL ASPECTS

Radiologists are well aware of the importance of proper film exposure and positioning. Similarly, technical expertise is crucial to the histopathologist. Having taken an adequate nontraumatized biopsy, it should be orientated on a suitable material, then placed in a clearly labeled container with the correct fixative and sent to the laboratory, accompanied by a request form showing the relevant clinical data and sigmoidoscopic findings. Orientation of the biopsy, on card, glass, or nylon mesh, is to assist the technical staff in cutting the biopsy perpendicular to its mucosal surface. The fixative used will depend on the investigation required. For example, most laboratories use solutions based on dilutions of formaldehyde, but tissue for electron microscopy requires its own special fixative and tissue for immunofluorescence needs to be flash-frozen.

Because many of the histological features on which a diagnosis is based are focal, it is customary to cut sections at different levels through the biopsy to improve sampling. Surawicz et al. (3) have shown recently that 90 sections from any one biopsy improves the yield of granulomas in cases of suspected Crohn's disease. However, most laboratories and pathologists could not cope with this work load, and each department must make its own compromise solution. Hematoxylin and eosin are the standard tissue stains. Others are seldom needed for routine diagnosis.

THE NORMAL BIOPSY

The normal rectal mucosa comprises crypts which extend from the surface to the muscularis mucosae. These are straight, parallel, unbranched tubes lined mostly by goblet cells. Near their surface, and on the surface between the crypts, nonmucus secreting absorptive cells are present. At the base of the crypts are the stem cells which replenish the crypt lining and also the cells of the amine precursor uptake and decarboxglation (APUD) system. Between the crypts is the lamina propria or connective tissue. This is sparse in the normal biopsy and contains blood vessels, macrophages, small numbers of eosinophils, mast cells, and plasma cells. Lymphocytes and even lymphoid follicles can be found (Fig. 1). Beneath the muscularis mucosae is the loose submucosa. This contains plexuses of veins and arteries as well as Meissner's plexus of autonomic nerves. An adequate biopsy should include both muscularis and some submucosa.

THE ABNORMAL BIOPSY

Many biopsies are abnormal but do not show characteristic features that permit the histopathologist to issue a diagnostic report. Barium studies in such patients may also show only limited nonspecific changes such as granularity of the rectal mucosa. Microscopy usually reveals increased numbers of inflammatory cells in the lamina propria and perhaps some separation of crypts. The proportion of acute and chronic inflammatory cells varies. The pathologist can do little more at this stage than report a proctitis in the absence of any other clues. The majority resolve and the etiology is never known. In those where symptoms persist, sequential biopsies often show a more specific disease pattern in time (e.g., ulcerative colitis, Crohn's disease, etc.)

In infective proctitis the picture is like the above, but the infiltrate in the lamina propria is predominantly of the acute type (i.e., polymorphonuclear neutrophils). They are often in focal aggregates and invade the epithelium of the mucosal surface and crypts (4) (Fig. 2). In most cases a repeat biopsy some weeks later will have returned to normal.

When the abnormal inflammatory infiltrate is minimal it is worth questioning the clinicians about traumatic instrumentation or the use of laxatives and enemas (5). A pure chronic inflammatory cell infiltrate is difficult to interpret in a single biopsy. It can represent the resolution of an acute episode of any form of inflammatory bowel disease.

ULCERATIVE COLITIS AND CROHN'S DISEASE

In the diagnosis of Crohn's disease and ulcerative colitis the pathologist, much like the radiologist, is armed with a series of patterns each with a different discriminating value (2,6). For example, the crypt abscess is a feature which scores only slightly in favor of ulcerative colitis as it is often seen in Crohn's disease. The granuloma, on the other hand, virtually excludes the diagnosis of ulcerative colitis. It is not, however, diagnostic of Crohn's disease. Tuberculosis and rarer conditions (e.g., an olegranuloma, a complication of the injection of haemorrhoids) must still be considered. The final diagnosis on any one biopsy is made after all the criteria have been evaluated. Certain pictures are diagnostic, and the majority will be highly suggestive of one or other of the two conditions. The number of patients in whom a definite histological diagnosis can be made will increase over a period of time as successive biopsies build up the characteristic morphology of one or other disease.

Ulcerative Colitis Despite its name, ulceration is seldom seen in a rectal biopsy. The typical picture corresponds more to the granularity and loss of mucosal pattern as described at sigmoidoscopy. The pattern is produced by an evenly spread heavy infiltrate of acute and chronic inflammatory cells in the lamina propria (i.e., plasma cells, polymorphs, and eosinophils). These separate the crypts which themselves may be dilated and their lumens filled by invading polymorphs, forming crypt abscesses (Fig. 3). The surface epithelium may be degenerate and the whole mucosa thickened as a result of the inflammatory infiltrate. Characteristically, the goblet cell population of the crypts is markedly depleted. There is also a florid vascular component with multiple dilated capillaries observed throughout the lamina propria. Goblet cell depletion and the diffuse mixed inflammatory cell infiltrate are perhaps the most helpful parameters to take note of in differentiating ulcerative colitis from Crohn's disease (2,6). When the biopsy includes muscularis mucosa and submucosa it can be seen that all the changes are limited to the mucosa, which is an important pathological feature of ulcerative colitis.

From the picture described, the pathologist can suggest ulcerative colitis as the most likely diagnosis. An attempt to exclude infective proctitis must always be undertaken by adequate microbiology. It is misleading to state that Crohn's disease can never present with the combination of changes noted above, but it is rare. It cannot be stressed too greatly that the features must be interpreted in their clinical and radiological setting with follow-up biopsies to confirm the development of the chronic disease pattern.

A biopsy taken in a resolving phase of ulcerative colitis will show that architectural disorganization of the crypts has commenced—a useful distinction between ulcerative colitis and Crohn's colitis when other features in this phase can be misleading. The goblet cell population has begun to return to normal and the inflammatory cell infiltrate often takes on a patchy distribution, both features seen more regularly in Crohn's disease. Thus, unless crypt disorganization is marked, the pathologist's report in this phase of ulcerative colitis may not be diagnostic.

In remission the biopsy picture of long-standing ulcerative proctocolitis is highly characteristic (Fig. 4). The pathologist can be dogmatic about the diagnosis. In this stage the involved segment is often seen radiologically as a straight, featureless tube. On microscopy there is florid crypt atrophy, with those remaining being short, bent, and branched. The lamina propria is devoid of inflammatory cells and the goblet cell population of the crypts has returned to normal. None of the other bowel diseases considered part of the differential diagnosis give this atrophic picture. Unfortunately, from the diagnostic point of view not all cases of ulcerative colitis progress to such a clear-cut picture. Although it is stated that the rectum will invariably remain abnormal after an attack of ulcerative proctocolitis, in practice this abnormality may be minimal and nonspecific. It is difficult to establish the diagnosis by biopsy in a patient with such a minimal residual abnormality. One needs a series of biopsies with accompanying radiological studies.

Cancer and precancer (dysplasia), although rare, are accepted complications of ulcerative colitis (7). They are just becoming accepted as complications of Crohn's disease (8) but are rarer still in this condition, and rectal biopsy is not considered part of the cancer screening program as it is for patients with chronic ulcerative colitis. Dysplasia is the histological marker that a cancer is already present or is more likely to develop in that particular tissue. It is recognized by cytological and architectural changes in the crypts, which can be graded as mild to moderate (low grade) or severe (high grade) (Fig. 5). Subtle changes can also be seen radiologically (9) and assist in guiding the endoscopist to the correct biopsy site, for it is the sampling error in the biopsy detection of dysplasia that limits its value as a means of cancer surveillance. The work by Riddell and Morson (10) shows that if multiple rectal biopsies are taken, dysplasia can be detected in up to 85–90% of patients who are harboring a cancer. This high figure is, however, disputed by others (11,12). A histological report of severe or high-grade dysplasia is at present the only indication for considering immediate prophylactic proctocolectomy (7,13). Recently, it has been suggested that finding dysplasia with a macroscopic lesion in the colon may also be an indication (12).

Polyps can occur in ulcerative colitis. Whatever the site, these may be adenomatous (neoplastic) or inflammatory. A similar situation exists for large bowel Crohn's disease. A biopsy of such lesions is important for cancer prevention, but the type of polyp means little in separating Crohn's disease from ulcerative colitis.

Crohn's Disease   The granuloma is perhaps the only absolute feature in a biopsy that distinguishes Crohn's disease from ulcerative colitis (Fig. 6). Unfortunately, it is not present in every case. Only 8–20% of rectal biopsies in Crohn's disease contain granulomas (14). Additional limitations to the value of rectal biopsy are the segmental nature of involvement of the bowel and the transmural inflammatory pattern, which can be deep to the grasp of biopsy forceps. Not only may the rectum be normal, but the most frequent pattern of disease is that limited to the ileum (15). However, rectal biopsy in such cases does have a role. Dyer et al. (16) found that 12.5% of rectal biopsies were diagnostic and 46% were abnormal when ileal disease only was present. In other studies diagnostic granulomas have been found in 3 of 7 (3) and 4 of 14 (17) patients with ileal disease only. Occasionally, a giant cell may be seen adjacent to a ruptured crypt. This does not constitute a granuloma and may be observed in ulcerative colitis.

Apart from the granuloma the other main diagnostic features for separating Crohn's disease from ulcerative colitis are transmural inflammation, lymphoid aggregates, and fissures. These are also some of the main features responsible for the diagnostic radiological appearances (narrowing of the bowel lumen, thickening of the wall, and rose-thorn ulcers). Unfortunately, they cannot be appreciated in biopsies, which are usually too superficial. However, in a typical case of rectal Crohn's disease a biopsy, even lacking a granuloma, is sufficiently different from ulcerative proctocolitis for the histopathologist to express a confident opinion. In the presence of a moderate mixed inflammatory cell infiltrate, the crypt architecture remains intact, with a normal or only minimally reduced goblet cell population. The inflammatory infiltrate which is present has a focal distribution between areas of virtually normal mucosa (Fig. 7). If the submucosa is present, the inflammation may be seen extending into it, with small clusters of lymphocytes adjacent to the bases of the crypts. Such a picture excludes ulcerative colitis and in the correct clinical context a confident opinion of Crohn's proctitis can be made. Tiny superficial clusters of histiocytic cells and lymphocytes without giant cells present (microgranulomas) are also an attribute thought to exclude a diagnosis of ulcerative colitis (17).

The diagnostic yield from patients with suspected Crohn's disease can be increased by examining serial sections through the biopsy. It is best reserved for selected cases, as it involves a significant increase in the work load on the laboratory and the reporting pathologist (3). When the features are less specific it is helpful to examine colonoscopic biopsies from several sites. The intermittent distribution of abnormalities is then valuable in distinguishing ulcerative colitis from Crohn's disease even though any one biopsy is unhelpful. The histological patterns in Crohn's disease, unlike those in ulcerative colitis, do not allow a correlation with disease activity and response to therapy. Again unlike ulcerative colitis, the detection of dysplasia in Crohn's disease as a precursor to cancer is not yet generally accepted. (8).

ACUTE FULMINATING COLITIS: TOXIC MEGACOLON

A special comment is needed about this complication of inflammatory bowel disease. It may occur in inflammatory large bowel disease of any cause but is more common in ulcerative colitis than in Crohn's disease (18). Because the transverse and right colon are usually the site of the dilatation, biopsies from the lower left colon and in particular a rectal biopsy may give misleading impressions, appearing virtually normal in the face of massive transverse colonic dilatation. The pathologist and radiologist should be aware of this trap. In these cases an x-ray will provide a more accurate picture of the impending disaster.

DIFFERENTIAL DIAGNOSIS

Short of seeing the diagnostic granuloma of Crohn's disease or the atrophic noninflamed mucosa of ulcerative colitis, it is always cautionary to consider several other diagnoses. Pathologists, like radiologists, must resist clinical pressure to overdiagnose on nondiagnostic material. The main differential diagnoses are as follows:

Infectious diarrhea
Pseudomembranous colitis
Ischemic colitis
Tuberculosis
Solitary ulcer syndrome
Irradiation proctocolitis
Diverticular disease
Irritable bowel syndrome

All bar the irritable bowel syndrome, and diverticular disease may have a diagnostic biopsy picture, but unfortunately on many occasions the features are less specific. The irritable bowel syndrome is associated with a normal rectal biopsy, as is diverticulitis. In the latter inflammation is usually limited to the diverticula and the adjacent mucosa is normal. The redundant folds of mucosa in diverticular disease can undergo limited prolapse and may become inflamed. The biopsy will then show the changes of mucosal ischemia, so it is important to know that diverticular disease was present. A normal biopsy is of some value in excluding ulcerative colitis but not, of course, Crohn's disease. Both conditions may coexist with diverticular disease (19).

As stated, all the other conditions have characteristic pathology which is well described in general textbooks and in the literature (1,4,20–22). It is relevant to emphasize only a few points here.

The typical picture of infectious diarrhea (Fig. 2a) depends at what point in the natural history of the disease the biopsy is taken. Usually, the biopsy will be taken a few days after the onset of diarrhea. At this stage the diagnostic focal acute polymorphonuclear infiltrate will have partially given way to a more diffuse chronic inflammatory cell infiltrate, so that the picture may be indistinguishable from acute active ulcerative proctocolitis. A stool culture is therefore mandatory before making a diagnosis of acute ulcerative colitis.

An infective colitis may of course be superimposed on ulcerative colitis. Furthermore, amoebae can be easily overlooked if not specifically sought. Although the examination of fresh stools and proctosigmoidoscopic aspirates is the method of choice for detecting amoebae, rectal biopsy still has a role. The organisms are often seen in the mucus debris on the surface of the biopsy, and technical care is therefore necessary to process any included debris. Fluorescent antibody techniques may be used to stain the organisms, but the simpler periodic acid–Schiff method colors the trophozoites magenta and is an adequate stain for routine purposes.

Pseudomembranous colitis (21) is perhaps the easiest biopsy diagnosis to make when a typical plaque is seen at sigmoidoscopy and on a biopsy (Fig. 8). However, the rectum can be spared or may simply show a picture similar to infectious proctitis (23). In such cases the demonstration of the fecal toxin of the etiological agent, *Clostridium difficile* (24), confirms active disease even when pseudomembranes are absent.

An immediate diagnosis of Crohn's disease is tempting when a granuloma is seen but clinicians, radiologists, and pathologists should always consider the likelihood of tuberculosis, particularly in patients from endemic areas. Irradiation proctocolitis is usually suggested from the history and the bizarre fibroblasts, nuclear changes, and mucosal vascular ectasia, which are easily recognized. In the solitary ulcer syndrome (22) the proctoscopic appearances of an anterior wall rectal ulcer make up the diagnosis with a histological picture of villiform mucosa and partial obliteration of the lamina propria by fibroblasts and ramifications of the muscularis mucosae (Fig. 9).

CONCLUSIONS Diffuse inflammation limited to the mucosa, goblet cell depletion, and the architectural distortion of the crypts are the main discriminating parameters for excluding Crohn's disease and making a confident diagnosis of ulcerative colitis. By contrast, a granuloma excludes ulcerative colitis. Focal inflammation with normal crypt alignment, a normal goblet cell population, and either a well-formed granuloma or "microgranuloma" allow a confident diagnosis of Crohn's disease.

On all occasions the pathology should be reviewed with the other clinical findings. This is especially important when the interpretation of the biopsy is difficult. It is nearly always possible to favor one diagnosis more than another and so help the clinician in the immediate management of the patient. A report reading "nonspecific proctitis" or "it may be Crohn's disease or it may be ulcerative colitis" should be avoided. Moreover, follow-up biopsies will resolve most of the difficulties.

Among the differential diagnosis of Crohn's disease and ulcerative colitis the exclusion of infectious proctitis is the most difficult, for stool culture may be negative in almost half the cases (25). Again, with good follow-up it is observed that in most infections the biopsy quickly returns to normal.

Despite stressing that every attempt must be made to distinguish Crohn's disease from ulcerative colitis, in one situation, with toxic megacolon imminent, the pathological overlap can be complete. Not only is the biopsy misleading as previously mentioned, but often no distinction can be made after examining the surgical resection (26).

REFERENCES

1. Morson, B.C., Dawson, I.M.P. (Eds.) (1972). *Gastro-intestinal Pathology*. Blackwell Scientific Publications, Oxford, Chap. 33.

2. Cook, M.G., Dixon, M.F. (1973). An analysis of the reliability of detection and diagnostic value of various pathological features in Crohn's disease and ulcerative colitis. Gut 14;255.

3. Surawicz, C.M., Meisel, J.L., Ylvisaker, T., et al. (1981). Rectal biopsy in the diagnosis of Crohn's disease: value of multiple biopsies and serial sectioning. Gastroenterology 81;66.

4. Price A.B., Jewkes, J., Sanderson, P.J. (1979). Acute diarrhoea: *Campylobacter* colitis and the role of rectal biopsy. J. Clin. Pathol. 32;990.

5. Meisel, J.L., Bergman, D., Graney, D., et al. (1977). Human rectal mucosa: proctoscopic and morphological changes caused by laxatives. Gastroenterology 72;1274.

6. Hywell-Jones, J., Lennard-Jones, J.E., Morson, B.C., et al. (1973). Numerical taxonomy and discriminant analysis applied to non-specific colitis. J. Med. 42;715.

7. Lennard-Jones, J.E., Morson, B.C., Ritchie, J.K., et el. (1977). Cancer in colitis: assessment of the individual risk by clinical and histological criteria. Gastroenterology 73;1280.

8. Craft, C.F., Mendelsohn, G., Cooper, H.S., et al. (1981). Colonic "precancer" in Crohn's disease. Gastroenterology 80;366.

9. Frank, P.H., Riddell, R.H., Feczko, P.J., et al. (1978). Radiological detection of colonic dysplasia (precarcinoma) in chronic ulcerative colitis. Gastrointest. Radiol. 3;209.

10. Riddell, R.H., Morson, B.C. (1979). Value of sigmoidoscopy and biopsy in detection of carcinoma and premalignant change in ulcerative colitis. Gut 20;575.

11. Evans, D.J., Pollock, D.J. (1972). In situ and invasive carcinoma of the colon in patients with ulcerative colitis. Gut 13;566.

12. Blackstone, M.O., Riddell, R.H., Rogers, B.H.G., et al. (1981). Dysplasia-associated lesion or mass (DALM) detected by colonoscopy in long standing ulcerative colitis: an indication for colectomy. Gastroenterology 80;366.

13. Butt, J.H., Lennard-Jones, J.E., Ritchie, J.K. (1980). A practical approach to the risk of cancer in inflammatory bowel disease. Med. Clin. N. Amer. 64;1203

14. Chambers, T.J., Morson, B.C. (1980). Large bowel biopsy in the differential diagnosis of inflammatory bowel disease. Invest. Cell. Pathol. 3;159.

15. Higgens, C.S., Allen, R.N. (1980). Crohn's disease of the distal ileum. Gut 21;933.

16. Dyer, N.H., Stansfeld, A.G., Dawson, A.M. (1970). The role of rectal biopsy in the diagnosis of Crohn's disease. Scand. J. Gastroenterol. 5;491.

17. Rotterdam, H., Korelitz, B.I., Sommers, S.C. (1977). Microgranulomas in grossly normal rectal mucosa in Crohn's disease. Am. J. Clin. Pathol. 67;550.

18. Javett, S., Brooke, B.N. (1970). Acute dilatation of the colon in Crohn's disease. Lancet 2;126.

19. Schmidt, G.T., Lennard-Jones, J.E., Morson, B.C., et al. (1968). Crohn's disease of the colon and its distinction from diverticulitis. Gut 9;7.

20. Day, D.W., Mandal, B.K., Morson, B.C. (1978). The rectal biopsy appearances in salmonella colitis. Histopathology 2;117.

21. Price, A.B., Davies, D.R. (1977). Pseudomembranous colitis. J. Clin. Pathol. 30;1.

22. Madigan, M.R., Morson, B.C. (1969). Solitary ulcer of the rectum. Gut 10;871.

23. Price, A.B. (1980). Pseudomembranous colitis. *In Recent Advances in Gastro-intestinal Pathology* (Clin. Gastroenterol., Suppl. 1). Wright, R. (Ed.) Saunders, Philadelphia.

24. Bartlett, J.G., Chang, T.W., Gurwith, M., et al. (1978). Antibiotic-associated pseudomembranous colitis due to toxin producing clostridia. N. Engl. J. Med. 298;531.

25. Jewkes, J., Larson, H.E., Price, A.B., et al. (1981). Aetiology of acute diarrhoea in adults. Gut 22;388.

26. Price, A.B. (1978). Overlap in the spectrum of non-specific inflammatory bowel disease—"colitis" indeterminate. J. Clin. Pathol. 31;567.

FIGURES 1 THROUGH 9

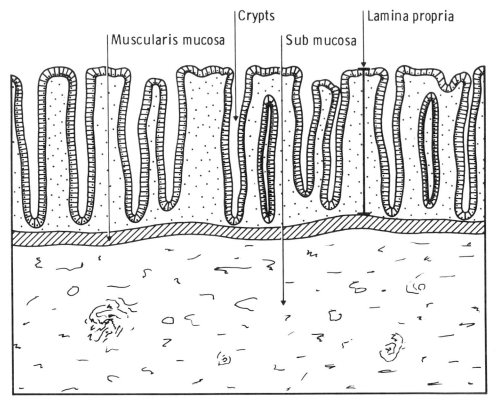

Figure 1a

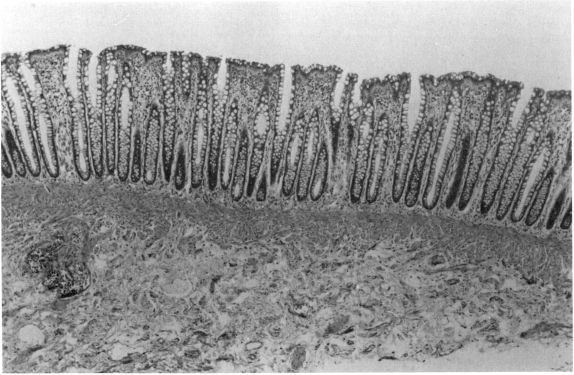

Figure 1b

Figure 1 The diagram (a) and section (b) show a normal biopsy. The crypts' alignment is regular. They are set close together with a small cellular infiltrate within the lamina propria.

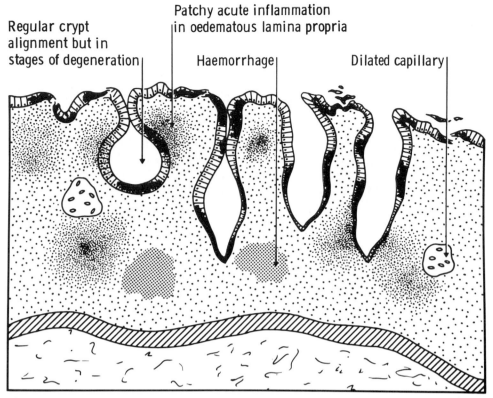

Regular crypt
alignment but in
stages of degeneration

Patchy acute inflammation
in oedematous lamina propria

Haemorrhage

Dilated capillary

Figure 2a

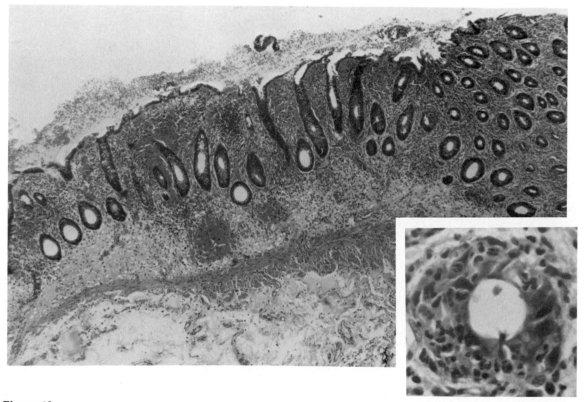

Figure 2b

Figure 2 In these illustrations of infective proctitis, marked edema has resulted in separation of the base of the crypts from the muscularis. The crypts remain aligned but can appear dilated as the individual lining epithelial cells degenerate and become attenuated. The inflammation is focal and contains a high proportion of polymorphonuclear leukocytes. The insert shows an incipient crypt abscess, a typical feature of infective lesions.

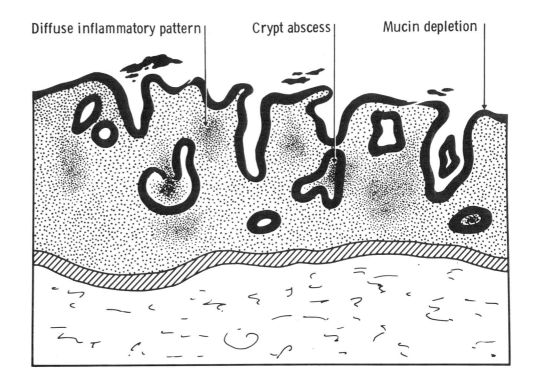

Diffuse inflammatory pattern   Crypt abscess   Mucin depletion

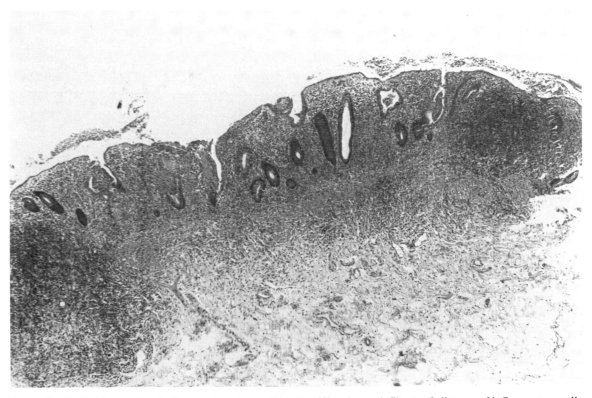

Figure 3   In the biopsy of typical acute ulcerative colitis, the diffuse heavy infiltrate of all types of inflammatory cells, the crypt abscesses, the goblet cell depletion, and crypt irregularity are a contrast to the picture seen in both infective proctitis and Crohn's disease.

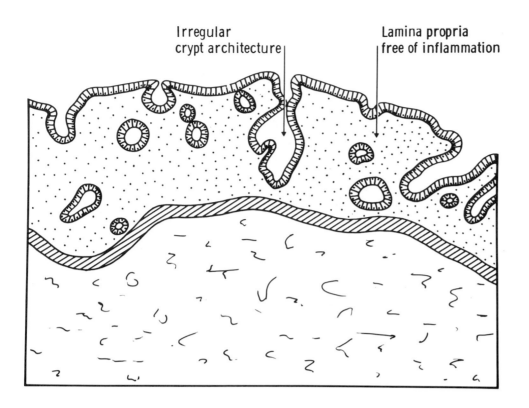

Irregular
crypt architecture

Lamina propria
free of inflammation

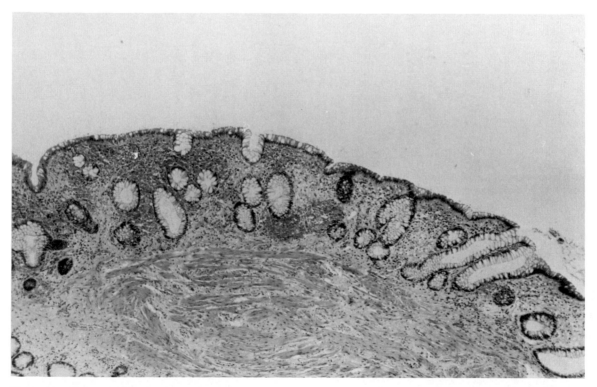

Figure 4   Crypt atrophy together with branched and angulated crypts in the abscence of inflammation is a feature virtually diagnostic of ulcerative colitis in remission.

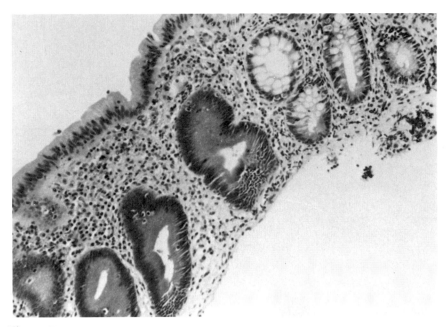

Figure 5a

Figure 5 These show mild (a) and severe (b) dysplasia, respectively. The degree of nuclear and cytoplasmic abnormality is clearly much worse in (b). The dysplastic epithelium forms a contrast to the few normal crypts present in both sections. Inflammatory epithelial changes can mimic dysplasia, which should therefore be assessed when disease is quiescent.

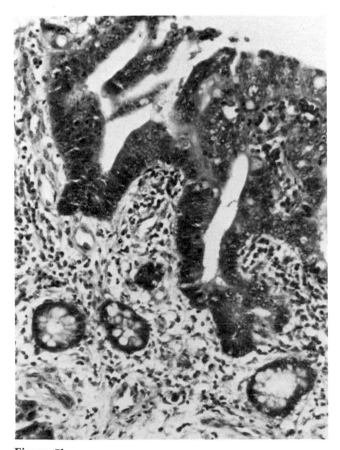

Figure 5b

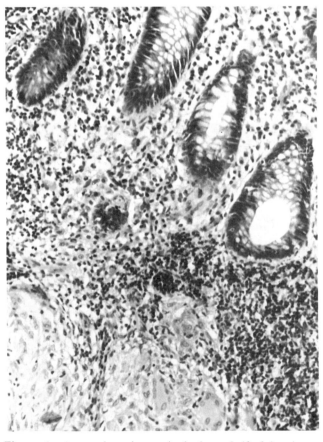

Figure 6 A granuloma is seen in the lower half of the picture.

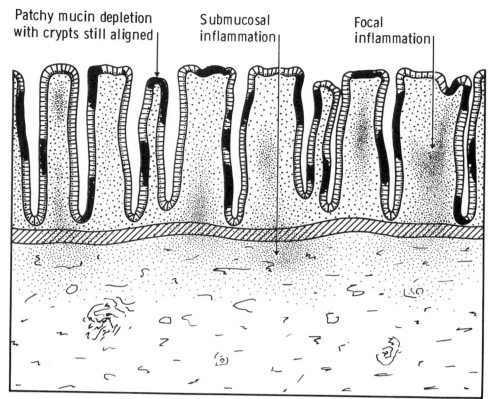

Patchy mucin depletion   Submucosal   Focal
with crypts still aligned   inflammation   inflammation

Figure 7a

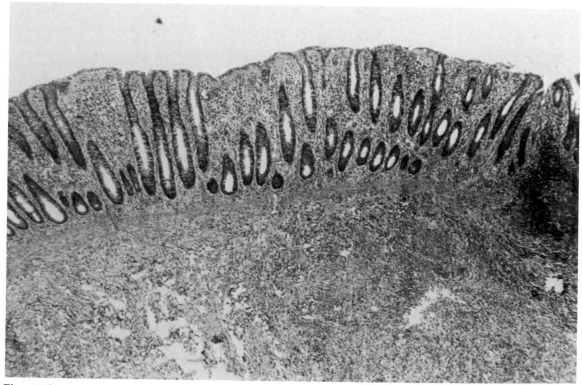

Figure 7b

Figure 7 These two illustrations demonstrate the major biopsy characteristics of Crohn's disease, excluding granulomas. The section (b) shows considerable submucosal inflammation, focal inflammation in the lamina propria, and a regular crypt pattern — a combination that is not seen in infective colitis (Fig. 2b) or ulcerative colitis (Fig. 3b).

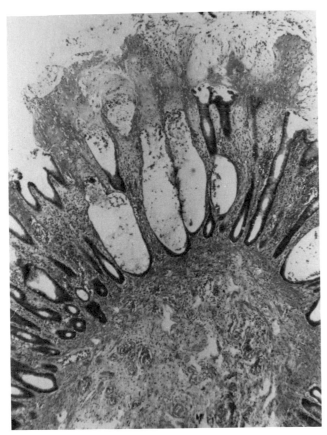

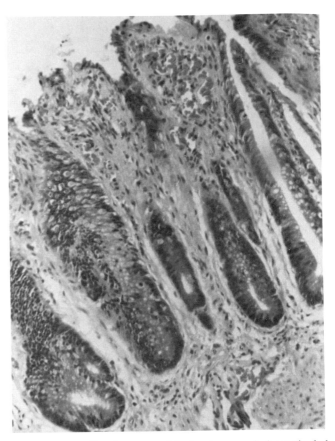

Figure 8 The typical "eruptive" lesion of pseudomembranous colitis. The luminal debris, mucin, and pus form the yellow plaque seen at sigmoidoscopy.

Figure 9a The fibrotic nature of the lamina propria intermingled with muscle fibers from the muscularis are typical of a biopsy from a case of the solitary ulcer syndrome. These changes may also be seen in ischemia. Mucosal prolapse with subsequent ischemia may form the basis of the changes.

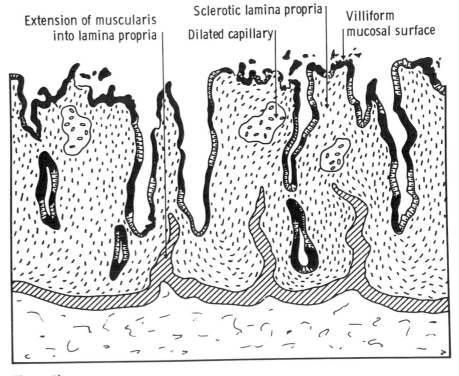

Figure 9b

Index

About the Authors

CLIVE I. BARTRAM is Consultant Radiologist at St. Mark's Hospital for Diseases of the Rectum and Colon and St. Bartholomew's Hospital, London, England, a position he has held since 1974. Dr. Bartram qualified as a Member of the Royal College of Physicians (M.R.C.P.) in 1968, and as a Fellow of the Royal College of Radiologists (F.R.C.R.) in 1972. In addition, he is a Member of the Society of Gastrointestinal Radiology and of the British Society of Gastroenterology, as well as a Fellow of the Royal Society of Medicine. Dr. Bartram was Visiting Professor in 1977 at the University of Pennsylvania, Philadelphia. Dr. Bartram has written and lectured extensively in his field, concentrating mainly on barium studies in colitis and neoplasia.

James P.S. Thomson is Consultant Surgeon and Dean of Postgraduate Studies, St. Mark's Hospital for Diseases of the Rectum and Colon; Consultant Surgeon, Hackney Hospital; Honorary Lecturer in Surgery, St. Bartholomew's Hospital Medical College; and Honorary Consulting Surgeon, St. Mary's Hospital, London, England. Mr. Thomson has written numerous articles and lectured widely particularly on the topics of surgery and benign neoplasia of the large bowel, condyloma acculata, and the dumping syndrome.

Ashley B. Price is Consultant Histopathologist, Northwick Park Hospital, London, and Clinical Research Centre, Harrow, Middlesex, England. He also regularly lectures at St. Mark's Hospital Postgraduate Courses and at the Leeds Course on Radiological Gastroenterology. Dr. Price is an editorial board member of both *Gut* and the *Italian Journal of Gastroenterology*.